FIGHTING CANCER *with* PLANTS *from the* RAINFOREST

A Guide to the Remarkable Healing Power
of 13 Anti-Cancer Plants

LESLIE TAYLOR, ND

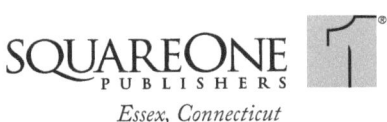

Essex, Connecticut

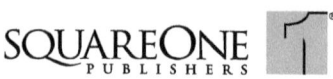

An imprint of The Globe Pequot Publishing Group, Inc.
64 South Main Street
Essex, CT 06426
www.globepequot.com

Copyright © 2026 by Leslie Taylor

The information and advice contained in this book are based upon the research and the personal and professional experiences of the author. They are not intended as a substitute for consulting with a healthcare professional. The publisher and author are not responsible for any adverse effects or consequences resulting from the use of any of the suggestions, preparations, or procedures discussed in this book. All matters pertaining to your physical health should be supervised by a healthcare professional. It is a sign of wisdom, not cowardice, to seek a second or third opinion.

All rights reserved. No part of this book may be reproduced in any form or by any electronic or mechanical means, including information storage and retrieval systems, without written permission from the publisher, except by a reviewer who may quote passages in a review.

British Library Cataloguing in Publication Information available

Library of Congress Cataloging-in-Publication Data available

Names: Taylor, Leslie author
Title: Fighting cancer with plants from the rainforest : a guide to the
  remarkable healing power of 13 anti-cancer plants / Leslie Taylor, ND.
Description: Essex, Connecticut : Square One, [2026] | Includes
  bibliographical references and index. | Summary: "Natural anti-cancer
  compounds and chemicals found in plants have long been a cornerstone in
  drug discovery; however, instead of waiting for the next generation of
  anti-cancer drugs, Dr. Leslie Taylor has compiled thirteen of the most
  effective rainforest plants containing active chemicals that have
  already been shown to target cancer cells. This book is designed to help
  readers understand how these compounds work and how they can be used
  directly to fight cancers"—Provided by publisher.
Identifiers: LCCN 2025041019 (print) | LCCN 2025041020 (ebook) | ISBN
  9780757005442 paperback | ISBN 9780757055447 epub
Subjects: LCSH: Cancer—Alternative treatment | Rain forest
  Plants—Therapeutic use | Cancer—Diet therapy | Materia medica,
  Vegetable | BISAC: HEALTH & FITNESS / Diseases & Conditions / Cancer |
  MEDICAL / Oncology / General
Classification: LCC RC271.H47 T395 2026 (print) | LCC RC271.H47 (ebook)
LC record available at https://lccn.loc.gov/2025041019
LC ebook record available at https://lccn.loc.gov/2025041020

CONTENTS

Preface v

How to Use This Book xv

Introduction 1

PART 1
Understanding the Power of Rainforest Plants

1. Why Rainforest Medicinal Plants Are Unique 8

2. The Power of Polyphenols for Cancer 14

3. The Difference between Plants and Drugs and the Research Behind Both 23

4. New Knowledge Results in New Treatments 32

5. Treating Cancer through the Main Cancer Pathways 42

PART 2
Harnessing the Power of the Plants

6. A Naturopathic Approach to Natural Anti-Cancer Remedies 80

7. Cancer Plans by Cancer Type 89

8. How to Prepare Your Own Natural Anti-Cancer Remedies 135

PART 3
The Anti-Cancerous Plants of the Rainforest

Anamu 198	Mullaca 274
Bitter Melon 207	Pau d'arco 284
Cat's Claw 217	Picão Preto 294
Chanca Piedra 226	Simarouba 304
Espinheira Santa 238	Suma 311
Graviola 252	Vassourinha 318
Guacatonga 267	

Conclusion   324

Resources   327

References   332

Index   333

About the Author   349

PREFACE

This book is long overdue, as I have wanted to write it for many years. Why? Because I am a cancer survivor who survived acute myeloid leukemia in my mid-20s by using herbal medicine and other natural healing modalities. My personal knowledge garnered in my own personal journey with cancer is that herbal medicine and medicinal plants can have a very beneficial effect for cancer patients; just like they did for me. This experience eventually propelled me into creating a company called Raintree Nutrition Inc. in Austin, Texas, in 1995. The establishment of this company resulted from finding a botanical drug that was being used in Europe as an adjunctive therapy for cancer. Once I determined the product was just a natural plant extract of a Peruvian rainforest plant called cat's claw (featured in this book), I knew I could import the plant directly from rainforests and sell it as an herbal supplement (for a lot cheaper than the herbal drug cost in the European Union [EU]). I also knew that a botanical drug, such as the one in the EU, would never be approved for use in the United States, and you'll learn why in this book.

I directed this company, which focused on the medicinal plants from the Amazon rainforest, for 18 years. Traveling down to the rainforest regions, I set up harvesting programs with Indigenous peoples and local communities in the Amazon for cat's claw and about a dozen other medicinal plants I learned about. I started researching and documenting all the herbal remedy uses of the plants, and I collected relevant scientific research performed on them. I created a database of information on these traditional uses and research, which was initially called the Rainforest Medicinal Plant Database on the Raintree website, and added to it as my research continued.

I wrote my first book on rainforest plants in 1998 called *Herbal Secrets of the Rainforest* on about 60 plants, which basically came from all the information in the database. Research on Amazonian rainforest plants took off, and many research organizations were publishing new studies on them. I published a new book in 2005 called *The Healing Power of Rainforest Herbs* to share all this new research on 76 medicinal plants from the Amazon. It's been so popular that it is still in print 20 years later and sold today (see the link in the "Resources" section, page 331).

Herbal supplements were and are regulated in the United States by the Food and Drug Administration (FDA) under a law called the Dietary Supplement Health and Education Act of 1994 (called DSHEA for short). Congress passed legislation to create the law, which was mostly intended to stop the FDA from blocking factual and important information from Americans that educated consumers on the benefits of healthy organic foods and food supplements. It was a huge consumer and natural products industry grassroots movement and a big fight in Congress to get the legislation approved. It established a new regulatory framework for dietary supplements by amending the Federal Food, Drug, and Cosmetic Act (FD&C Act) and prohibited the FDA from regulating supplements in the same fashion as drugs or to prohibit new supplements from being approved by them prior to being marketed.

The challenge for those in the natural product industry was in educating those in Congress that herbal medicine systems have existed for thousands of years, and that these treatments worked. As it turned out, Congress agreed that consumers of herbal supplements should be entitled to that information and manufacturers should be able to provide this information to their customers. Along the same lines, if there was scientific research that could explain these traditional uses, there should be some legal way to disclose that information as well. Back then, vitamin and mineral natural products were called food supplements, and plant products were called herbal supplements; and the legislation lumped them all together using the term "dietary supplements" (after much discussion).

Since I started Raintree just a year after the FDA started issuing the first regulations to enact DSHEA, I made sure I followed all regulations. The Federal Trade Commission (FTC), the agency that regulates advertising of all products sold in the United States, also weighed in on the new law and published a guidance document to the natural products industry on specific ways manufacturers could refer to traditional uses and scientific research when advertising and marketing their products. Writing these books and compiling the plant database were a part of that. The first regulations were in keeping with Congress's intent in providing factual, non-misleading information on the traditional uses of plants used as herbal remedies, and how to comply with sharing research in an allowable manner as well as how to refer to "third-party documentation" on both. Many other natural product companies did the same, and dietary supplement sales boomed.

Soon after starting my company, I ended up with two product lines: a retail product line of mostly single plant capsules and extracts, and a practitioner line of more remedy-specific multi-plant formulas that combined different plants together. I formulated products based on the research and the traditional uses of how they were used in herbal medicine systems. I also knew the type of information I could provide to a health practitioner was more extensive than what could be shared in the consumer market under DSHEA. Since rainforest plants were not known very well, I had a lot of teaching to do.

The company made the rounds exhibiting at all the natural products conventions where we educated retail customers as well as manufacturers on the benefits of rainforest plants. Some of these became major herbs of commerce and are now available under many different company labels. I always encouraged competition because these were wild-harvested plants that had direct rainforest conservation benefits. Sustainable harvesting of medicinal plants in the Amazon directly competed with the profits of lumber companies chopping down the rainforest. That was another principle my company was founded on.

We also made the rounds in all the alternative/integrative physician, naturopathic, chiropractic, and other alternative health industry conventions and symposiums. We ended up with many practitioner clients using the formulas in their practices, and even some veterinarians who were using them with animals. Some of the formulated products were easy. For example, there's more fungi and mold in a rainforest than anywhere else on earth, so picking some effective plants with those actions for a formula for candida and other fungal infections was easy. Other multi-plant formulas were developed upon request by different practitioners who had hard-to-treat patients, or some kind of condition that did not have any effective products to treat it. Oftentimes I created a formula for a practitioner, encapsulating it myself, and offered it for free just to see if it would help. Some worked quite well; the practitioner would tell their colleagues, and patients would tell their friends and relatives. I then had to add it to the product line because I couldn't continue handling all the requests by hand encapsulating the formula.

Some of these formulas became so popular through word-of-mouth referrals that even the practitioners couldn't keep up. Many of them were moved to the retail line of products (usually with a new name and more limited information in accordance with the DSHEA regulations). The FDA's enforcement of its regulations, however, changed frequently over time. It clearly demonstrated the concept that if something really works, you don't have to advertise it or push it. Just allow it to flow into the market with people sharing their experience using these products. In fact, Raintree did no advertising at all other than exhibiting at conventions. I also set up a company policy that allowed a full refund, with no questions asked, if whatever the customer bought didn't work as they thought it would.

In 2000, out of the blue, I received a phone call. It was from a cancer researcher working for a large pharmaceutical company. He found me because I was the only company in the United States that was using a plant that he had been researching for the past eight years. I only used it as an ingredient in one of my practitioner formulas for intestinal parasites. He explained that his research team had tested the plant in animals with remarkable results on different cancer types. They had also identified a group of chemicals in the plant that were responsible for its anti-cancerous actions. He revealed they had picked one chemical out of more than 20 they had found that had the strongest action against tumors in animals. He then said he had spent more than six years just trying to copy that one chemical to reproduce it in their lab.

He explained that they were unsuccessful after many attempts mainly because of a polarity issue (an electrical charge) and the unique manner in which these chemicals were made inside the plant. I listened carefully as he talked. I could hear the passion, frustration, and even sadness in his voice, especially when he told me he had been instructed to shove all of his research in a drawer and move on to something else. The fact was, if they could not copy the chemical in the plant, they could not change it enough to patent it, so that they could then test it as a new possible drug. If they were having so many problems just copying it, then trying to change it while keeping the same action would be even harder and more time consuming—and costly. Despite the plant chemicals showing promise, if a potential drug wasn't possible, they had to move on.

I think he just felt the need to tell someone because his company never let him publish the remarkable animal studies they had conducted using

PREFACE

the plant. Since my company was the only one currently using the plant, he thought I should know. This isn't unusual either since new cancer drugs are highly profitable. Drug research is competitive and expensive; and many drug companies keep quiet about what they are studying until they have a patent in place. I could tell he was in his profession because he really wanted to make a difference, and I think he hoped I could use the information somehow. The plant is called graviola, and yes, it's found in this book.

I thought about it for several weeks, mulled it over, prayed about it, examined all the DSHEA limitations, evaluated the risks, and prayed some more. One of the issues was that this plant was widely used as a parasite remedy in rainforest areas, but there were no traditional remedies using it to fight cancer. At the time, there was only one test-tube study published on the plant showing it killed various cancer cells, which wasn't all that consequential. Another issue was treating cancer with chemotherapy drugs is a big and profitable industry with many powerful players involved around the world. Competing with that in any way was asking for trouble.

Being a cancer survivor, and my journey with Raintree evolving as a type of spiritual journey rather than a hard-core profit-driven company like I've had in the past, I just couldn't ignore the information (or how I acquired it). I knew it would be difficult creating a single plant product because all I could say to anyone was that it was a parasite remedy and refer to that type of research. So, I began formulating my first rainforest formula for cancer for the company's practitioner line. I selected some other plants that were traditionally used for cancer and had the best research on them. To avoid any DSHEA prohibitions on product names, I called the formula "N-Tense" and described it as "a combination of the rainforest's most potent and powerfully intense plants in one synergistic formula." In the initial practitioner information, I could refer to the anti-cancer research on the individual plants specifically.

Practitioners tried the formula on their patients, and we all learned a lot. It worked great for some types of cancer, and not so great on others. Some types of cancers disappeared, some just stopped growing, and some had no effect at all. I made some adjustments to the formula based on the feedback and developed a second formula for non-tumorous cancers; and upon many requests, I made a liquid extract that could be used topically for skin cancer. All those formulas made the practitioner rounds again. And once again, after about a year, word-of-mouth referrals came in from practitioners and patients telling others about their experiences, which required me to offer the products directly to consumers. The practitioners couldn't keep up with demand.

Now, I want to stop here before going any further and repeat what I've always said . . . none of these plants or formulas I created are the be-all and end-all "Cure for Cancer." Cancer is a complicated disease. Every type of cancer is different. All humans are different, and many things about our health status, immune status, genetic makeup, and even our diets are different. That means that no one will have the exact same results with any natural product (or drug) even if they have the same type of cancer. This was clearly evidenced as the practitioners used the plants and formulas with their patients. I've also always said that cancer is a life-threatening disease and people should review all their conventional and alternative options (and there are many) to design an individualized game plan specifically for them. Nothing I've written about these plants or in this book suggests you should avoid conventional treatment and rely just on these plants. I specifically don't recommend it. And my personal experience has been that conventional cancer treatments don't work for all either. I turned to herbal and natural therapies after I had exhausted all conventional medicine options, and they'd given up on me and sent me home "to put my affairs in order."

That said, I'll continue. Eventually, some person who tried the multiple plant formula was interviewed on a Texas-based program on the Christian Broadcast Network. He said something like "God Bless Leslie and Raintree—my cancer is now gone." I got to meet the folks at the Texas Department of Health the next day. I never saw the TV program or knew who was interviewed, but I got to hear all about it from them. After a long day of discussion and thorough review of my products, website, and literature, they found no medical claims or DSHEA violations and left. But the dance had begun . . . I was on their radar. I did change the name of the plant database from the Rainforest Medicinal Plant Database to the Tropical Plant Database to appease them.

About a year later, I was interviewed by an alternative health organization that published a newsletter and wanted to talk about N-Tense. Since the formula was proprietary and only offered by my company, I asked them to focus their article on the new information about graviola instead, and they agreed. By this time, graviola was offered as a natural product under a couple of labels from the word-of-mouth education in the marketplace and probably from the plant database information. New anti-cancer research had also been

PREFACE

published on it by a different U.S. research group who had determined how it worked against cancer, and another company had launched a topical product for head lice with graviola. A new research group made progress by copying the one graviola chemical. I still had no graviola single plant product—just the multi-plant formula. Their article on graviola was rather sensationalized, and it went viral (and I was glad it wasn't just on my proprietary formula). It fueled even more research on graviola by other research organizations, and in many countries, several major supplement manufacturers launched graviola products in capsules and liquid extracts. And yes, it prompted another Texas Department of Health visit (turning up the volume for the dance).

After a couple more television and radio interviews/testimonials by various cancer patients and a few practitioner articles written about their experiences with the formula or graviola over the next few years, the Department of Health dance became more heated. They started demanding I remove the Tropical Plant Database from the website, even though it met federal DSHEA regulations on third-party documentation (and Texas had no laws or regulations over dietary supplements to enforce). I scheduled a meeting with the head of the department who was making this demand. Her bias and dislike of any and all dietary supplements was palpable, and I knew the dance would continue no matter what I did. I decided to move from Texas and landed in Carson City, Nevada. I was tired of the dance that never ended, especially since if I spent a lot of money to sue and win, it would just perpetuate the dance in other ways based on this department head's bias.

During these years, the FDA changed various enforcement procedures concerning the marketing and dissemination of factual information about dietary supplements that basically took any education mechanism out of the law. Some of these didn't even write a new regulation; FDA enforcement actions changed based on their new interpretations of existing regulations. The end result concerning traditional uses, which is in place today, is that no natural product company can refer to any traditional use if the traditional use names an actual disease or condition (like constipation or diarrhea) without facing FDA reprisals. They then made the same determination about referring to third-party documents like research on the product or the natural ingredients in a dietary supplement. If the researcher studied any disease or condition, they declared it cannot be listed, linked to, or referred to in the marketing of a natural product without reprisals.

I spent years during my direction of Raintree Nutrition changing product labels, product names, product literature, product webpages, and the Tropical Plant Database repeatedly to keep up with new regulations and enforcement actions that evolved over the years. I had several discussions with the FDA as the rules changed. They disliked the Tropical Plant Database as much as the Texas Department of Health did. In 2012, I moved the plant database to its own website and then jumped through the new hoops regarding how product companies could link to factual, non-misleading third-party documentation through their allowable series of multiple links and pop-up disclaimers to get there.

In late 2012, I was presented with a new dilemma. The FDA had detained a large shipment of rainforest plants coming into the United States from the Amazon during Raintree's normal import procedures without declaring a reason. My FDA attorney was flabbergasted by the ensuing conversation. He told me the FDA was demanding changes to my product pages and the plant database—not under DSHEA (which I complied with), but under the newer (and almost unlimited) authority that was given to them in the Homeland Security Act to protect the food supply from terrorism. This was the first time he had even heard of this concern about terrorism; DSHEA was the law of the land regarding herbal supplements, and my website was in compliance with those regulations. In fact, the specific changes the FDA wanted on the product pages would make them less safe because they demanded I remove the information on possible contraindications and drug interactions, which was the only thing I quoted from my book/database pages.

When my attorney called them back to relay this information, he still met resistance. He finally asked them, off the record, "What does she need to do to get this shipment released?" They told him that I needed to take the plant database offline. My attorney advised that I fight it since DSHEA regulations should take precedence, and this was the first time this new homeland security law was being used. I recognized this was just the start of a new dance that I had danced before in Texas, and even if I won, the dance would continue in other ways.

The fact is, however, the information in the plant database had reached tens of millions of people everywhere. It had helped fuel research on these rainforest plants in laboratories and universities around the world. I know that because I see the plant database cited as a reference in numerous

PREFACE

researchers' published studies. I believed it was an important source of valuable information on rainforest plants that exists nowhere else helping many people looking for natural remedies to address their health concerns. That's why the FDA wanted it removed. Most of the regulations or enforcement actions they had developed over the last 20 years was to limit information on herbal supplements to keep consumers in the dark about the benefits they may have—despite this being the opposite of Congress's intention in having passed the law.

So it really wasn't that much of a dilemma after I thought long and hard about it. I decided that the information was more important than me selling herbal supplements. I had created a large international market for many rainforest plants, and I had no doubt that they would continue to sell. I decided I would continue to provide the factual information on them as I always have. I shut down Raintree Nutrition in late 2012. I moved the plant database back to the Raintree website and published all the recipes on the multi-plant product pages so anyone could make them themselves. I also added back all the information that I had removed to stay in compliance with regulations as a seller of products. Under the law, if I sell no supplement products, I am no longer under the authority of the FDA or DSHEA. It is now a publisher's website called Rain-Tree Publishers, and it will continue to be the best place to learn about rainforest medicinal plants, their benefits, and how to use them. I have written several articles on this subject in 2018. See the "References" section (page 332) for the links.

I have spent many years consulting with practitioners helping their cancer patients with rainforest plants based on my knowledge on the subject. And as remarkable as the effects of graviola may be, as you will learn, there are other rainforest plants that show just as much promise. Today, there is a wealth of new information on these plants because drug companies are now studying some of them in their quest for new chemotherapy drugs. You'll read about one in the book that is in Phase II clinical trials now. See espinheira santa, page 238.

In addition, scientists are now using new testing methods in cancer research that actually explain how these plants and/or their active chemicals are achieving anti-cancer actions on a molecular level to target cancer cells—to kill them, stop them from growing, and/or prevent them from spreading. This type of research has now been conducted on almost all the plants in this book. It is really fascinating, and much of it confirms or helps explain my practical experience with the plants. Some of this new research is explaining how these plants or their natural chemicals are now being combined with frontline chemotherapy drugs to reduce side effects and/or toxicity to healthy cells the drugs cause and how that is working on a molecular level. It's been quite inspiring reading so much new research on the plants I've used for so many years.

I really wished that I might find the cure for cancer as I was trekking through the Amazon rainforest over many years, but I haven't. I don't think there will ever really be one cure for all. Cancer is just too complex. Our bodies are complicated and uniquely different. I did, however, find some really important medicinal plants that are making a real difference in some people's lives. The intention of writing this book is to share this information with you, share my personal experiences using them, and share how I combined them together for different kinds of cancer to get better results. Some of the natural chemicals in a few of the plants in this book will likely be turned into new chemotherapy drugs—they are in progress now.

History shows, however, from the time they find an anti-cancerous chemical in a plant to the time a new cancer drug is sold, it can take between 30 and 50 years. These natural plants with their unique chemicals are available now, and unfortunately, too many of us don't have the time to wait. This is why a plant like graviola has been used as a natural herbal remedy around the world. In 2018, a federal law was passed that allows cancer patients the "right to try" unapproved drugs for diseases like cancer. Shouldn't Americans have a right to try natural remedies for cancer in the same manner?

Hopefully you'll learn in this book the best way to use graviola and other rainforest plants like graviola—how to combine them with other plants, or to use other plants that might be more effective on certain cancers. I believe it's time to share that knowledge in a meaningful way. It is my sincere hope that you might find information in this book that will make a difference in your own personal journey if you are fighting cancer—and for some, the hope to carry on and keep fighting the battle with new ammunition and resources.

HOW TO USE THIS BOOK

In the United States, cancer is an industry. Like any other industry, there's always an eye on profits, strategies to minimize risks (and lawsuits), and marketing strategies to increase sales. Just like any other business. The average frontline oncologist has one primary objective—to provide at a minimum the "standard therapy protocols" based on the type of cancer you have and what stage it's in. They are trained in these protocols, which have been approved by the companies employing them. There is nothing really for them to decide. The standard level of care is outlined for them, the chemotherapy drugs are selected for them already, and whether to add other therapies (and when), like radiation and/or immunotherapy, is already in the standard protocols that the Food and Drug Administration (FDA) has blessed. Following these standard protocols is the key to avoid getting sued for malpractice, so they're pretty much written in stone.

For that reason, your oncologist has probably never heard about any of the plants in this book and most probably doesn't want to know. They are limited to prescribing standard therapies and drugs within set protocols, so they rarely take the time to follow any cancer research on unapproved drugs or plants. In fact, the standard protocols they follow also require them to ask their patients for a list of all natural products and herbal supplements they are taking. Then, the majority routinely tell their patients to discontinue all supplements since there is never enough human research (which costs tens of millions of dollars) on them to prove they won't interfere with the drugs the oncologists are prescribing. Again, this protocol is more about reducing their liability. I've heard of quite a few oncologists who fire any patient (refuse to treat them) if they do not agree to discontinue any and all herbal/dietary supplements. So, the first thing you should know is that you shouldn't attempt to use this book to educate your oncologist about natural remedies for cancer that you may want to take.

You will learn in chapter 3 why there will never be any significant human studies on a whole plant as an herbal remedy (which contains more than 300 natural chemicals working synergistically together in mostly unknown ways) like you'll find in this book. You'll also learn why this type of research will never be performed inside the United States. In a nutshell, no U.S. company can profit from conducting this type of research—the FDA cannot approve a whole plant used as an herbal remedy (much less a multi-herb formula) as a drug or an herbal drug that makes medical claims for something like cancer under their current regulations. No product = no profits = no research.

You will also learn in chapter 3 that herbal remedies have been used in herbal medicine systems around the world for millennia (and much longer than our rather young by comparison pharmaceutical industry, which emerged in the late 19th and early 20th centuries). The birth of the drug industry was first all about studying herbal and natural remedies and trying to figure out how or why they were working. For example, the pain-relieving willow bark tea remedy resulted in the extraction of a chemical called aspirin, which resulted in an aspirin drug.

The early 1900s saw a move toward chemically synthesizing and purifying these natural compounds, leading to more precise and potent medications and eliminating the need for harvesting any natural materials. All the published research on the plant starts with testing the plant to see if scientists can confirm an action that explains the herbal medicine use. Then the individual chemicals inside the plant are tested individually, looking for any chemical that may explain that action. If the researchers find such individual chemicals, then they'll typically do animal studies to confirm that action and more studies to determine how it is achieving that action on a molecular level. If all goes well, they'll start to figure out how to copy the one chemical providing the strongest action and synthesize it in their labs with the goal of changing it slightly so they create a new and patentable chemical with the same action. This is the process of creating a new drug and the type of research that is published along the way.

You'll see me referring to many research studies in Part 3 of this book that have been published on the anti-cancer plants featured herein. You need to keep in mind, however, that none of the plants or the multi-herbal

HOW TO USE THIS BOOK

formulas discussed in this book will ever be drugs, or ever have the type of research conducted on them that drugs do in the United States. A rainforest medicinal plant usually has a minimum of 300 active plant chemicals. While a researcher can test an individual chemical, it doesn't explain how it will behave in the presence of 299 other active plant chemicals. Oftentimes, it can create entirely different active chemicals when it joins and binds to another active chemical. Other reactions are also common. For example, one active chemical can be tested with very low bioavailability (the ability of being digested and entering the blood stream so it can go to work) when tested individually, but in the presence of other natural chemicals in the plant, it greatly enhances bioavailability.

Surprisingly, new research on the gut bacteria in the gut microbiome reports that when some plant chemicals with low bioavailability make it to the bacteria in the colon intact, the gut bacteria use them as food and/or some bacteria create new active chemicals with them as well. And most notably, one single plant may have between 10 and 110 different anti-cancer chemicals that work in many different ways to kill cancer or inhibit its progression, spread, and invasiveness. No one has gone through the extensive research required to determine how all those anti-cancer chemicals are working together synergistically. But looking at the research may help to explain why the whole plant is so effective, or why it's effective for so many different types of cancers.

So, the main way you should use this book is to always keep in mind that you are learning about effective natural remedies made from rainforest plants. I've personally sold the featured plants and/or formulas from 1995 through 2012. After I closed my company in December 2012, other herbal manufacturers in the United States, Eastern and Western Europe, and Australia began making the cancer formulas (and others) and selling them under their own labels with the formula information I uploaded on the Raintree website. These plants and formulas have been anti-cancer remedies for 25 years or more. Some of the plants featured herein have an even longer history of use as cancer herbal remedies; pau d'arco's uses for tumors, for example, were first reported in 1873, and many other plants herein were due to NCI's screening of plants for cancer use beginning in the 1960s.

The published research referenced in the book will be available on the Raintree website, and links will be provided at the end of each plant's details in the book. There has been so much research on rainforest plants in the last 10 years that including them in this book would double the book's size. These referenced research files will include the initials *HS*, *IVT*, *IVA*, *REV*, *INS*, and *NEW* to describe the published studies. *HS* refers to research conducted in humans; *IVT* refers to *in vitro* research conducted inside of test tubes; *IVA* refers to *in vivo* research conducted in animals; *REV* refers to a review article that evaluates and summarizes multiple studies on the same subject; *INS* refers to *in silico* research (newer computer modeling including molecular docking studies); and *NEW* refers to new biological testing methods that determine genes and signaling pathways, and molecular pathways of actions that were developed during and after the Human Genome Project (discussed in chapter 4).

While *in vitro* test-tube research is common, it usually isn't considered important until the same actions are confirmed in animals. Even then, how something acts in animals may not completely relate to how it might act in humans. The newer research methods and computer models are quite interesting because some of them can accurately predict how a plant extract or plant chemical might act in humans. Again, all of this is interesting and may help people understand why the plant and formulas work, but you are still learning about herbal remedies for cancer that will never have enough research to convince any classically trained oncologist of their true value.

That they continue to be sold after 25 years by word-of-mouth referrals and without any marketing by a manufacturer disclosing what they actually do is quite compelling and, to a practitioner like me, more compelling than any published research in the pursuit of a new chemotherapy drug. If something continues to flow into the market because it actually works (and not because of any dissemination of any research or even disclosure of what the formula or plant might do) speaks volumes.

INTRODUCTION

We have been fighting the "war against cancer" from the moment we declared it in 1971, and we are still not winning. Cancer is still a leading cause of death worldwide, accounting for nearly one in six deaths. Globally, new cancer cases were estimated at more than 20 million with around 10 million deaths due to cancer. Currently, here in the United States, more than 2 million new cancer cases are diagnosed each year with more than 600,000 cancer deaths—and unfortunately, those numbers continue to increase. The most common new cases of cancers found here are breast, lung, colorectal, and prostate cancers.

Most of Western medicine research is still looking for new cancer cures based on the use of highly selective pure single chemicals with a strong specificity for their targets. One chemical to kill one type of cancer cell. Cancer, however, is a multifaceted disease that in most cases deserves a multifaceted therapeutic approach. We now know that cancer has the unique ability to change many chemical processes, genes, and signaling pathways (how chemical substances interact and "talk" with each other) and involve many cascading chemical reactions of genes and their proteins and other substances, which allow cancer cells the ability to grow, multiply, and thrive. In fact, it's estimated that cancer can modify or change the function of more than 400 different genes. Cancer can even create complex chemical defense mechanisms that allow them to hide from the immune system, promote more nutrients to fuel their rapid growth, resist chemical agents meant to kill them, and turn off the "kill switch" that tells them to die after making a copy of itself.

One single chemotherapy drug or chemical has very little chance to affect so many things that have gone wrong. That's why we're losing the war. While conventional cancer protocols usually now include administering more than one cancer drug at a time (usually two to three drugs are now used in combination), it has still not resulted in any real cures because, again, cancer has too many (up to 400) ways to avoid two to three chemicals. Drug resistance after chemotherapy is typically the norm.

Can plant-based medicines hold the key? Absolutely. Instead of just one molecule/chemical, a medicinal plant can have up to 400 different natural plant chemicals. All these chemicals can have similar or very different actions and have a much better chance at affecting many more of the processes controlled by cancer. For example, one anti-cancer plant featured in this book (see graviola, page 252) contains more than 60 different plant chemicals that can kill cancer cells in 15 different ways. With so many chemicals working in different ways, the cancer cells will have a much harder time creating defense mechanisms against them all. The plant can also affect 17 different chemical substances that cancer changes to create the main defense mechanisms to defend itself, other natural compounds that reduce the blood supply to tumors, and yet even other compounds that prevent the tumor from metastasizing by robbing it of the energy it needs in five different ways. You'll find, as you read about the rainforest medicinal plants in this book, that every one of them has these kinds of abilities to affect cancer on many different levels.

Now consider how traditional medicine systems usually combine three to seven medicinal plants together for remedy-specific formulas to treat a myriad of diseases and conditions. Some may be chosen to directly impact the condition, while others are chosen to treat the symptoms in the meantime. With anti-cancer herbal remedies, the most effective will be able to affect the largest number of changes that the cancer causes (to promote its survival) and to kill it efficiently. And this can be quite cancer specific. The manner in which prostate cancer promotes its own survival will be quite different from how lung cancer protects itself and promotes its growth. Thankfully, you'll also learn how we now have new research and testing methods that help explain what the plants and their active natural chemicals are doing on a molecular level to address and affect cancer in hundreds of different ways. When plants are combined into remedies, there are now thousands of active chemicals going to work in many different ways that have a much better chance of affecting the hundreds of ways cancer can thrive.

How to combine the anti-cancer plants of the rainforest together based on specific cancer types is the key to these remedy-specific formulas' abilities

INTRODUCTION

to fight cancer more efficiently. The most effective way to treat cancer may well be to address all these many factors and determine the right combination of medicinal plants—based on the type of cancer one has to fix and the known changes the cancer has caused—while shutting down the specific defense mechanisms cancer uses that limit the effectiveness of traditional chemotherapies. In fact, you'll find information in the book about how mainstream cancer researchers are now combining some of the natural plant chemicals detailed in this book with their chemo drugs for just that purpose. They are also reporting how these natural plant chemicals can selectively target just cancer cells without much toxicity to healthy cells.

This book is divided into three parts: Part 1 explores the new advances in cancer research made to design new, more effective drugs to fight cancer; why plants thriving in the rainforest offer real hope in these endeavors; and how to combine them together for greater efficacy. Chapter 1 explains why rainforest plants are so unique, how and why they create highly active plant chemicals to thrive in an intense and stressful environment, and how humankind has been harnessing and harvesting these remarkable natural plant defensive chemicals for effective new drugs. Based on extensive screening programs conducted between the 1960s and 1980s, the National Cancer Institute (NCI) targeted more than 3,000 plant chemicals with anti-cancerous actions, and 70% were found in rainforest plants. Since that time, more than 25,000 plant chemicals have now been identified with anti-cancerous actions through computer modeling and new testing methods, and yes, the majority grow in the rainforest or tropical climates.

Several rainforest plants and their active chemicals have already been targeted for this purpose and are detailed in this book. Scientists around the world are conducting ongoing research concerning the benefits of combining these natural defensive plant chemicals with various gold-standard cancer drugs. They are reporting that the combination can increase the efficacy of the chemo drug, lower the toxicity to healthy cells, and even overcome or prevent drug resistance.

Information on these defensive plant chemicals is detailed in chapter 2, which provides information on a large classification of plant compounds called polyphenols. Rainforest plants (as well as most fruits and vegetables) produce these natural chemicals to prevent and overcome the damage resulting from negative growing conditions. In fact, you'll learn that all plants produce these types of compounds and understand why poor diets, lacking in fresh fruits and vegetables, are now considered to play an important role in increasing our risks of getting cancer and a number of chronic diseases now plaguing our current society. The lack of polyphenols in the average American diet is now also linked to developing chronic inflammation. The chapter provides important information concerning the link between chronic inflammation with cancer, which many readers may not realize. You'll learn in this book that new data reveals that one in six human cancers could be attributed to chronic inflammation. It is also estimated that appropriate diet and lifestyle modifications could prevent more than two-thirds of human cancers worldwide, and diet is responsible for 10–70% (on average, 35%) of human cancer mortality.

Chapter 3 discusses the scientific methods and procedures drug researchers employ to turn a plant into a new drug. You'll learn that there are plant-based drugs that are manufactured and prescribed in other countries for specific diseases and conditions (including cancer) and why they'll never be approved in the same fashion in the United States. This information reveals how a plant-based drug is usually some patented extraction process of a natural plant, rich in many plant chemicals. For this reason, much of the published research on the plants reviewed to write this book was published in other countries that manufacture, sell, and prescribe these plant-based drugs. In the United States, these plant products are sold as herbal supplements; mention of any medical claims as to what to use them for is not allowed. As a result, far less research is being conducted on natural plant products in the United States because product manufacturers are not permitted to share the research to educate their customers.

The information provided in chapter 4 explains why and how these new plant testing methods were created and reveals how a huge international collaborative research program was conducted to study every gene in the human body. The information obtained in gene research revealed the wonderfully complicated chemical cascades that happen when a gene is activated to do its job. It involves a chain reaction of up to 100 other substances (proteins, enzymes, and other molecules) in the body, which also interact with other genes and their substances. This allowed scientists to create a "road map" of how genes functioned.

INTRODUCTION

Then, many of the major players in the research collaboration began studying the genes in people with various types of cancer and other diseases to create other important road maps, which revealed what substances had changed in the gene function chemical cascades. This chapter will tell you how this new information changed the face of cancer research, cancer treatment, and drug development forever. Not only did it help explain how their current drugs were working on a molecular level, but it also provided new chemical targets in these chain reactions of cascading chemicals they could use to design new drugs. The chapter also provides information on what the main catalysts are that start a healthy cell in the body to mutate or transform into a cancer cell, the evolution of cancer, and how our cancer drugs have evolved over the years.

Chapter 5 outlines the real benefits of these new road maps. It attempts to describe in an easy-to-understand manner the pathways that cancer uses to transform and survive the immune system and other programmed processes of life and death, as well as the survival mechanisms cancer uses to promote rapid growth and spread to distant sites by changing certain substances in the cascading chemical reactions. We know so much more with these new road maps! This chapter also provides an overview of the new chemical targets being used for cancer treatment today, highlights which drugs (new and old) are trying to use these targets to treat cancer, and which rainforest plants and/or plant chemicals have been reported to change these same chemical substances/targets.

Part 2 discusses harnessing the power of the plants. Chapter 6 provides the naturopathic protocols I developed almost 20 years ago. I used these protocols to develop several multi-plant formulas for cancer, trained and worked with alternative health practitioners helping cancer patients, and lectured and taught in various alternative health venues. Chapter 7 provides a specific plan for different cancer types. I share the actual formulas I developed, and provide information on which specific plants I used to combine with them for various types of cancer and the results I saw. In chapter 8, I share how I would change these formulas today based on all of the new research that has been conducted on these rainforest plants since I first developed them. This type of information cannot be found anywhere else but this book. It will tell you how to make a specific formula for the type of cancer you have and give you the option to prepare the remedy in capsules, teas, or various types of extracts along with how to take them.

Part 3 of the book is all about the rainforest plants that I have used for many years to help fight cancer. It provides important new information on 13 rainforest medicinal plants and focuses on what is known today on how they might fight cancer. The information for each plant includes a brief summary of where the plant is found, its traditional uses, and which uses have been validated by research. It describes all anti-cancerous research conducted on the actual plant, identifies which active chemicals in the plant demonstrated anti-cancer actions (which might explain actions demonstrated in the plant), and then reviews all the research and information on those active plant chemicals (and if any are the subject of new drug research).

New information on the plants is provided in a section that describes how the plant and/or its chemicals are working on a molecular level to affect cancer, which cancer pathway is being affected, and/or which specific chemical targets within that pathway were changed. Also provided is information on what other researched benefits and actions have been demonstrated in research, which a cancer patient might find to be helpful. As always, the plant data in this chapter provides information on safety, availability of products, dosages, possible contraindications, and possible drug interactions for each rainforest plant.

PART 1

Understanding the Power of Rainforest Plants

1
WHY RAINFOREST MEDICINAL PLANTS ARE UNIQUE

Rainforests hold the highest biodiversity and sheer number of novel chemicals on the planet. Acre for acre, they contain more species of plants and animals and, yes, even bacteria, mold, fungi, and virus species than anywhere else on earth. There is something special about the plants that grow in the Amazon and other rainforests in the world. The Amazon is teeming with life, and its biodiversity is unequaled. One hectare (2.47 acres) of Amazon rainforest land may contain more than 750 types of trees and 1,500 species of higher plants. Comparing that to a hectare of typical temperate forest in the United States, which has a half dozen tree species or fewer, really does define *high diversity*. With each plant and tree containing between 300 and 400 plant chemicals—that's a lot of chemicals!

Plants' Survival Instincts Helping Humankind

Literally all living things have inbred survival instincts. It is part of the cellular makeup of all species on earth. In highly mobile species like humans and other animals, the main survival instinct and mechanism is "flee, fight, or hide." Even bacteria and virus species have learned to flee or hide from immune cells and chemical agents attacking them, as well as to fight them by mutating or changing their own physical structure to defend against them. With stationary plants rooted to the ground and incapable of physically fleeing from danger, their survival instinct is controlled by wonderfully complex and rich chemical defense mechanisms that have evolved over eons. Plants have either created a defense mechanism against what might harm them, or they have succumbed and become extinct.

In the species-rich rainforest, there are many species of fungi, mold, bacteria, viruses, parasites, and insects that attack and kill plants. It is of little wonder that rainforest plants contain so many potent and active chemicals: the plants are in a constant battle for survival in an environment literally teeming with life that is constantly evolving. From soil-borne root rot (a virus) that attacks tender herbaceous plants, to the fungi and mold smothering the life out of huge canopy trees, or to the incredible number of insects devouring any defenseless leaf in the forest, rainforest plants have learned to adapt, create chemical defenses against attack, and survive.

Within this rich arsenal of defensive chemicals are antibacterial, antiviral, antifungal, antiparasitic, anti-mold, and insecticidal chemicals with tested potent actions. This is the mechanism the plants use to survive, grow, and flourish, as well as to fight the many disease-causing organisms that attack them. It is likely that, within these diverse chemicals created to protect the plants from disease, at least a handful or more will be harvested and put to use protecting humans and animals from the same types of disease-causing organisms.

All plants contain some of these defensive chemicals, but rainforest and tropical plants have much more than cultivated plants. The growing conditions in the tropics are just more intense and stressful. High humidity (which promotes more mold and fungi), intense heat and too much sunlight at the top of the canopy with too little sunlight on the forest floor, and periods of monsoon-like rains followed by dry periods in the typical rainy-dry seasons of the tropics all contribute to the tropical plants' need to increase production of plant chemicals to protect themselves from all these other stress factors.

Due to annual flooding washing away top soils (along with their nutrients), rainforest soils are notoriously nutrient deficient. Rainforest plants and huge trees had to create adaptive chemical mechanisms to store the nutrients they need for growth and fertility inside themselves and not rely on uptake from soils as normal plants do. And let's not forget about the bugs! Without a cold season to kill off crawling bugs as well as bacteria, viruses, and fungi, the diversity of pests that tropical plants are exposed to is much higher in the tropics than anywhere else in the world. When botanists say a particular plant has "adapted" to grow in the tropics, this adaptation is usually all about the plant having increased its natural production of protective chemicals enough to survive in these more extreme growing conditions.

Cultivated plants, which encompass the fruits and vegetables in our diet, are grown with the idea that all these stressors should be minimized and controlled to enhance productivity and therefore profits. You will learn in the next chapter that rainforest plants and cultivated plants do share some of the same defensive chemicals (called polyphenols); however, rainforest plants have much more of these polyphenols, as well as a wide variety of novel and unusual defensive chemicals that cultivated plants just don't create.

Many scientists have studied these rainforest defensive plant chemicals for their anti-cancerous, antibacterial, antiviral, antifungal, anti-inflammatory, and antiparasitic actions in their search for new drugs for many years. It is of little wonder that the U.S. National Cancer Institute identified 3,000 plants that are active against cancer cells more than 30 years ago, and 70% of these plants were found in the rainforest. Today, more than 25,000 identified plant chemicals have been shown to possess potent anti-cancer activities with the majority still found in tropical plants growing around the world. In fact, more than 47% of current anti-cancer drugs on the market are natural products, their derivatives, or natural product synthetic mimics that come from tropical plants.

TRADITIONAL MEDICINE SYSTEMS RESULT IN TRADITIONAL REMEDIES

The people in the rainforest, led by the shamans, medicine men, and herbal healers, have learned over thousands of years how to harness the power of these rainforest plants to protect themselves from the same harmful pathogens and to treat other common diseases. These plants have been their only pharmacy in the remote jungles of the Amazon. Their knowledge is irreplaceable.

For example, years ago, scientists evaluated a jungle shaman's "dysentery remedy" in the Amazon rainforest. It was a crude plant extract that contained seven plants. Now, one must remember, dysentery in the Amazon can be attributed to any number of different bacteria, amoebas, and parasites common in the area (and commonly shared in the close communal living environments of Indigenous groups). The Indian shaman doesn't have the ability to send blood or stool samples to a laboratory to find out which specific organism is causing the dysentery in his village, but he must still select the appropriate plants to treat his patients. Maybe this is why a shaman usually selects a handful of plants (about four to seven) to brew into a remedy, instead of just one.

When the 7 different plants in the dysentery remedy were analyzed, at least 12 different known antibiotic chemicals, 5 anti-amebic chemicals, and 7 antiparasitic chemicals were found between all the plants in the shaman's formula. The 12 different antibiotic chemicals in the extract were found to kill bacteria in at least 5 different ways; these ways are called biological pathways of action. The shaman didn't really need to know which "bad bug" was the culprit, in what mainstream medicine would call his "shotgun" approach. But does this really matter either? This particular remedy, containing a total of several thousand individual plant chemicals, had at least 31 active chemicals that hit the top 10 or so main bugs that might cause dysentery. (And yes, you'd think your doctor was completely nuts if he sent you home with 31 prescriptions, so maybe "shotgun" is an appropriate analogy within your doctor's limitations.)

If the dysentery bug was an easily mutating bacteria like staph, how likely would it be that this one organism could survive long enough to create a defense against 12 different antibacterial chemicals coming at it in at least 5 different ways simultaneously? These drug-resistant strains of bacteria are certainly more prevalent in First World nations in which single-chemical antibiotics are regularly employed than in poor tropical countries in which mainly plant-based remedies are used. Maybe it will take a broadly scattering shotgun to fight these tricky and quickly mutating organisms, instead of a single-chemical bullet. Food for thought, for sure!

The herbal remedy and traditional uses for the plants featured in this book will provide a quick summary. More in-depth knowledge of how rainforest healers use them, as well as herbal remedies in other traditional medicine systems, have been published in my other book, as well as the free online Tropical Plant Database. I authored both to memorialize the traditional uses of rainforest plants. This puts the knowledge in the public purview, which prevents the plants from being patented for any particular use discovered by Indigenous uses in any country. See the links provided in the "Resources" section (page 327) to access the book and Tropical Plant Database.

Traditional remedies aren't found just in the rainforest; plants have been used as medicine since the beginning of human history. Evidence of medicinal plant use by neanderthals who lived 40,000 years ago were reported in *Nature* magazine in 2017. Texts from ancient Sumeria, India, Egypt, China, and others contain recipes for medicinal plant preparations for the treatment of disease. Today, medicinal plant use remains widespread, and a significant portion of the world's population utilizes natural herbal remedies as the primary mode of health care. In the United States, nearly 20% of Americans surveyed were found to utilize herbal supplements to treat health conditions in 2012; today it has been estimated to be 50%. In developing or economically disadvantaged nations, herbal remedies for diseases and conditions are used 80% of the time as frontline health care.

The World Health Organization (WHO) has long accepted that traditional medicine and herbal remedies have been central to people's health and well-being across cultures and countries for centuries. The WHO established the Global Traditional Medicine Centre (GTMC) in 2022 to increase that knowledge, encourage and/or fund research to help scientifically validate traditional remedies, and provide guidance to member nations on regulatory, safety, and efficacy information on them.

Pharmaceutical companies around the world use this type of knowledge extensively. It helps them target specific plants to study in their search for novel chemicals for drugs. For example, if they want to develop a new drug for arthritis, they start with the plants that are traditionally used to treat arthritis and inflammation. Then they begin looking for anti-inflammatory and pain-relieving chemicals in the plant remedy that are responsible for the traditional use. Chapter 3 provides more detailed information on this process.

New Cancer Research on Rainforest Plants

The exciting news in cancer research, which you'll learn about in the pages of this book, is that rainforest plants and their active plant chemicals are now being harvested by drug companies for their ability to prevent and overcome cancer's ability to create defense mechanisms to avoid our gold-standard cancer drugs. Yes, just like all other organisms, cancer has the ability to "flee, fight, or hide" from cancer drugs as well as natural immune processes in the body meant to find cancer cells and kill them. You'll learn more about this research in Part 3. The compelling news in new cancer research has shown that it is possible to combine some active defensive plant chemicals, which have antioxidant actions, with oxidative cancer drugs (designed to kill cancer cells through oxidation) to positive effect. This research reports that these defensive chemicals do not act like antioxidants in cancer cells, only in healthy cells. More astonishing, however, is that studies have been conducted on this combination therapy in cancer patients and animals. These plants and/or their defensive chemicals are showing the ability to reduce or eliminate cancer drugs' toxic effects on healthy cells, enhance the efficacy of the cancer drug, and prolong drug treatment with fewer side effects.

The rainforests of the world are, and will continue to be, of great importance and one of the main areas where this cancer research likely will take place. These rainforest plants are powerhouses of active and beneficial plant chemicals and can be prepared into effective herbal remedies. They are the true wealth of the rainforest, and they can be the pharmacy to the world.

Many of the defensive and healing chemicals that plants make to survive and thrive fall into a classification of natural plant chemicals called polyphenols. They have fascinated scientists for many years with their wide array of beneficial actions and are the subject of a huge body of research. Turn the page to the next chapter to learn more about the power of polyphenols.

2

THE POWER OF POLYPHENOLS FOR CANCER

Scientists have long known that the polyphenols in plants can benefit humans in many of the same ways they benefit, protect, and heal plants. Polyphenols are the subject of a huge amount of research; more than 70,000 studies have been published on polyphenols since the mid-1980s, and research continues today at a fast pace. The healing power of polyphenols to positively affect our health is incredible, and thankfully more health-conscious consumers are learning of their many benefits.

Remember when coffee was once supposed to be bad for you and doctors told you to avoid it, mainly because of the heart-stimulant actions of caffeine? Then, suddenly, it was good for you. The same thing happened with chocolate and red wine, which once were supposed to be avoided and are now considered almost health foods. What happened? It was all the new research on the powerful health benefits of polyphenols. Coffee, chocolate (especially dark chocolate), and wine (especially red wine) are all significant sources of these powerful healing polyphenols. That polyphenols can overcome the negative effects of the caffeine in coffee, the high fat and calories in chocolate, and the alcohol content in wine, and still provide a net effect that is beneficial to our health speaks to the real power of these polyphenols.

As discussed in the previous chapter, all plants contain polyphenols, and the human body has evolved to rely on fruits and vegetables in the diet to obtain these important substances we need to stay healthy. In addition to coffee, wine, and chocolate, polyphenols also are found in green tea and the oils of plant seeds and fruit seeds. This is one of the reasons why olive oil and green tea are now widely thought of as "healthy"—they are rich in polyphenols. Even common spices like cinnamon and cloves, culinary herbs like oregano and thyme, and many medicinal plants are significant sources of beneficial polyphenols, which can be greater than those found in vegetables.

The polyphenol content of the foods we eat varies significantly based on many factors. Some powerful polyphenols are water soluble and are very sensitive to heat. The high heat generated in cooking fruits and vegetables can significantly lower the polyphenol content, which is why many nutritionists recommend having lots of raw fruits and veggies in our diets—it's all about the powerful and beneficial polyphenols in these raw foods.

This is pretty well established in conventional medicine systems (based on a significant body of research); for example, dietary recommendations instruct that we should be consuming at least five to seven servings of fruits and vegetables daily. Extensive research has established that the lack of polyphenols in the diet significantly increases the risks of getting cancer and a number of chronic diseases that plague our society today; unfortunately, many Americans might not be aware of this.

As the research on diet-derived polyphenols evolved, studying how the average American diet has changed over the years, it has become obvious that the polyphenols in our diets don't stand a chance in counteracting all the bad stuff we're eating these days. This includes all the highly processed foods, full of human-made chemicals, and the high-fat, high-calorie, and high-sugar content in fast foods, cereals, and snacks that are in the American diet today, just to name a few. Sadly, when researchers started examining diets in Americans in terms of polyphenols, coffee and chocolate were the main sources, and fruits and vegetables came in dead last.

In general, research on polyphenols indicate they have antioxidant, anti-inflammatory, anti-cancerous, and cancer-preventative actions, and many have anti-microbial actions. The main benefit of polyphenols, which help protect us from our dietary choices, is the strong antioxidant actions all polyphenols possess.

What Is a Free Radical?

There are two main types of free radicals: reactive oxygen species (ROS) and reactive nitrogen species (RNS). These substances are reactive because they are missing an electron. The human body is an oxygen-based system, as is most all life on the planet, including plants. Oxygen is an element indispensable for life. Inside the body, however, some oxygen, with the help of a catalyst, splits into single atoms with unpaired electrons. Electrons like to be in pairs, and these atoms, called free radicals, scavenge the body for other electrons so they can become a pair. As they travel through the body in search of a new electron, they cause damage to cells, proteins, and DNA, and interrupt or change cellular signaling (how cells in our body interact and "talk" to each other) through a process called oxidation.

Consider what happens when the fats or oils we use to cook with are exposed to too much oxygen—over time they become rancid. The rancidity is actually oxidation of the fat molecules. When fat molecules (called lipids) in our bodies are exposed to too much ROS, they also become rancid and are damaged in a similar manner. And when cooking oils are heated to high temperatures to fry foods, oxidation is rapid and ROS is created. We're actually adding more ROS to our diets when we eat fried food.

Free radicals, and specifically ROS, are a way of life in both humans and plants. ROS are formed as a natural byproduct of the normal metabolism of oxygen, and they even play important roles in how cells communicate (called cellular signaling). Basically, free radicals are a byproduct of many different chemical processes going on simultaneously inside our wonderfully complex biochemical-driven bodies.

In addition to metabolizing oxygen, another large source of free radicals produced inside our bodies is the natural chemical process of how we metabolize our foods. Turning food into the cellular energy that all our cells need to function is a complex biochemical process. Free radicals are waste products generated from various chemical reactions that occur in this natural food metabolism process. Therefore, how much we eat and what we eat can be significant factors that raise our ROS levels. For example, free radicals are naturally formed each time we metabolize an ingredient in our food. Highly processed and fast foods contain many human-made chemical preservatives and additives, and each ingredient will create free radicals as it is metabolized in our bodies. One popular fast-food chain listed 19 ingredients in their french fries, not just potatoes, oil, and salt. Consider how much more ROS is generated, metabolizing all those ingredients!

Free radicals are created inside our bodies through these natural processes, and catalyst substances in our environment can create even more ROS. External catalysts that generate free radicals can be found in the food we eat, the medicines we take, the air we breathe, and the water we drink. These substances include fried foods, highly processed foods, high-fructose sugars, alcohol, tobacco smoke, pesticides, exposure to X-rays, chemicals and environmental toxins, and air and water pollutants. All these substances can significantly raise the levels of ROS and free radicals in our bodies to unhealthy levels.

The levels of internally produced free radicals also increase from immune cell activation, inflammation, mental stress, excessive exercise, ischemia, infection, cancer, aging, diabetes, and obesity, which takes us over the edge of balance and into the state of oxidative stress. Free radicals can also provoke inappropriate or overexpressed immune responses and cause autoimmune conditions and greatly increase cellular-aging processes.

What Is an Antioxidant?

In the simplest of terms, the most basic definition of an antioxidant is a substance or molecule that lends one of its own electrons to a free radical that is seeking one to make a pair. When the free radical has a new set of paired electrons, it becomes a stable molecule and is no longer reactive and causing cell damage. Remember, free radicals are radical because they are missing an electron. This process of an antioxidant lending an electron is usually called "quenching free radicals."

Our Built-In Antioxidant System

Because ROS generation is a natural process, our bodies have a natural built-in antioxidant system that is supposed to disable these free radicals as they are created and keep them at healthy levels. This is a perfect example of one of the amazing ways our bodies maintain their delicate balance. Through other biochemical processes, our bodies produce chemicals that are the main antioxidants that make up our built-in antioxidant system. These include chemical enzymes called superoxide dismutase (SOD), catalase, glutathione peroxidase, and glutathione reductase, which are considered our first line of defense.

We also produce other substances that are non-enzyme antioxidants that participate in our built-in antioxidant system. These include chemicals we produce inside our bodies such as lipoic acid, glutathione, L-arginine, coenzyme Q10, melatonin, uric acid, bilirubin, metal-chelating proteins, and transferrin.

Vitamin and Mineral Antioxidants

While these natural built-in antioxidants are main players in our antioxidant system, they need help from various vitamins and minerals that aid in the biochemical process to produce them, activate them, and help them do their job. These include vitamins A, E, and C, as well as the minerals selenium, manganese, copper, and zinc, which we're supposed to be getting from the foods we eat. These vitamins and minerals are the subject of thousands of studies on their antioxidant actions and the roles they play in the body and within our antioxidant system.

Plant Polyphenols with Antioxidant Actions

Plants, like humans, need oxygen to survive, and they also create their own species of reactive oxygen molecules (ROS) during their metabolism of the oxygen they breathe. For this reason, plants produce natural antioxidants and polyphenols in their cellular processes to keep ROS in check and at healthy levels, just as we do. These plant chemicals are also an important component in a plant's built-in defense mechanisms that protect the plants from negative growing factors (discussed in the previous chapter). These natural compounds also help heal the damage from browsing animals and insects chewing on them (the equivalent of wounds in humans) and help plants recover from various bacteria, mold, fungi, and plant viruses that damage them.

In addition to lending electrons, polyphenols have a unique way to provide antioxidant actions that our natural antioxidant system cannot. The main thing that makes a polyphenol a polyphenol is its shared unique molecular structure. This structure allows it to attach or bind to other substances in the body easily, and even with other polyphenols. The binding action of polyphenols can happen inside plants to make more healing and antioxidant chemicals when the plant needs them, and these bonds can happen and new chemicals are formed inside our bodies during digestion. These types of chemicals are called metabolites—a product of metabolism.

Unbelievably, while scientists have confirmed there are more than 8,000 unique polyphenols, they estimate that between 100,000 and 200,000 metabolites of polyphenols are created in plants, animals, humans, and even microbes like bacteria.

Using its binding abilities, polyphenols can suppress the formation of ROS by binding with and inhibiting two enzymes involved in the production of ROS. Plant antioxidants can also trigger the body's natural production of antioxidants and send them to cells that are being damaged by oxidative stress by binding with signaling molecules. Much as chemical messengers signal the immune system to send healing agents to the site of an injury, plant antioxidants can signal the body's antioxidant system to send healing antioxidants to the site of oxidative stress, as well as encourage the production of more body-produced antioxidant chemicals.

What Is Oxidative Stress?

Basically, the hallmark of a Western diet is the lack of essential nutrients we need, including natural vitamins, minerals, and polyphenols that keep our natural antioxidant system humming along and doing its job of keeping free radicals in check. Havoc ensues when our antioxidant system falters, and the result is oxidative stress. If the antioxidant system doesn't recover, then chronic oxidative stress ensues. You may be surprised to learn that one of the main deregulations and effects that free radicals cause is the level of inflammation in our bodies. Oxidative stress and chronic inflammation go hand in hand and have surfaced as the "root of all evil" when it comes to cancer and chronic diseases. Free radicals and inflammation are uniquely intertwined since inflammation promotes the creation of free radicals and free radicals promote inflammation—they are reacting together in a self-perpetuating cycle that leads to chronic inflammation and chronic oxidative stress.

What Is Chronic Inflammation?

Tens of thousands of research studies have been published on chronic inflammation and oxidative stress and the roles they play in numerous diseases. We now know that inflammation and oxidative stress can be a cause or a contributing factor to a wide range of diseases, including almost every chronic disease. From heart diseases, diabetes and other metabolic disorders, Alzheimer's disease, and cancer to high cholesterol levels, autoimmune diseases, and even obesity—chronic inflammation and oxidative stress are playing significant roles. Many of these studies reveal that when you reduce oxidative stress and chronic inflammation, it has a beneficial impact on these conditions.

Better yet, if you manage your levels of oxidative stress and chronic inflammation with polyphenols, you can avoid developing these many conditions. Polyphenol compounds with antioxidant and anti-inflammatory actions have surfaced in all this research as the most important natural plant compounds available to us that have the ability to help prevent these diseases. Since the inflammation is normally being orchestrated and delivered by immune cells, this self-perpetuating cycle is also associated with deregulations in our immune system and may be associated with autoimmune diseases and changes in normal immune function. Chronic inflammation is estimated to contribute to the cause of approximately 25% of all human cancers.

The whole subject of free radicals—how diets specifically increase free radicals, how chronic oxidative stress and chronic inflammation are associated with many diseases, and how dietary changes can be beneficial—is explained in much more detail in several books I have written. Information is provided in the "Resources" section on page 327.

Polyphenol Benefits for Cancer Prevention and Treatment

It is scientifically validated that free radicals and/or the oxidative stress they cause can activate cancer genes and mutate healthy cells into cancerous ones. It is also well established that free radicals can damage DNA in various cells in our bodies. This DNA damage can be the catalyst in a healthy cell mutating into a cancerous cell. For that reason, one of the main roles our natural built-in antioxidant system plays is to protect us from cancer by preventing the DNA damage free radicals cause. Many plant polyphenols have been reported in research to protect cells from mutating into cancerous cells (called "antimutagenic"), and some have even been documented with the ability to repair the DNA damage caused by free radicals through their antioxidant actions. This has resulted in many studies around the world reporting that polyphenol-rich diets, as well as many individual polyphenols and other antioxidant chemicals in plants, can provide cancer-preventative actions.

About 30–35% of new cancer cases are linked to diet, and chronic inflammation is estimated to contribute to approximately 25% of human cancers. There is strong evidence that what we eat can either help prevent or promote cancer. The Mediterranean diet is one of the more popular diets being studied for cancer prevention and treatment. In countries where people eat less red meat, drink wine, consume dairy in moderation, and eat lots of fresh fruits, vegetables, and olive oil, cancer rates tend to be much lower. Fruits and vegetables contain many beneficial polyphenol compounds that have antioxidant, anti-inflammatory, and anti-cancer effects.

If you're fighting cancer, it's important to change any unhealthy eating habits that might have contributed to getting cancer in the first place. This knowledge, thankfully, is going more mainstream; many books written on "cancer diets" and "anti-inflammatory diets" as well as cookbooks on the subject are now available in the marketplace. Spend some time finding a good one that will be easier for you to follow at first. And remember to stick to whole foods without too many food preservatives and additives to lower exposure to free radicals, which are generated every time each ingredient in your meal is metabolized on a molecular level.

Summary

Cancer develops in three main stages: initiation, promotion, and progression. Oxidative stress plays a role in all of these stages. In the initiation stage, reactive oxygen species (ROS) can cause DNA damage by creating mutations and changing the DNA structure. In the promotion stage, ROS can lead to abnormal gene activity, prevent cells from communicating properly, and interfere with cellular communication, which can result in more cell growth or less cell death. Finally, during the progression stage, oxidative stress can cause even more DNA damage in the cells that have already been affected and promote inflammation inside the cancer cells, which promotes cancer's growth, movement, and migration.

The multiple actions polyphenols can have against cancer involve several factors that affect how cancer cells survive, grow, develop, move, form new blood vessels, respond to hormones, detoxify, and create defense mechanisms. These findings strongly suggest that polyphenols have anti-cancer effects because they can change the way cancer cells behave and change the chemical signaling messages they send and receive. Specifically, natural polyphenols can help fight cancer by affecting cell growth, removing harmful substances, boosting antioxidant enzymes, and triggering the death of cancer cells or stopping them from growing. Rainforest plants like those found in this book are a rich source of diverse and even novel polyphenols that these plants produced to protect and heal itself from the intense growing conditions in the rainforest that won't be found in the typical cultivated fruits and vegetables in average diets.

In fact, you'll read about the polyphenols found in some rainforest plants featured in Part 3 that are so powerful that they can selectively hunt down cancer cells and selectively kill them without any damage to healthy cells. Others are reported to actually relieve the oxidative stress in healthy cells caused by chemotherapy drugs while simultaneously increasing ROS and oxidative stress inside cancer cells. The last five books I've written on rainforest plants have a chapter on polyphenols because they are an integral part of the powerful and effective health benefits these unique rainforest plants provide, and this book is no exception.

3

THE DIFFERENCE BETWEEN PLANTS AND DRUGS AND THE RESEARCH BEHIND BOTH

It is estimated that more than 60% of the approved drugs and new drug developments for cancer and infectious diseases are from natural origin. The use of natural compounds as a potential source of antitumor agents has been deeply studied in many cancer models, both *in vitro* and *in vivo*. While many drugs have originated from biologically active plant chemicals, and many plants' medicinal uses can be attributed to various active chemicals found in them, there is a distinct difference between using a medicinal plant and a chemical drug.

The difference is one that scares most conventionally trained doctors with no training in plants. Drugs usually consist of a single chemical, whereas medicinal plants can contain 300 or more chemicals. It's relatively easy to figure out the activity, side effects, and drug interactions of a single chemical, but scientific investigation of medicinal plant products is challenging because of their immense complexity and variability to map all the complex interactions and synergies that might be taking place between all the various chemicals found in a plant, or a traditionally prepared crude plant extract, containing all these chemicals. And when you're talking about combining plants into a multi-plant formula, like those discussed in this book, the complexities grow exponentially.

Synergy of Multiple Chemicals in Multiple Plants

In some instances, a particular plant chemical's activity is enhanced or increased when it is combined with another chemical or chemicals that occur naturally in the plant. This is now scientifically termed as "synergy." An example of synergy is the rainforest plant cat's claw (see page 217). First, the crude extract of cat's claw was shown to boost immune function. Then, specific alkaloid chemicals in the plant were tested and scientifically documented (and patented) to be the "active constituents" that provided this effect. Scientists discovered much later, however, that if they extracted just the alkaloids, these alkaloids were less potent at stimulating immune cells than they were when combined with other chemicals in the crude extract (called catechin tannins). Adding the tannin chemicals to the alkaloids increased the immune-stimulating effect of the alkaloids by almost 40%. In this instance, a drug made using only the alkaloids would be less effective than using the whole plant that contained both alkaloids and tannins.

Single Chemical–Single Action Drugs

Based on the classic pharmacological dogma "one drug–one target," monotherapy has been the traditional approach, not only to treat diseases but also to find new active drugs against a chosen target. The U.S. drug industry often misses the boat in this regard. Their motivations, however, are different because our drug approval processes here are different. Crude plant extracts or whole plants in capsules or tablets cannot be patented or approved as drugs in the United States. The drug researcher's goal is to come up with a single chemical with good biological activity—one that can be changed in some way (without losing activity), so that it can be patented as a novel chemical and then be synthetically manufactured into a new patented drug. Sometimes, the isolated chemical might not be quite as effective as the crude extract in which it was found, but the researchers have the ability to deliver more of the chemical therapeutically by increasing the dosage of the single chemical.

Sometimes, they can even improve on the activity of the plant chemical by modifying it in some way, which also makes it patentable. Even if patents were not an issue, the drug company still would not be able to provide enough scientific data on how so many naturally occurring plant chemicals work individually, much less in combination with one another, to get a crude plant extract approved as a drug under our current drug regulations and approval processes.

This is also why so many drugs that use a plant chemical are typically much more toxic and/or have many more side effects than using the plant in which they discovered the plant chemical. The synergy of many chemicals working together may prevent any toxicity or side effect of any single chemical. For example, a plant might have two chemicals that create oxidative stress, while containing 20 or more other chemicals that provide an antioxidant effect. Overall, using the plant relieves oxidative stress. If the drug researchers chose one of the oxidative chemicals to copy, without all the other antioxidant chemicals in the plant, their new drug molecule would cause widespread oxidative damage to all cells thereby increasing its toxicity and side effects.

Many Chemical–Many Use Plants

The other concept of using herbal medicines that typically causes a traditionally trained physician's eyes to roll back in their head is how one single medicinal plant can treat so many different and diverse health conditions. It's simply because a medicinal plant has so many different and diverse active chemicals that are affecting so many things. Again, cat's claw is a great example. This rainforest vine has one group of chemicals that reduces inflammation effectively as an arthritis remedy; others that boost immune function; and yet even more that increase oxidative damage in cancer cells while preventing oxidative damage in healthy cells (which reduces chemotherapy drugs' toxic effects to healthy cells). Additionally, the vine has several direct ways that it actually kills other cancer cells using other active chemicals it possesses. To a physician, when you look at all the active plant chemicals in play, it would be the equivalent of writing 30 or more prescriptions of single-chemical drugs, which, of course, they simply would never do.

Herbal Drugs in Other Countries

Outside of the United States, herbal drugs are much more common and available. Herbal drugs are available in Germany and several other countries in the European Union, India, China, Brazil, and some African and Southeast

Asian countries. Many of these drugs are simply a chemical or chemicals extracted from plant materials and put into a capsule, tablet, or liquid. One such example is the plant chemical called cynarin, which occurs naturally in the common artichoke plant. In Germany, a cynarin drug is manufactured and sold to treat hypertension, liver disorders, and high cholesterol levels. The drug is simply this single chemical, or an artichoke extract, that has been concentrated and chemically manipulated to contain a specific amount of this one chemical; such a preparation is called a standardized extract.

This drug is manufactured by pharmaceutical companies and sold in pharmacies in Germany with a doctor's prescription. The medical purpose of the plant-based drug (like lowering cholesterol or treating liver disorders) can be relayed to users of the drug when prescribing the product. Usually, some proprietary extraction process is created to extract the active chemicals or standardize them to a certain level, which can be patented by the manufacturer. This gives them the ability to recoup their research dollars that validate the medical claims they make for their patented products.

No Herbal Drugs—No Medical Claims in the United States

In the United States, artichoke extracts are available as dietary supplements and sold in health food stores. Some U.S. artichoke products are even standardized to contain a specific amount of cynarin, yet they can still be purchased here as a natural product without a prescription (and for a lot less money than in Germany). There may be little to no difference between the cynarin drug produced in Germany and the artichoke standardized herbal supplement made in the United States considering that the same amount of cynarin is being delivered, dose for dose. No medical claims or uses can be made for the U.S. product, however, and the product company cannot tell customers what to use it for if it names any medical condition like liver disorders or high cholesterol.

The U.S. law of the land is that drugs treat diseases and conditions and all dietary/herbal supplements can only "nutritionally support healthy organs or systems." Worse still, even if there is a large body of research and knowledge validating how a natural product affects, benefits, or treats a particular disease or condition, the U.S. company cannot mention it to their customers in the marketing of their product. If the research names any disease or condition, it cannot be used to tell customers what to use it for (which is considered a "medical claim"). Instead, Americans see—on artichoke products, for example—phrases like "supports healthy digestion" or "nutritionally supports healthy cholesterol levels."

For that reason, no supplement manufacturer can justify spending any research dollars to prove that a dietary supplement might treat any disease or condition. They could never even mention the expensive research, as it would make a disallowed "medical claim" and subject them to civil and criminal penalties.

Research Differences for Pharmaceutical Drugs versus Herbal Drugs

These factors also result in how plant research is performed around the world. For example, in the United States, cancer researchers will test crude plant extracts in test tubes to determine if the plant can kill cancer cells. When they find a good candidate, they immediately look at the plant's chemistry to see if any known anti-cancer natural compounds are present. Next, they look at new and novel chemicals that the plant might contain and they start testing all those chemicals individually in test tubes. Once that is completed, they usually pick just one chemical that has the greatest anti-cancer effect. They then begin testing that natural plant chemical in laboratory animals to determine effective dosages, toxicity, and side effects.

If successful, they try to change the chemical enough so that it can be patented as a new chemical with the same anti-cancer action. At that juncture, all research on the plant or plant chemical stops and everything focuses on their new patented chemical that they hope to eventually turn into a new chemotherapy drug after much more research in animals and then humans. Their goal is not to prove that the plant or a plant chemical can kill cancer cells or treat cancer. All of their money goes into creating a new profitable drug and validating scientifically it can treat cancer and how.

Plant research is conducted differently in countries that have approved plant-based drugs. Much more research is conducted on the plant and various extraction methods to extract the most active chemicals. Research with animals starts much earlier and is more extensive on various plant extracts (both liquids and those that are dried in some fashion to a powder to create tablets and capsules). Their goal is to come up with a patented extraction method to use that makes their plant drug patentable. In some countries, there are several drugs available utilizing the same plant but different manufacturing/extraction methods. Because they can make medical claims for their products, they spend much more on research to confirm and validate the medical claims, which can be recouped when they begin selling their new herbal drug. They begin funding human clinical trials much earlier as well.

Remember, here in the United States, herbal supplements cannot treat or cure any disease or condition. This fact alone makes any expensive research to prove that a plant can treat a disease a losing proposition and unprofitable. For that reason, very little research is conducted on plants, plant extracts, and herbal remedies in the United States. Especially, if the research doesn't yield a patented product, how does a research company recoup those expensive research dollars if anyone could use their research to sell unpatented products and compete directly with them? With the Food and Drug Administration (FDA) position of "only approved drugs can treat diseases and conditions," all the research dollars given to U.S. government agencies and universities for health research are spent on everything else *but* confirming traditional medicine uses of herbal remedies or validating any medical claim on herbal supplements. In the United States, there is simply no one left with the motivation (or budget) to research how any plant or herbal supplement might treat any medical condition like cancer.

Other countries that regularly approve and use herbal drugs fund the majority of research on plants and plant-based drugs in the world. The countries leading this type of research are China, India, and Germany. Oftentimes, government agencies will partially or fully fund plant-based drug research in other countries. Some have programs that routinely test herbal remedies to determine their efficacy and possible development into new herbal drugs to lower their countries' health care costs. For these reasons, much of the research on the plants in this book that is discussed herein have been conducted outside of the United States. It's usually always the case.

Results of Recent Research

Results of this research has revealed that the multi-component nature of medicinal plants makes them particularly suitable for treating complex diseases such as cancer and offers great potential for exhibiting synergistic actions. One reason for this could be that many diseases (especially cancer) are caused by multiple factors, not just one. Cancer can change many genes in the body, so multiple chemicals/drugs are required to address them.

There are mechanisms underlying synergistic therapeutic actions of herbal medicines: different medicinal plants can affect the same or different parts of the body, helping each other work better; they can help the body absorb plant chemicals and drugs more effectively by affecting enzymes and transporters in the liver and intestines; they can help fight cancer by overcoming the many different ways cancer cells resist treatment; and they can reduce side effects and make drugs more powerful by interacting with each other.

Small-Molecule Drugs

A naturally occurring plant chemical is sometimes referred to as a small-molecule drug due to its potential therapeutic properties and ability to interact with various biological targets. A small-molecule drug is really defined as a low molecular weight, organic compound that can be synthesized or derived from natural sources. These drugs are characterized by their ability to easily penetrate cell membranes and interact on a molecular level with specific biological targets like enzymes or proteins and other chemical substances in signaling pathways, making them effective for treating various diseases.

Many of the plant chemicals discussed in this book that have been turned into new cancer drugs are defined as small-molecule drugs. They usually act by binding to specific enzymes or receptors, or blocking or enhancing certain biological and signaling pathways. They can work by interacting with proteins, DNA, or other small molecules within the body. They also have the ability to have multiple mechanisms of action by affecting multiple pathways that may have been changed by cancer.

The FDA approves, on average, 30 small-molecule drugs annually. Many of these drugs are taken orally rather than injected or infused, and usually at least half of those approved annually have a use for cancer.

Targeted Cancer Therapies

Many of the small-molecule drugs developed for cancer can also be defined as "targeted therapies." This is a type of cancer treatment that uses drugs or other substances to precisely target specific molecules on or in cancer cells, disrupting their growth and survival. Unlike chemotherapy, which broadly affects rapidly dividing cells, targeted therapy focuses on the specific characteristics that make cancer cells different from normal cells. Molecular targeted therapeutic agents used in cancer treatment may exhibit different functions and characteristics. According to the chemical target, these drugs work by finding specific parts of the cell, like surface markers, growth factors, receptors, or pathways that control things like cell growth, cell death, spread, and the formation of new blood vessels.

As you read about the anti-cancer plants detailed in Part 3, you'll learn about which molecules are being targeted by various chemicals in the plant, and how those chemicals interact on a molecular level to treat cancer. Chapter 4 will explain the remarkable advances in cancer research that were made to discover all these new molecular targets that helped create these new targeted therapy drugs for cancer.

Targeted drugs have become a main treatment for cancer because they are more effective and safer than traditional chemotherapy. The first targeted drug, imatinib, was approved by the FDA in 2001. Since then, more small-molecule targeted drugs have been developed to treat cancer. By the end of 2020, 89 such drugs had been approved by both the FDA in the United States and China's National Medical Products Administration (NMPA).

Cancer tumors grow quickly and need more blood supply. To do this, they create more blood vessels in a process called *angiogenesis*. They can use about 30 different molecules across six signaling pathways to make this happen. If one pathway is blocked by a drug or plant compound, the tumor often just switches to another. While we do have drugs that slow tumor growth by blocking blood supply, we now know angiogenesis is complex, involving many pathways and interactions. This has shifted research from targeting one molecule at a time to using combination therapies (two to three drugs administered together) or multi-target agents (like plant-based compounds) that hit several pathways at once to reduce resistance. Natural remedies like N-Tense, made from eight plants, may contain 800–1,600 active chemicals. These could potentially impact all six pathways. Scientists haven't yet figured out exactly how all these chemicals work, interact, or are broken down by the body—but maybe we don't need to know everything to see their benefit.

Summary

As you will learn in the next chapter, cancer isn't just one disease; it's a complex condition where many molecular pathways and cell processes go wrong. Each type of cancer has its own unique characteristics, and at least one key feature of cancer is usually altered. Despite these differences, all cancers share a common trait: uncontrolled growth and invasion. This invasive ability to spread is what makes cancer so dangerous and, in many cases, is still a major challenge, leading to illness and death. Only when we can reverse cancer's uncontrolled growth and invasion will we be able to "win the war on cancer."

Molecular targeted therapies are revolutionized therapeutics that interfere with specific molecules to block cancer growth, progression, and metastasis and offer our best hope today. And the powerful chemicals found in plants are once again leading the way for these new therapies. Many small-molecule targeted therapies approved by the FDA have demonstrated remarkable clinical success in the treatment of a myriad of cancer types including leukemia and breast, colorectal, lung, and ovarian cancers.

4

NEW KNOWLEDGE RESULTS IN NEW TREATMENTS

The main way a healthy cell starts the transformation into a cancer cell is by introducing it to a carcinogen (a substance known to cause cancer, usually through gene mutation or gene functioning). Carcinogens are basically the triggers or catalysts that begin the transformation process. We've known this for many years. These carcinogens include the following:

• Physical carcinogens such as ultraviolet and ionizing radiation linked to skin cancers and others;

• Chemical carcinogens such as asbestos, components of tobacco smoke, alcohol, aflatoxin (a food contaminant), arsenic (a drinking water contaminant), and a whole host of other man-made chemicals that are in our foods and environments;

• Biological carcinogens such as infections from certain viruses, bacteria, or parasites. These include, but are not limited to

 o *Helicobacter pylori*, a bacteria that can cause stomach ulcers and is linked to stomach and bowel cancers.

 o Human papillomavirus, which can cause cervical cancer.

 o Hepatitis B and C viruses, which can cause liver cancer.

 o Epstein-Barr virus, which can cause lymphomas and lymphatic cancers, nasopharyngeal cancers, and stomach cancers.

Cancer-causing infections are responsible for approximately 30% of cancer cases in low- and lower-middle-income countries. These statistics are around 10% in higher-income nations like the United States because we find and treat these infections more often and more effectively.

In addition to carcinogens and infections, the data reports around one-third of new cancer cases and deaths from cancer are caused by diet and lifestyle factors due to tobacco use, high body mass index (obesity), alcohol consumption, low fruit and vegetable intake, and lack of physical activity. These statistics also contain a few carcinogens found in cigarette smoke and air pollution, which are risk factors for lung cancer. They are included in lifestyle factors statistics because we decide to smoke and we decide where we live. It is estimated that appropriate diet and lifestyle modification could prevent more than two-thirds of human cancers, and diet is responsible for 10–70% (on average, 35%) of human cancer mortality.

Preventing Cancer

The number one thing that our government can do to help win the war on cancer is to clean up our food supply and environment from known man-made carcinogenic chemicals. There are about 350,000 man-made chemicals that are registered for production and use, and about 2,500 new chemicals are created and registered annually. The majority of older chemicals were never required to be tested as carcinogens, and many have proven to be carcinogens over the years and linked to causing various cancers. Many U.S. foods contain known carcinogenic chemicals that were banned in other countries. These include common preservatives and colorants we use in foods, endocrine-disrupting and growth hormone chemicals used in growing animals and to increase milk production, and nitrates and nitrites in processed meats, as well as chemicals used in fertilizers, pesticides, and plant growth regulators, just to name a few.

Our government can and should remove the chemicals from our food supply that are known carcinogens immediately (just like other First World nations did). The National Cancer Society (NCS) has a published list of more than one hundred known man-made chemical carcinogens and even more likely carcinogens, and they could start there. Following the research that resulted in banned chemicals in other countries (which may not be on the NCS list), others should be added as well. For example, a common stabilizer used in many food products in the United States is named brominated vegetable oil (called BVO and contains a chemical called bromine). Bromine is an endocrine disruptor chemical (see later in this section), and BVO is known to cause behavioral, developmental, and reproductive issues; neurological problems; and thyroid, heart, and liver problems (with a possible link to liver and thyroid cancers). BVO was banned in India in 1990, the European Union (EU) in 2008, Japan in 2010, and the United States just banned it in July 2024 with Canada following suit in August 2024. The United States should be the leader in protecting our food, not the last. The regulation allowed manufacturers one year to comply, so BVO remained in American foods until August 2025. We can do better than this, and we need to find out why we're not. Following the money is a good place to look first.

There are also many chemicals that are now known to be "endocrine disruptor chemicals" (EDCs), which aren't considered direct carcinogens, and there are a lot of them. These chemicals can affect estrogen and androgen hormones in humans, which are now being linked to hormonal cancers like breast and prostate cancers and possibly explain why these cancers are on the rise. A well-known example of a man-made EDC is Bisphenol A (BPA), commonly found in plastic products like food containers and beverage cans. Other examples include chemicals called phthalates (used in plastics and fragrances), certain pesticides, and some flame retardants. Other common ones are the EDCs given to cows to increase milk production. The EDCs accumulate in milk (and milk products like cheese) and are linked to hormonal cancers.

Our milk and cheese products are banned from import into several other countries for this reason. These particular EDCs are also considered one of the reasons why children in the United States are reaching puberty at a much younger age than in the past and in other countries. EDCs in our foods, body care products, and environment are also now considered to be a possible cause of America's declining fertility rates. These types of chemicals need to be on the government's radar to fund or conduct independent and unbiased research to assess what effect they really are having on humans developing cancer and affecting or causing other conditions instead of allowing manufacturers who make the chemicals perform very limited and biased research.

Man-made chemicals found in our food, body care products, and plastics—and now polluting our water, air, and soils—are contributing factors making our fight against cancer monumentally difficult; cancer (and chronic disease) is on the rise, and it's occurring at a much younger age. We don't have a chance of winning the war until we address one of the main root causes.

What Can We Do?

Just as important, changing our lifestyle to limit the exposure to known cancer- and inflammation-causing substances like those found in pesticides, cigarettes, plastics, highly processed foods, high fructose corn syrup found in many popular beverages, and many known chemical carcinogens decreases the likelihood of getting cancer. You should start reading food labels and look for foods with the least number of chemical preservatives, stabilizers, colorants, and other man-made chemicals.

Rule of thumb . . . if you can't even pronounce the name of an ingredient in a food product, put it back on the shelf or take the time to look it up. Strategies to limit exposure to known EDCs and carcinogens include the following: eating organic food as much as possible; choosing conventionally grown foods with the least amount of pesticide residue and washing everything well; eating food that is as close to whole as possible; avoiding plastic food packaging (and never putting plastic packaging in microwaves); and cooking in stainless steel or cast iron instead of nonstick pots and pans.

If you already have cancer, it's even more important to make these dietary and lifestyle changes because even more cancer cells are being created by these factors while you're trying to kill them.

The Complicated Cancer Cell

Cancer is not a simple disease involving a single gene but, instead, a complex disease involving interactions between many genes that control many substances and processes in the body. The instigator is usually a carcinogen, an EDC, inflammatory chemicals, and other processes that break the DNA strand in a gene or multiple genes. The DNA holds the programming of genes and recruits many other molecules and protein substances in the body to start a complicated cascading chemical reaction to perform the gene's programming and function. For example, just one gene that controls a type of inflammation that responds to an injury like a sprained ankle recruits more than 100 different substances in the body to perform its function of making the ankle swell with fluid. This fluid contains the healing molecules to repair it while the swelling stabilizes and protects it. This process affects more than a dozen other genes when substances are recruited that are created by those other genes. It is all very complicated, lots of stuff is going on, and it's hard to explain to someone without some medical knowledge.

It gets even more complicated when cancer mutates multiple genes, or starts changing various substances in all the cascading chemical reactions of the many genes affected. Depending on the cancer type, cancer can affect between 300 and 500 genes! The changes in the genes promote the transformation of a healthy cell to a cancerous one, enable it to multiply more times and faster than healthy cells, create defense mechanisms, and enable it to grow and metastasize. The next chapter will attempt to explain all that, hopefully, as simply as possible.

The Evolution of Cancer and Cancer Treatments

A tumor usually starts when a normal cell changes due to the activation of proto-oncogenes and the blocking of tumor suppressor genes. Proto-oncogenes control how fast cells grow, when they divide, and when they die. When these genes are turned on incorrectly, the cell stops acting like a normal cell and starts behaving like a cancer cell. These changes make the cell able to grow on its own without the usual signals that would stop it. It's basically like turning the death switch off, which allows the cell to avoid normal programmed death (called apoptosis), allowing the tumor to keep growing. The tumor grows even faster because of angiogenesis, which is the process of making new blood vessels. These new blood vessels supply the tumor with extra oxygen and nutrients it needs to fuel rapid growth, help it spread to nearby tissues, and allow it to move to other parts of the body.

Early cancer research and resulting treatment mostly involved giving a cancer patient a drug or chemical that was known to kill cancer cells. It was largely ineffective because the toxic substance killed healthy cells as well as cancer cells. They just hoped it would kill enough of the cancer cells before they had to stop the therapy due to the life-threatening side effects of killing too many healthy cells. While this may have delayed death from the cancer and prolonged their life by a few months, many patients died of the side effects (renal failure and heart failure were common) before the cancer killed them. Many cancer patients (myself included) would tell you, however, that those last few months the drug therapy gave them weren't worth much since they dealt with numerous side effects that negatively affected their quality of life.

Next, they began injecting the anti-cancer drug/substance directly into tumors, helping to minimize the toxicity to healthy cells. This method is still sometimes used and has evolved to the use of special infusion pumps worn outside the body that continuously drip the drug into the tumor site. While this does help prevent toxicity to healthy cells in other vital organs, it still wasn't highly effective or efficient to cure cancer—mostly because cancer can creatively mutate to create defense mechanisms to prevent the drug from killing it.

Then they developed other less toxic drugs that did not kill cancer cells directly but only injured them. This was supposed to trigger the body's immune system to attack the injured or damaged cancer cells and remove them from the body—creating apoptosis (see page 36) within the cell. These types of drugs are still widely in use today. While they are better than the first cancer drugs, there are still some problems and limitations. First and foremost, these drugs injure all cells, not just cancer cells, and most come with significant side effects from injuring and eventually causing healthy cell death.

The other main problem is that every cell has an innate survival code (fight, flee, or hide) that creates unique defense mechanisms to prevent things from killing it. Cancer cells have evolved to be really creative in these defense mechanisms. They can fight the drug by creating their own intercellular pump (called a P-glycogen pump). These pumps push the drug out of the cell as fast as the infusion drug pumps it in or the chemotherapy drug goes through the bloodstream. Once they create these intercellular pumps, they are completely resistant to that drug, and even other chemotherapy drugs subsequently used against it. This creates what's called multi-drug-resistant tumors. However, this is only one out of five different ways that cancer cells use to become resistant to drugs.

In addition to directly fighting, cancer cells can also flee from the drug, moving into adjacent tissues and even distant sites. Cancer cells can instigate internal changes within their cells, or affect other genes, and their cascading chemical reactions can hide from various immune cells and processes that are meant to identify a cancer cell and kill it.

The chemotherapy pump therapy (as well as some less toxic common chemotherapy drugs) does buy the cancer patient more time with less toxic effects, which provides a higher quality of life; however, it almost always eventually results in quickly growing drug-resistant tumors that recur, and many can cause death quickly. Not every cancer cell can develop an intercellular pump quickly enough before it is killed, but some do. So, while the therapy may have eradicated the initial tumor, there will still be some percentage of cells (2–5%) that survived with a pump. That's why they say the patient is "in remission" rather than cured. When the surviving cells eventually create a new multi-drug-resistant tumor—sometimes years later and sometimes at a completely different place in the body—they say the patient is out of remission or the cancer has returned. The rule of thumb is that an oncologist will not say you're cured until at least five years of cancer-free progression without any recurrences. Some types of cancer extend that to 10 years of cancer-free progression before they say the therapy was curative.

Important New Information Results in New Cancer Treatments

One of the most important advancements in understanding cancer and creating new therapies resulted from the completion of the Human Genome Project (HGP). The Human Genome Project was primarily funded by the U.S. government, with significant contributions from international collaborators like the United Kingdom, France, Germany, Japan, and China. The project officially began in October 1990 and was completed in April 2003. This huge international collaborative research effort successfully mapped and sequenced the entire human genome. It identified every human gene and provided a road map of the DNA in genes that control the gene's purpose, actions, and interactions. The main type of chemical produced, controlled, or activated by genes are called proteins.

New whole genomic testing methods were developed to easily and quickly test all the genes in a human. They started with healthy individuals and then began testing groups of people with the same type of chronic disease and cancer. This new data revealed specific genes and common gene mutations that were implicated in many diseases. New road maps revealed the intricate complicated interactions between genes and many substances and molecules in the body and how cancer was able to change them in their fight to survive. Medical knowledge of how our bodies work in health and in disease grew exponentially. As expected, the knowledge then extended to what was causing some diseases and how to better treat them.

This new information has forever changed cancer research, cancer treatment, and new cancer drug development. In their research with cancer, the data revealed that the prevention or progression of human cancer depends on the integrity of a complex network of defense mechanisms in which 300–500 genes have gone wrong. Because we had the road map of how these genes work, and what substances were recruited in the complex cascade of substances the gene uses, we had a better idea what was needed to fix it or combat it.

Some cancer advances from the genome project include the following:

- The International Cancer Genome Consortium (ICGC) was launched to coordinate large-scale cancer genome studies in tumors from 50 different cancer types and/or subtypes by mapping the genomes of hundreds of thousands of cancer patients. Through this, scientists were able to rapidly uncover cancer driver genes, and to discover drugs for those, at unprecedented speed.
- Other large-scale studies like the UK Biobank have since sequenced the genomes of hundreds of thousands of volunteers to study disease associations by linking their genetic data with detailed health records. They focused on many chronic diseases and other common health problems like hypertension and obesity.
- The Cancer Genome Atlas (TCGA), a landmark cancer genomics program, molecularly characterized more than 20,000 primary cancer and matched normal samples spanning 33 cancer types.
- Before the HGP was finished, a new international group of researchers began to study the Human Gut Microbiome since it was shown in HGP that bacteria in the gut microbiome can significantly affect the expression of the same protein-coding genes in humans that were found in HGP. This research, mostly conducted in the EU, studied healthy and sick volunteers' gut microbiomes, which linked to the same proteins that were causing illnesses like cancer and chronic diseases in the Biobank data.
- New testing methods were developed to test the DNA from blood or other bodily fluids, which allows for monitoring cancer progression and detecting minimal residual disease; this can be crucial for treatment decision-making.

- Other biological testing methods developed improved approaches to predict increased risk and earlier detection of cancer.
- Some cancer patients (especially breast and prostate) are now routinely screened for specific genes or abnormal genes (mutations) discovered in the project that make cancer more invasive or metastasize more quickly, which helps create a more effective treatment.
- Three FDA-approved cancer gene therapies are now available that transfer genetic material into cells to correct those abnormal genes.
- Gene transfer is a new treatment (currently in clinical trials) that introduces new genes into a cancerous cell or the surrounding tissue to cause cell death or slow the growth of the cancer.
- New immunotherapy drugs have been developed (approved, in trials, and under development) based on the new understanding of genes regulating the immune system that help the immune system recognize and kill cancer cells.
- The knowledge of all the human genes and their functions created new opportunities for discovering and developing novel drugs, changing research strategy and how researchers approach drug discovery.
- The road maps created in the project and in the ICGC project have provided novel chemical targets that can be used to develop more effective but less toxic drug therapies. A few have been approved or are in trials, and many more are under development.
- New ways of combining chemotherapy drugs have been developed based on road maps showing which genes (and the proteins they produce) the cancer uses to grow, spread, and protect itself.
- Extensive databases were created to hold all the information comparing a healthy genome to the genomes of a large number of patients with various illnesses, including cancer and all chronic diseases.
- New computer modeling techniques were developed, called *in silico research* and *molecular docking studies*, which queried these databases to speed up and lower the cost of new drug discovery.
- New biological testing methods were developed to quickly test the cascading chemical reactions employed and/or changed by cancer cells, as well as to identify what was repaired or changed by new molecules, drugs, and plant chemicals as possible new therapies.

NEW KNOWLEDGE RESULTS IN NEW TREATMENTS

- In 2011, the National Cancer Institute established the Clinical Proteomic Tumor Analysis Consortium to better understand cancer through proteogenomics—a method integrating both proteomics and genomics. Proteomics is the study of the entire set of proteins (the proteome) expressed in a cell, tissue, or organism, analyzing their functions, interactions, and modifications to understand biological processes and diseases. It's important because proteins are the workhorses of cells, and understanding their activity is crucial for diagnosing, treating, and preventing diseases, especially cancer.

SUMMARY

The Human Genome Project provided a blueprint for understanding the human body and its genetic makeup. This knowledge is crucial for understanding how genetic mutations can lead to cancer and for developing targeted therapies that exploit these mutations. The HGP's findings led to the development of new cancer drugs that target specific genetic abnormalities in cancer cells, such as those that affect growth, division, or spread. It also facilitated the development of new diagnostic tools that can identify genetic mutations that predispose individuals to cancer or that are present in specific types of cancer. The HGP continues to be a valuable resource for researchers around the world, and new discoveries are constantly being made that further our understanding of cancer and its genetic basis.

All of this new data on genetic signaling has provided new molecular targets (proteins, enzymes, and such that are recruited to conduct the gene's purpose/role) that can be used to specifically target cancer cells by looking for the chemical substances and changing their expression, or enhancing or silencing their signals. These substances also include non-coding genetic material, which is also important and can act as a regulatory element, helping to turn genes on and off or change their signaling.

These new molecular targets are further detailed in the next chapter and will provide how they treat cancer, which current cancer drugs are utilizing the targets, and which plants and plant chemicals provide similar actions.

5

TREATING CANCER THROUGH THE MAIN CANCER PATHWAYS

Cancer develops in several steps, and during this process, it gains six key abilities that set it apart from normal cells. These six features help scientists understand how cancer works, which results in a better understanding of how to treat cancer. Cancer does the following:

1. Keeps signals turned on that tell cells to grow.

2. Ignores signals that tell cells to stop growing.

3. Avoids programmed cell death.

4. Lives and divides forever.

5. Grows new blood vessels to get nutrients.

6. Spreads to other parts of the body.

These traits are what make cancer cells different from normal cells. Behind these main features of cancer are several important factors: unstable genes, which cause changes in DNA that help cancer cells develop these features faster; inflammation, which supports many of the cancer traits; changing how cells use energy; and avoiding attacks from the immune system. Cancer isn't just made of cancer cells. Tumors also include normal cells that are pulled in and help the cancer grow. These supporting cells form what's called the "tumor microenvironment" and also play a role in cancer's development and its survival.

Cancer research was affected by the Human Genome Project (HGP). This was an international research project designed to map out and sequence all the genes in the human body. During the research, they discovered many complicated chemical interactions and crosstalk between the genes controlling inflammation and the genes controlling the manufacture and action of all the immune cells in the body. This provided road maps of the many interactions and provided new chemical targets and therapies. (See chapter 4 for more information.) These road maps shed light on specific new ways to address, stop, or change the six core abilities that cancer develops. For example, one of the newer classifications of cancer drugs produced from this knowledge is now called *immunotherapy*. Several new immunotherapy cancer drugs have been approved and are used today, others are in clinical trials, and many more are under development.

Signaling Pathways

This crosstalk between the different genes (and the substances they create) is termed "signaling pathways." For example, when inflammation occurs somewhere, there are chemicals in the body that sense it. These sensing chemicals then signal the IL6 gene, which makes a protein called IL-6. The gene coded the protein to look for inflammation and take certain actions in response. This protein then sends a signal to specific immune cells to go to the site of inflammation; this signals other chemicals like ligands, enzymes, and other substances that are either pro-inflammatory or anti-inflammatory, which recruit other healing chemicals, trigger lymphatic flow, and lots of other things to deal with the inflammation. Signaling pathways intersect and exchange chemicals, and much more.

The end result is that many of these signaling pathways and resulting signaling messages are now known, and we know what specific chemicals are in the message. More important, we're now learning which of these many chemicals we might change in a signaling pathway to block, prevent, or change signals that are creating negative results. For example, instead of blocking the production of IL-6, which is necessary for other cells, we can interrupt the signal sent by a cancer cell that is asking for more IL-6 to be sent to promote its growth. We can accomplish this by targeting any substance in the signaling pathway that is being used to send this message.

The good news is that signaling messages sent by cancer cells are usually chemically different than normal cells and normal signaling pathways. If we know which chemical (or combination of chemicals) in the cancer cell's pathway is different, we can use that chemical to specifically target cancer cells without any toxicity to healthy cells. This results in cancer drugs that are much less toxic. When you read about drugs, plants, or plant chemicals in this book that "selectively target cancer cells," it's usually targeting a chemical in a signaling pathway that is different than healthy cells, a chemical that is much higher (or overexpressed, meaning the signal is stronger) in a cancer cell than healthy cells so they are affected first, or a specific chemical that's only found in the cell wall or inside of a cancer cell.

The first four key abilities that cancer has are working within a specific cancer pathway called the Apoptosis Pathway.

THE APOPTOSIS PATHWAY

Apoptosis is defined as *programmed cell death* and is essential for eliminating unnecessary, damaged, or infected cells in the body. It is considered a vital component of various natural processes inside the human body including normal cell turnover, proper development and functioning of the immune system, embryonic development, and chemical-induced cell death. Inappropriate apoptosis (either too little or too much) is a factor in many human conditions including neurodegenerative diseases, autoimmune disorders, and many types of cancer. The ability to modulate the life or death of a cell is recognized for its immense therapeutic potential.

Every cell in the body has a genetic code that tells it what to do, how to behave, how many copies of itself to make, and when to die. Some cells live much longer than others. For example, skin cells have a very short life span, while those found in major internal organs live much longer. When it's time to die, a tightly controlled, cascading chemical chain of events begins. It involves many chemical substances reacting together. These include chemical signaling molecules, proteins, enzymes, ligands, and other substances. This chain of events causes the cell to commit suicide by breaking down its own components in a controlled manner, package them up in small bundles, and signal specific cells in the immune system to clean them up by removing them from the body.

In cancer cells, mutations can effectively prevent the cell from responding to communication signals that would normally initiate apoptosis. It turns off the suicide switch that every cell is programmed with and allows the cancer cells to replicate forever and form tumors. There are two main signaling pathways for apoptosis: the extrinsic death receptor pathway and the intrinsic mitochondrial pathway. The extrinsic pathway begins outside a cell, when conditions in the extracellular environment determine that a cell must die. For example, when immune cells recognize that bacterial, viral, and cancer cells need to be eliminated, the extrinsic pathway goes to work. The intrinsic pathway begins when an injury occurs within the cell and the resulting stress activates the apoptotic pathway. Many chemotherapy drugs work through the intrinsic pathway.

Death by Oxidative Stress

Oxidative stress is caused by an unstable molecule, called a free radical, creating damage to other molecules within your body's cell structures. This includes proteins, cell membranes, and DNA. Some chemotherapy drugs are designed as pro-oxidants and meant to create what is called an "oxidative burst" within a cancer cell. This injures the cell by causing oxidative stress, which is supposed to send signals to trigger the normal apoptosis process. This was thought to be better than outright killing the cancer cell because this pathway works usually without causing too much inflammation. The problem with chemotherapy drugs, however, is that the oxidative burst occurs in all cells and not just a cancer cell. The burst is so large and affects so many cells that it easily overcomes the innate antioxidant system. Many different organs (especially the heart) can be injured by this oxidative stress. Immune cells are highly susceptible to this oxidative burst, which is why these drugs suppress (or destroy) the immune system. Since the apoptosis process needs immune cells to clean up the aftermath, the process can be hampered or incomplete, resulting in side effects. Since this is happening in many cells and not just cancer cells, there is a lot of aftermath that needs to be addressed.

All of this aftermath (the packets immune cells created, and dead and dying cells that weren't processed properly because there weren't enough immune cells) travel in the blood and lymphatic fluid through organs meant to filter all this debris out including the liver and kidneys. One main side effect of oxidative-type cancer drugs is called "tumor lysis syndrome." That's when all of this debris gets stuck in the kidneys and it starts damaging them. It can also get stuck in the liver and damage that organ as well. This debris can also slow down and clog up the lymphatic fluid and/or get stuck in the lymph glands through which the fluid travels. The lymphatic system is the main bodily system designed to filter debris and remove it in the apoptosis pathway. This is thought to be one way cancer can metastasize; a cancer cell is just injured and moves into the lymphatic fluid without an immune cell breaking it down and packing it up first. The injured cancer cell has internal processes to repair itself during the journey and starts creating a brand-new tumor wherever it lands, even far away from the original tumor.

Reactive oxygen species (ROS) connect to and influence a wide array of cellular signaling pathways involved in processes like cell survival, proliferation, differentiation, and apoptosis, as well as pathways crucial for inflammation and immune responses. Key pathways affected by ROS include the NF-κB, MAPK, PI3K-Akt, and Keap1-Nrf2-ARE signaling pathways, with ROS acting as signaling molecules at various concentrations.

Drugs: The main cancer drugs in use that treat cancer through this oxidative burst are carboplatin, cisplatin, doxorubicin, epirubicin, etoposide, imexon, and methotrexate.

Plants: The plants in this book that have shown the ability to increase the oxidative burst in cancer cells but provide an antioxidant benefit to healthy cells include bitter melon, cat's claw, espinheira santa, graviola, guacatonga, mullaca, picão preto, and simarouba. Taking any or a combination of these plants listed here with the chemotherapy drugs listed earlier has shown to reduce the oxidative damage these drugs cause to healthy cells.

The Intrinsic Apoptosis Pathway

Cancer cells evade apoptosis (programmed cell death) by altering the genetic pathways that trigger cell death, often by overexpressing anti-apoptotic proteins, downregulating pro-apoptotic proteins, or mutating key genes involved in the apoptotic signaling cascade. Remember, cancer can mutate or change 300–500 genes depending on the cancer type! This effectively prevents the cell from responding to communication signals that would normally initiate apoptosis. It turns off the suicide switch that every cell is programmed with and allows the cancer cells to replicate forever and form tumors. Key substances involved in the communication pathways that happen in the intrinsic pathway include anti-apoptosis genes and chemicals such as p53, Bcl-2, Bcl-x, Bcl-xL, Bcl-xS, Bcl-w, and BAG, and pro-apoptosis chemicals such as Bcl-10, Bax, Bak, Bid, Bad, Bim, Bik, and Blk.

P53

P53 is a tumor suppressor protein that plays a crucial role in preventing cancer development. It is encoded by the TP53 gene. P53 acts as a guardian of the genome, detecting and responding to DNA damage. When DNA damage occurs, p53 induces cell cycle arrest to allow for DNA repair; or triggers apoptosis to eliminate damaged cells; and activates genes involved in antitumor immune responses. Mutations in the TP53 gene can lead to a loss of p53 function, which increases the risk of cancer development and survival. This is because p53's tumor-suppressing abilities are impaired or completely silenced, allowing damaged cells to proliferate and form tumors. The TP53 gene is mutated in approximately half of all human cancers, including those of the breast, colon, lung, liver, prostate, bladder, and skin. Some of the cancers with high TP53 mutation rates include ovarian cancer, colorectal cancer, lung cancer (both small cell and non–small cell), breast cancer, head and neck cancer, and esophageal cancer. Understanding the role of p53 in cancer has led to the development of therapeutic strategies aimed at restoring p53 function in cells with p53 mutations and targeting p53 pathways to induce apoptosis or inhibit tumor growth. Given that avoiding apoptosis is one of the prominent hallmarks of cancer, an ideal therapeutic strategy to effectively kill cancer cells is to restore p53 function, which will eliminate the cancer through apoptosis.

Drugs: Chemotherapy drugs that affect p53 indirectly through signaling pathways include cisplatin, temozolomide, doxorubicin, and gemcitabine.

Plants: Rainforest plants that restore p53 function directly or indirectly (through signaling pathways) include anamu, bitter melon, chanca piedra, espinheira santa, graviola, guacatonga, mullaca, pau d'arco, picão preto, simarouba, suma, and vassourinha. This represents 12 out of the 13 rainforest plants in this book; obviously rainforest plants have a unique advantage in flipping the p53 "kill switch" back on as a main mechanism of action in treating cancer!

Bcl-2 Inhibitors

The B-cell lymphoma 2 (Bcl-2) protein plays a role in cancer by preventing programmed cell death in cancer cells. It is overexpressed in many cancers, including B-cell lymphoma, leukemia, myelomas, and brain, breast, lung, and pancreatic cancers. It can also contribute to drug resistance. Bcl-2 inhibitors are a class of drugs designed to interfere with the function of the Bcl-2 protein. This disruption of Bcl-2's function restores apoptotic pathways, allowing cancer cells to undergo programmed cell death again. Only cancer cells are manipulating this gene and its cascading array of chemical actions in this way. Therefore, as you read about the plants in this book, those that have this effect are reported in research to be selectively toxic only to cancer cells.

Drugs: There is one Bcl-2-inhibitor drug approved for lymphomas and leukemias: Venetoclax. Three others are currently in human clinical trials, and several others are in the pipeline.

Plants: Anamu, espinheira santa, graviola, pau d'arco, picão preto, suma, and vassourinha have Bcl-2-inhibitor actions.

BCL-xL Inhibitors

BCL-xL inhibitors target the BCL-xL protein, a key anti-apoptotic protein involved in regulating cell death. These inhibitors are being investigated for potential use in cancer treatment. BCL-xL overexpression is associated with drug resistance and disease progression in many cancers including solid tumors like lung, breast, ovarian, colorectal, and pancreatic cancers, as well as blood-type cancers like T-cell acute lymphoblastic leukemia.

Drugs: Currently, there are no FDA-approved drugs that specifically target BCL-xL. There are three new drugs in human clinical trials presently.

Plants: Espinheira santa, pau d'arco, and vassourinha have BCL-xL-inhibitor properties.

MCL-1 Inhibitors

The anti-apoptotic family member myeloid cell leukemia-1 (MCL-1) acts as a master regulator of apoptosis in various human cancers. Inhibition is a promising therapeutic strategy in cancer treatment, particularly for blood-type cancers that have developed resistance to other treatments. MCL-1 is an anti-apoptotic protein that promotes cell survival, and its overexpression is often associated with drug resistance and poor prognosis in various cancers. Targeting MCL-1 with inhibitors can help overcome these barriers and enhance the efficacy of other cancer treatments. MCL-1 inhibition has shown promise in treating multiple myeloma, acute myeloid leukemia, and non-Hodgkin lymphoma.

Drugs: There are three new MCL-1 drugs in human clinical trials now (AZD5991, S63845, and ABBV-467), and several others are under development.

Plants: Chanca piedra, espinheira santa, graviola, and pau d'arco have shown MCL-1-inhibitor actions in cancer research.

Bax Activation

The activation of the pro-apoptotic protein Bax plays a crucial role in cancer cell death. When activated, Bax can induce mitochondrial outer membrane permeabilization (MOMP), leading to the release of molecules that trigger apoptosis (programmed cell death). In cancer cells, Bax activation can be a key step in overcoming apoptosis resistance, a hallmark of cancer, and is a target for cancer therapy. Activating the Bax protein can be beneficial in treating certain types of cancer including colorectal, lung, breast, pancreatic, and ovarian cancers, as well as acute lymphoblastic leukemia.

Drugs: Venetoclax is classified as a Bcl-2 inhibitor, but by blocking Bcl-2's anti-apoptotic function, it allows Bax to become activated, which triggers apoptosis.

Plants: Anamu, bitter melon, espinheira santa, graviola, pau d'arco, picão preto, simarouba, and suma can activate Bax.

Bak Activation

Bak activation, specifically its role in MOMP, is crucial for apoptosis, the programmed cell death process that helps eliminate damaged or cancerous cells. In cancer cells, however, this process can be dysregulated, leading to resistance to chemotherapy and other treatments. Activation of Bak has shown very promising results in lung cancer (non–small cell lung cancer and small cell lung cancer) as well as breast cancer, colon cancer, lymphoma, multiple myeloma, pancreatic cancer, and osteosarcoma.

Drugs: While no drugs are directly and exclusively labeled for Bak activation by the FDA, some approved medications can indirectly induce Bak activation through various mechanisms. Several small-molecule drugs are approved for cancer research that specifically activate Bak, but none have been approved yet.

Plants: Graviola has shown the ability to activate Bak in research.

Noxa

Noxa, a protein encoded by the PMAIP1 gene, plays a crucial role in cancer cell death, particularly in response to anti-cancer treatments. It acts by neutralizing anti-apoptotic proteins like MCL-1, promoting the activation of pro-apoptotic proteins like Bax and Bak. This leads to the release of cytochrome c from mitochondria, triggering the apoptotic cascade. Noxa is involved in the development and progression of several cancers, including gastric cancer, breast cancer, and pancreatic cancer. Research indicates that Noxa expression can be altered in these cancers, impacting their behavior and response to treatment.

Drugs: Some drugs can induce Noxa expression as an indirect consequence of their mechanism of action, which can lead to apoptosis. For example, certain chemotherapeutic agents like cisplatin, paclitaxel, and bortezomib can induce Noxa expression. Despite these indirect effects, there isn't a drug specifically designed to directly target Noxa itself to induce cancer cell death.

Plants: Mullaca was reported to induce Noxa expression.

THE EXTRINSIC PATHWAY

The substances involved in the extrinsic pathway are different and include Fas, TNFR1, DR53, DR4, DR5, TNF-alpha, TRAIL, caspase-3, and caspase-8. Several of these genes and resulting substances in the signaling cascade have become new targets to create new drugs to treat cancer (or explain why older chemo drugs were working).

TNF Inhibitors

Research suggests that tumor necrosis factor (TNF) inhibitors might have antitumor effects in specific cancers or when used with other treatments. Studies are investigating their use for melanoma, lung cancer, breast cancer, and lymphoma, with some showing promising results or potential to enhance other therapies. They may also play a role in stabilizing disease in certain advanced or recurrent cancers like breast cancer, ovarian cancer, and renal cell carcinoma.

Drugs: There are no TNF-inhibitor drugs approved to treat cancer. Common TNF-inhibitor drugs approved for autoimmune and inflammatory conditions include adalimumab, infliximab, etanercept, certolizumab, and golimumab.

Plants: Based on research, cat's claw, graviola, and suma have TNF-inhibitor actions.

Caspase-3

Caspase-3 is a caspase protein that interacts with caspase-8 and caspase-9. It is encoded by the CASP3 gene. It is a crucial executioner molecule in the apoptotic pathway, responsible for orchestrating the dismantling of cellular components during programmed cell death. Activating caspase-3 can trigger cancer cell death, making it a target for new drug development. Cancers that may benefit from caspase-3 activation (through apoptosis) include melanoma, colon, ovarian, gastric, and breast cancers.

Drugs: While no drugs are specifically and solely FDA approved for caspase-3 activation, some FDA-approved drugs can indirectly activate or affect caspase-3.

Plants: Anamu, cat's claw, espinheira santa, graviola, mullaca, pau d'arco, picão preto, simarouba, and suma can activate caspase-3. Chemicals in espinheira santa and graviola have been turned into small-molecule drugs to activate caspase-3.

Caspase-8

Caspase-8 is another crucial initiator caspase in the extrinsic (death receptor) pathway of apoptosis. When death receptors on the cell surface of a cancer cell are activated, caspase-8 is recruited and activated, triggering a cascade of caspase activation leading to cell death. Cancers that may benefit from caspase-8 activation (through apoptosis) include ovarian cancer, glioblastoma, lung adenocarcinoma, and many of the epithelial cancers (which form in the lining of various organs and body surfaces).

Drugs: While no drugs are specifically and solely approved for activating caspase-8, some FDA-approved drugs have been shown to indirectly activate or influence caspase-8 as part of their mechanism of action, particularly in the context of cancer treatment. Bortezomib and lenalidomide, used in multiple myeloma treatment, are examples of drugs that activate caspase-8.

Plants: Rainforest plants that activate caspase-8 include bitter melon, cat's claw, graviola, mullaca, pau d'arco, and simarouba.

PARP Inhibitors

Poly(ADP-ribose) polymerase (PARP) cleavage, often a hallmark of programmed cell death, is a complex process with implications for cancer treatment. It can be induced by various factors, including DNA damage, and serves to inactivate PARP and prevent further DNA repair, ultimately contributing to apoptosis or necrosis within a cancer cell. PARP inhibitors, which prevent PARP from repairing DNA, are used in cancer therapy to enhance the effectiveness of other treatments or induce synthetic lethality in cancers with DNA repair deficiencies. PARP inhibitors are most effective in treating cancers with mutations that affect DNA repair, such as BRCA mutations. Specifically, they are used in advanced or metastatic cancers like breast, ovarian, prostate, and pancreatic cancers. Ovarian, fallopian tube, and primary peritoneal cancers also benefit from PARP inhibitors.

Drugs: Olaparib, niraparib, rucaparib, and talazoparib treat cancer by inhibiting PARP.

Plants: Research indicates that bitter melon, espinheira santa, and pau d'arco can also inhibit PARP.

TrxR Inhibitors

Thioredoxin NADPH Reductase (TrxR) is an enzyme chemical found in the cascading chemical reactions that control apoptosis. TrxR inhibitors are being explored as potential cancer treatments because they disrupt the antioxidant defenses of cancer cells, leading to increased oxidative stress and cell death. By inhibiting TrxR, these inhibitors can impair the cancer cells' ability to manage reactive oxygen species (ROS), which are normally scavenged by the thioredoxin system. This can lead to a buildup of ROS, triggering apoptosis in cancer cells. The overexpression of TrxR1/Trx1 has been shown in breast, ovarian, colorectal, lung, pancreatic, and gastric cancers.

Drugs: Cisplatin, carboplatin, doxorubicin, and auranofin (approved for rheumatoid arthritis and in clinical trials for cancer) inhibit TrxR.

Plants: A chemical in mullaca (withangulatin A) has reported to be a very effective TrxR inhibitor, which may result in a new cancer drug in China.

TREATING CANCER THROUGH THE MAIN CANCER PATHWAYS

ENERGY INHIBITORS

Cancer cells need much more cellular energy than healthy cells do because they are growing and dividing at a much faster pace. Disrupting a cancer cell's energy stores can slow down its growth at a minimum, and when significantly impaired, it can no longer sustain its cellular processes and the cell dies. Energy inhibitors are applicable to all types of cancers. Because cancer cells need so much more energy, they are affected first before healthy cells are. Some of the plants listed in this section have also shown to be selectively attracted to high energy cells and seek them out. New chemical targets to inhibit energy to cancer cells include the following:

ATP Inhibitors

Adenosine triphosphate (ATP) is the main energy-carrying and storage molecule found in the cells of all living things. It is often called the "energy currency" of the cell. It stores energy in the bonds between its phosphate groups, releasing this energy when needed for various cellular processes. Cancer cells are considered high-ATP cells. They need much more ATP energy to fuel their rapid growth since they are dividing and replicating at a much faster rate than a normal cell. When a cancer cell creates an intercellular pump to pump out chemo drugs from their cells before the drug can kill them, it requires even more ATP energy to fuel that pump.

Drugs: Several drugs that inhibit ATP are approved for uses other than cancer. At least two are being considered for new approvals for cancer (bedaquiline and gboxin), and several new ATP-inhibitor drugs are in the pipeline. Two under development are based on acetogenin plant chemicals discovered in graviola (see page 252).

Plants: Anamu, bitter melon, graviola, and mullaca are ATP inhibitors with graviola providing the strongest effect.

Mitochondrial Complex I Inhibitors

These inhibitors target cancer cells by interfering with their energy production process. These inhibitors disrupt the electron transport chain, forcing cancer cells to rely on glycolysis, which is the primary energy source in many cancers. This shift in metabolism can lead to cancer cell death or growth inhibition.

Drugs: While several mitochondrial complex I inhibitors are being explored for cancer therapy, including IACS-010759 and metformin, no complex I inhibitor is currently approved by the FDA specifically for cancer treatment. IACS-010759 has undergone clinical trials for various cancers, while metformin (a diabetes drug), has shown some promise in cancer research.

Plants: Graviola and many of its acetogenin chemicals are strong mitochondrial complex I inhibitors, which is why cancer researchers are developing new drugs by these chemicals.

Glycolysis Inhibitors

Inhibiting glycolysis, the process cancer cells use to generate energy (which converts glucose into ATP), is a promising anti-cancer strategy. Cancer cells often rely on glycolysis, making them vulnerable to inhibitors that disrupt this pathway. Glycolysis inhibitors can kill cancer cells, especially those with mitochondrial defects or in hypoxic (low oxygen) conditions, and can also sensitize cancer cells to other treatments, like chemotherapy and radiotherapy. Glycolysis inhibitors directly inhibit the enzymes involved in the glycolytic pathway, reducing ATP production and disrupting the energy supply for cancer cells.

Drugs: Several glycolysis inhibitors are being investigated for cancer treatment, including 2-Deoxy-D-Glucose (2-DG), 2-Cyano-3-(4-hydroxyphenyl)-2-propenoic acid (CHC), 3-Bromopyruvate (3-BrPA), and Dichloroacetate (DCA). While some have shown promising results in preclinical studies, their clinical application is limited due to factors like low specificity and potential side effects.

Plants: Bitter melon, cat's claw, graviola, and pau d'arco have shown the ability to inhibit glycolysis without side effects.

LDH-A Inhibitors

Lactate Dehydrogenase A (LDH-A) is an enzyme that is crucial for glycolysis and is being explored for potential anti-cancer applications. Less glucose is absorbed in cancer cells when this enzyme is inhibited, which lowers cellular energy.

Drugs: There is only one LDH-A-inhibitor drug approved to treat oxalate kidney stones. It has also been widely studied in cancer but is not approved to treat cancer yet. Several natural plant chemicals have been studied by cancer researchers, but no new drugs have been approved yet.

Plants: Cat's claw and graviola have shown the ability to inhibit LDH-A.

GLUT1 Inhibitors

A gene recruited by cancer cells that has a signaling pathway used for proliferation is called GLUT1. It is a newer chemical target in new cancer drug development. Some types of cancer cells can overexpress this gene, which allows cells to absorb more glucose (sugar). This provides more energy to fuel their rapid replication and proliferation. These cancers include head and neck squamous carcinomas, breast cancer (including triple-negative), ovarian, brain, and non–small cell lung cancers. Inhibiting GLUT1 decreases tumor cell proliferation and damages the tumor cell through lack of energy. This can trigger apoptosis when enough glucose is blocked.

Drugs: One new GLUT1-inhibitor cancer drug (BAY-876) is in FDA-approved human cancer trials, and others are in the pipeline.

Plants: Anamu, bitter melon, graviola, and mullaca are GLUT1 inhibitors.

THE INFLAMMATION/IMMUNE PATHWAY

Chronic inflammation is a condition where the body's immune system keeps attacking and damaging tissues over a long period. It involves immune cells like macrophages, neutrophils, and eosinophils, which contribute to inflammation. Research shows that chronic inflammation can be a major cause of cancer and can speed up aging. It is also linked to many age-related diseases, such as diabetes, heart disease, and autoimmune disorders. Chronic inflammation creates oxidative stress, which weakens the body's ability to fight off damage. The excess free radicals produced can harm cell membranes, proteins, and even DNA, which can lead to cancer and other age-related diseases. Understanding how free radicals affect diseases could help scientists use antioxidants in preventing cancer and aging.

There are many complex interactions between the genes that control inflammation and the genes that manage immune cells in the body. For normal cells to turn into cancer cells, changes like mutations in tumor-suppressor genes, DNA changes (like DNA methylation), and protein alterations are needed. These changes disrupt the normal balance of cells and can trigger inflammation, which may lead to cancer. Inflammation is the body's natural defense against injury and involves immune responses and chemical signals. Many types of cancer have higher levels of inflammation, which is linked to cancer development. Inflammation plays a key role in various stages of cancer, including its beginning, growth, spread, and how the immune system reacts to the tumor. Immune cells in tumors interact with cancer cells in a complicated way, and scientists are working to understand these interactions. Chemicals that cause inflammation, like cytokines, free radicals, and certain enzymes, create an environment that supports tumor growth.

This environment is made up of immune cells like macrophages, B cells, T cells, and natural killer cells, which normally fight cancer. Certain cells (like Tregs and type 2 macrophages), however, can stop the immune system from working properly, leading to long-term inflammation and a tumor-friendly environment. Over time, the immune cells and the enzymes they produce can actually help the tumor survive, grow new blood vessels, and prevent immune cells from fighting the cancer.

Mounting evidence suggests that chronic inflammation can cause many chronic diseases and cancer. Today, the data suggests that at least one in seven malignant tumors diagnosed worldwide results from chronic inflammation and infection (which causes inflammation). Oxidative stress from poor diets (not enough antioxidants in the diet) causes chronic inflammation, and then that inflammation creates more oxidative stress, setting up a vicious cycle. Being obese or overweight causes chronic inflammation and resulting oxidation (I describe the phenomenon in my aptly named book, *Avenca: Nature's Secret for Weight Loss* (2021), which focuses on the rainforest plant known as avenca). More than 100 different substances in the body are recruited and interact in several different signaling pathways to create inflammation in the body. And these substances can be the first trigger to cause a healthy cell to begin the transformation into a cancer cell.

The three main inflammation pathways are Nuclear factor kappa B (NF-κB), Mitogen-activated protein kinase (MAPK), and Janus kinase/signal transducers and activators of transcription (JAK-STAT). Other signaling pathways include but are not limited to IκB/NF-κB and JNK/AP-1/.

Two of these pathways, NF-κB and STAT3, have emerged as major regulators of cancer, including cell transformation, tumor cell survival, proliferation, invasion, angiogenesis, and metastasis in cancer cells. Within these signaling pathways, many chemical substances create cascading chemical reactions, including immune cells, proteins, and enzymes. Thus, agents that can impact these pathways and resulting substances are the new targets to prevent and treat cancer as well as many inflammatory diseases. Some of these include AP1, COX1, COX2, cyclin D1, cyclin D3, CDK4, CDK6, cyclin E, and c-Jun NH2 kinase, as well as cytokines, called *interleukins*, that the immune system uses to respond to inflammation. Downregulating some pro-inflammatory cytokines, such as PGE2, NO, IL-1β, IL-6, and TNF-α, or upregulating some anti-inflammatory cytokines (Interleukins 4, 10, 11, 19, 35) can be targets for intervention.

The signaling pathways between inflammation and immune function intersect in many ways, and sometimes they use the same pathways. Inflammation can cause negative effects to immune function, and immune cells can cause inflammation; cancer uses both to thrive. Therefore, these have been combined together to describe strategies and chemical targets to address both. The specific signaling pathways and individual chemicals identified in both pathways are shown in the following sections.

IL-6 Inhibitors

Interleukin-6 (IL-6), one of the major cytokines in the tumor microenvironment, is an important factor that is found at high concentrations and known to be deregulated in cancer. Its overexpression has been reported in almost all types of tumors. IL-6 is implicated in various stages of tumorigenesis, including the initiation, growth, and progression of different cancers.

Drugs: Commonly used IL-6-inhibitor drugs include tocilizumab, sarilumab, siltuximab, and satralizumab.

Plants: Research indicates that cat's claw, graviola, mullaca, and suma can reduce IL-6 levels.

IL-1β Inhibitors

IL-1β can promote tumor growth and metastasis by influencing angiogenesis (formation of new blood vessels) and the tumor microenvironment.

Drugs: The main IL-1β-inhibitor drugs in use include anakinra, canakinumab, and rilonacept.

Plants: Mullaca and suma can also reduce IL-1β levels.

JAK/STAT3 Inhibitors

The JAK-STAT signaling pathway plays a crucial role in cancer by regulating cell proliferation, survival, and immune responses. Dysregulation of this pathway can contribute to tumor progression, immune evasion, and drug resistance. Targeting JAK-STAT is a promising therapeutic approach for various cancers. JAK-STAT activation can promote cancer cell growth, survival, and migration, leading to tumor progression and proliferation. The pathway can also influence immune responses, potentially suppressing antitumor immunity and allowing cancer cells to evade immune surveillance. JAK-STAT3 inhibitors show promise in treating several cancers including leukemia, pancreatic cancer, head and neck cancers, breast cancer, prostate cancer, renal cell carcinoma, colorectal cancer, and esophageal cancer.

Drugs: Several JAK inhibitors are in clinical development or have been approved for other diseases, offering potential therapeutic avenues for cancer treatment. JAK inhibitors like ruxolitinib have shown promise in treating some blood cancers (leukemias, myelomas, and lymphomas) and may have utility in solid tumors as well.

Plants: Bitter melon, cat's claw, graviola, pau d'arco, and suma have been described as JAK-STAT3 inhibitors in clinical research.

NF-κB Inhibitors

Nuclear factor-kappaB (NF-κB) is a protein that controls the activity of certain genes, and it plays a key role in cancer development as well as inflammation. Many cancer-causing agents and viruses can activate NF-κB, leading to changes in the cell that help cancer grow. NF-κB helps cancer cells grow, survive, and spread; causes inflammation; and forms new blood vessels. Blocking NF-κB can be an important way to treat or prevent cancer, and this has been shown with steroids, painkillers, and certain natural and man-made compounds. New treatments targeting specific parts of the NF-κB pathway have also shown promise in fighting cancer in quite a few clinical studies. NF inhibitors have shown potential in treating various cancers, including lymphomas, leukemias, and breast, prostate, lung, pancreatic, cervical, and gastric cancers.

Drugs: There are no NF-κB drugs approved specifically for cancer. One drug for rheumatoid arthritis (auranofin) is an NF-κB inhibitor.

Plants: Cat's claw, chanca piedra, espinheira santa, graviola, mullaca, picão preto, and vassourinha have shown the ability to inhibit NF-κB.

TREATING CANCER THROUGH THE MAIN CANCER PATHWAYS

Inhibition of the MAPK Signaling Pathway

The MAPK (mitogen-activated protein kinase) pathway is a crucial signaling pathway directly involved in regulating cell growth, proliferation, and survival of cancer cells. It plays a significant role in many cancers, and dysregulation of this pathway can lead to uncontrolled cell growth and tumor formation. The MAPK pathway is a key target for cancer therapies, and various inhibitors have been developed to block its activity and prevent cancer cell growth. These inhibitors can be used to treat various conditions, including cancer, by blocking the activity of mutated proteins within the pathway. MAPK inhibitors are beneficial in treating cancers with specific mutations in the MAPK pathway, notably those involving BRAF and KRAS. Inhibiting the MAPK pathway has been used to treat melanoma, lung cancer, colorectal cancer, and thyroid cancer, as well as low-grade serous ovarian carcinoma, pancreatic and adrenocortical cancers, and certain pediatric gliomas.

Drugs: Capivasertib, fruquintinib, momelotinib, pirtobrutinib, quizartinib, repotrectinib, and ritlecitinib are among the FDA-approved drugs that target the MAPK pathway.

Plants: Bitter melon, chanca piedra, and espinheira santa are the plants that can target this important pathway.

AP-1 Inhibitors

Activator Protein-1 (AP-1) plays a significant role in cancer development and progression. Dysregulated AP-1 activity is associated with tumor cell proliferation, invasion, metastasis, and resistance to therapy. AP-1 is a potential target for cancer therapy, and research is ongoing to develop inhibitors and combination therapies that target AP-1 to improve cancer treatment outcomes. Because AP-1 is often overactive in cancer cells, inhibiting it can potentially suppress tumor growth, induce apoptosis, inhibit metastasis, and sensitize cancer cells to chemotherapy. Overexpression of AP-1 is found in many cancers, including breast, ovarian, liver, skin, bone, lung, endometrial, and colorectal tumors.

Drugs: There are no approved AP-1-inhibitor drugs yet, but quite a few are in the pipeline and/or in various stages of clinical trials.

Plants: The rainforest plants shown to inhibit AP-1 include bitter melon, chanca piedra, guacatonga, and mullaca.

The Angiogenesis Pathway

Angiogenesis, the process of new blood vessel formation, is critical for various physiological functions in the body. When cancer activates this pathway, however, it contributes detrimentally to both cancer development and cancer progression. A quickly growing and dividing cancer cell needs more energy than a normal cell, so it signals for more blood vessels to form to provide the needed oxygen and nutrition the blood provides. Consequently, therapies that target these processes and reduce angiogenesis are crucial in the fight against cancer. Angiogenesis can be activated by cancer cells through several signaling processes and pathways (VEGF, VGFA, PDGFR, HIF-1α, SPHK-1, RAF/MEK/ERK, and AKT/GSK-3β). This process is triggered by chemical signals released by tumor cells, stimulating the growth of new blood vessels from existing ones.

Drugs: Approved drugs include axitinib, bevacizumab, cabozantinib, everolimus, lenalidomide, lenvatinib mesylate, pazopanib, ramucirumab, regorafenib, sorafenib, sunitinib, thalidomide, vandetanib, and ziv-aflibercept. They are not used as a frontline therapy, however; rather, they are just added to one or more other chemotherapy drugs intended to kill cancer cells directly.

Plants: Bitter melon, chanca piedra, espinheira santa, graviola, mullaca, picão preto, simarouba, and vassourinha have been reported to have anti-angiogenic actions.

The Proliferation Pathway

Cancer is often seen as a disease where the normal control of the cell cycle is lost. Normally, cell growth, signals from outside the cell, and the condition of the DNA are carefully checked at different stages of the cell cycle. Cancer can start when the balance of proteins that control the cell cycle is disturbed, causing cells to grow and divide abnormally. Because of this, stopping the cell cycle in cancer cells is an important approach to treating cancer. Natural chemicals from plants that can affect how the cell cycle works are getting a lot of attention, especially because research shows they can both slow down cell division and help trigger cell death (apoptosis).

When a normal human cell makes a copy of itself (replicates), there are four phases it goes through: G1 phase, S phase, G2 phase, and M phase. Cells increase in size during G1 phase, which is followed by DNA replication in S phase. Protein synthesis and the production of substances called microtubules occurs during G2 phase, which is then followed by mitosis (M phase). Normal cells have checkpoints at different stages of the cell cycle to monitor for DNA damage and ensure proper replication. Cancer cells often lack or have faulty checkpoints, allowing them to divide even with damaged DNA. This damage can allow cancer cells to rewrite their own DNA code in this process. This damage can cause what are known as *aberrant signaling pathways*. For example, cancer cells may have mutated (changed) genes that regulate cell division, leading to abnormal signaling pathways that promote continuous cell growth. Unlike normal cells that have a limited lifespan, cancer cells can proliferate indefinitely due to the disruption of what are called cellular senescence mechanisms found in the DNA code.

One of the hallmarks of cancer is aggressive proliferation of cells. In a normal cell, a fine balance between growth signals and antigrowth signals regulates how many times and how often a cell makes a copy of itself (proliferates). This fine balance is lost in cancer cells, however, which often show uncontrolled growth due to the loss of both growth-controlling factors. Cancer cells can acquire the capability to generate their own growth signals, and they can also become completely unresponsive to antigrowth signals.

Numerous factors regulate the natural progression of a normal cell. Some of these factors, such as cyclins, are upregulated in cancer cells, causing the cells to replicate uncontrollably. Cyclins are the regulatory proteins that control the cell cycle, while other factors such as COX-2 and c-Myc play a supporting role. The most commonly affected cyclin in cancer cells is cyclin D1, an important cell cycle regulator that plays a role in transition of the cell from the G1 phase to the S phase. Cancer cells show overexpression of this cyclin D1, and thus it has been linked to the development and progression of cancer.

Cell cycle checkpoints are crucial for maintaining genomic stability, and their malfunction is a hallmark of cancer. Cancer cells often develop mutations that disrupt checkpoint function, leading to uncontrolled cell division and genomic instability. These defects can make cancer cells more susceptible to certain therapies that target checkpoint pathways, while simultaneously making them resistant to others. For example, Chk1 is a kinase that regulates the G2/M checkpoint. Inactivation of Chk1 can lead to mitotic catastrophe in cancer cells.

Checkpoint inhibitor drugs: Ipilimumab, nivolumab, pembrolizumab, atezolizumab, avelumab, durvalumab, and cemiplimab.

Checkpoint inhibitor plants: Anamu, bitter melon fruit, cat's claw, chana piedra, espinheira santa, graviola, guacatonga, mullaca, picão preto, simarouba, suma, and vassourinha. For more information see the "Cell Cycle Arrest" section that follows.

Cell Cycle Arrest

The cell cycle refers to the process of cell growth and division and consists of four main phases: the G1 phase, S phase, G2 phase, and M phase. Among them, the G1 phase is the preliminary stage of DNA synthesis and determines whether the cell can enter into the S phase. If the cell stops in the G1 phase (i.e., when it is in a dormant state), it is called the G0 phase. The S phase is the synthesis of DNA, where the cell carries out DNA replication. The G2 phase is the preparatory stage when the cell is ready to enter into the dividing phase. The M phase is also known as mitosis, wherein the cell carries out division and makes a copy of itself. In tumor cells, the cell cycle is disturbed. Some tumor cells may enter into a state of endless proliferation, leading to the continuous enlargement of the tumor. Therefore, many anti-cancer drugs inhibit the proliferation of tumor cells by interfering with the tumor cell cycle.

There are several mechanisms to arrest cell cycles, including upregulating the expression of proteins that play key roles (including p53, p21, and p27) or inhibiting the expression levels of cyclin D1 and cyclin-dependent kinase (CDK) 4 and 6. Other methods include inhibiting microtubules. This can suppress or block cell cycle progression, and results in apoptosis.

Plants capable of arresting cancer cell cycles:

- Anamu can arrest the normal cell cycle (at G2/M) as tumor cells divide and replicate, which triggers the normal apoptosis process.

- Prostate cancer treated with bitter melon in animals and test tubes experienced S-phase cell cycle arrest by modulating cyclin D1, cyclin E, and p21 expression. In breast and liver cancer cells, bitter melon fruit juice was reported to cause cell cycle arrest in the G0/G1 phase.

- Cat's claw alkaloids arrest the cell cycle at the G0/G1 stage in acute lymphoblastic leukemia cells, triggering apoptosis.

- Chanca piedra induced S-phase and G1-phase cell cycle arrest and apoptosis in leukemia and ovarian cancer cells; and in G2/M phase in liver cancer.
- Espinheira santa has shown to induce tumor cells to arrest in the G1 phase mainly by inhibiting the expression levels of cyclin D1 and cyclin-dependent kinase (CDK) 4 and 6.
- Graviola has shown to induce cell cycle arrest and apoptosis in the G0/G1 phase, the G1/S phase, and G2/M phase depending on the cancer type.
- Guacatonga caused cell cycle arrest at the G2/S phase, which initiated apoptosis by affecting two molecular targets (p53, p16). In other cancer types, a guacatonga main chemical caused G1/S cell cycle arrest by reducing ERK phosphorylation and cyclin D1 expression levels.
- Mullaca causes cell death in the G2/M cell cycle phase for some cancers and in the G0/G1 cell cycle phase in other types of cancers.
- Picão preto caused cell cycle arrest in leukemia cells in the G1/S phase and in the G2/M phase in liver cancer cells.
- Simarouba caused cell cycle arrest in the G2/M phase.
- Suma caused cell cycle arrest in liver cancer in the S phase.
- Vassourinha induces G1 cell cycle arrest in colorectal and lung cancers.

Cancer Stem Cells (CSCs)

CSCs are thought to possess stem cell-like properties, including self-renewal and the ability to differentiate into various cancer cell types. They are often more resistant to conventional cancer treatments like chemotherapy and radiation, contributing significantly to treatment failure and cancer recurrence. Many of the "microscopic cancer cells left behind" after conventional therapies, which oncologists talk about, are CSCs. Researchers have discovered two ways (so far) that CSCs can be killed. First, many CSCs have unique or specific metabolic requirements. Inhibiting enzymes involved in their metabolism can selectively target CSCs and kill them. Second, CSCs also rely on certain signaling pathways (like Wnt, Notch, STAT3, and Hedgehog) for survival and self-renewal. Inhibitors targeting these pathways can disrupt CSC function.

Drugs: Salinomycin and Dasatinib. In human trials: Napabucasin (BBI608) is an oral CSC inhibitor copied from a natural chemical discovered in pau d'arco (see page 284), CA3, CSC-6.

Plants with metabolic modifying actions specific to CSCs: Anamu, bitter melon, espinheira santa, graviola, pau d'arco, simarouba, and vassourinha.

Plants altering CSC-specific signaling pathways: Anamu, bitter melon, cat's claw, chanca piedra, espinheira santa, graviola, guacatonga, mullaca, pau d'arco, picão preto, simarouba, suma, and vassourinha.

Microtubule Inhibitors (MTIs)

Microtubule inhibitors (MTIs) are drugs that target microtubules, vital components of the cell's internal structure and involved in various cellular processes, including cell division. MTIs are frequently used in cancer treatment due to their ability to disrupt the cell division process of rapidly growing cancer cells. MTIs are used for many different types of cancers, including leukemias, lymphomas, and breast, ovarian, lung, prostate, testicular, and head and neck cancers.

Drugs: Vincristine, vinblastine, paclitaxel, ixabepilone, eribulin, cabazitaxel, and fosbretabulin.

Plants: Anamu and espinheira santa are described in clinical research as microtubule inhibitors.

PAK1 Inhibitors

The p21-activated kinase 1-dependent pathway (PAK1) plays a significant role in cancer development and progression, particularly in processes like cell growth, motility, and survival. PAK1 is often overexpressed or hyperactivated in various cancers, and its downstream signaling can promote tumor growth, metastasis, and drug resistance. Its involvement in growth factor signaling, metastasis, angiogenesis (blood vessel formation), and drug resistance makes it an attractive therapeutic target for cancer treatment. PAK1 is overexpressed or hyperactivated in several cancers, including breast, liver, kidney, pancreatic, and colorectal cancers.

Drugs: There are currently no FDA-approved PAK1-specific inhibitor drugs available. Preclinical and clinical studies are under way for various PAK1 inhibitors in the treatment of a range of diseases, particularly cancers.

Plants: Bitter melon, pau d'arco, and simarouba can inhibit PAK-1.

P2X7 Inhibitors

The P2X7 receptor, activated by ATP, plays a significant role in breast cancer, promoting cell migration, invasion, and tumor growth. It is upregulated in aggressive breast cancer subtypes and triple-negative breast cancer, and its inhibition has been shown to reduce breast cancer–induced bone metastasis. In addition to breast cancers, based on research to date, some cancers that may benefit from P2X7 inhibitors include glioblastoma, non–small cell lung cancer, acute myeloid leukemia (AML) neuroblastoma, and pancreatic, colorectal, thyroid, and gastric cancers.

Drugs: There are no P2X7-inhibitor drugs approved yet specifically for cancer. Several are in various stages of development including human trials. One existing drug (ivermectin) has shown potential as a P2X7 inhibitor in research.

Plants: Anamu and cat's claw have evidenced P2X7-inhibitor actions.

c-Myc Inhibitors

c-Myc inhibitors are molecules that specifically target the c-Myc protein, a key regulator of cell growth, proliferation, and differentiation, and are being developed as potential cancer therapeutics. These inhibitors work by disrupting c-Myc's activity, leading to reduced cell growth and potentially inducing tumor regression. c-Myc inhibitors show promise in treating several cancers, including neuroblastoma, small-cell lung cancer, breast cancer, pancreatic cancer, and various lymphomas.

Drugs: There are currently no FDA-approved drugs that directly inhibit c-Myc, although numerous research efforts are under way to develop such therapies. Many compounds have shown promise in preclinical and early clinical trials, but these have not yet reached the final stages of FDA approval.

Plants: Rainforest plants that have shown the ability to inhibit c-Myc include bitter melon, espinheira santa, guacatonga, mullaca, simarouba, and vassourinha.

EGFR Inhibitors

EGFR inhibitors block the epidermal growth factor receptor (EGFR) protein, which can be overexpressed or mutated in some cancer cells, leading to uncontrolled growth. EGFR inhibitors are particularly effective in EGFR-mutated non–small cell lung cancer where mutations in the EGFR gene lead to abnormal cell growth. Other cancers with EGFR mutations include colorectal cancer and head and neck cancers. EGFR is also expressed in cancers of the ovary, cervix, bladder, prostate, esophagus, stomach, brain, endometrium, and pancreas.

Drugs: Gefitinib, erlotinib, afatinib, cetuximab, osimertinib, and panitumumab.

Plants: Anamu, bitter melon, espinheira santa, and graviola.

TOPO I Inhibitors

Topoisomerase 1 is a newer target for new chemotherapy drugs to disrupt DNA replication and transcription. DNA topoisomerase I inhibitors are a class of medications that target the enzyme topoisomerase I, which is involved in DNA replication and transcription. These inhibitors work by preventing topoisomerase I from cleaving DNA strands, leading to DNA damage and ultimately cell death. This mechanism makes them particularly effective against cancer cells, which have higher levels of topoisomerase I activity than normal cells. These cancers include small cell lung cancer, sarcomas, leukemia, and colorectal, ovarian, pancreatic, cervical, and glioblastoma cancers.

Drugs: Irinotecan and topotecan.

Plants: Pau d'arco and picão preto.

TOPO2A Inhibitors

Topoisomerase II alpha inhibitors are a class of drugs that target the enzyme topoisomerase II alpha (TOPO2A), which is crucial for DNA replication, transcription, and chromosome segregation. These inhibitors work by stabilizing the transient DNA breaks introduced by TOP2A gene, leading to the accumulation of DNA damage and ultimately cell death, particularly in cancer cells. Inhibiting TOPO2A has shown to be beneficial in leukemias, sarcomas, lymphomas, and lung, colorectal, ovarian, pancreatic, cervical, liver, testicular, and glioblastoma cancers.

Drugs: Etoposide, teniposide, doxorubicin, idarubicin, epirubicin, and mitoxantrone.

Plants: Graviola was shown in research to inhibit TOPO2A.

(Note: TOPO2A is the enzyme that is produced by the TOP2A gene.)

Telomerase Inhibitors

Telomerase inhibitors are being explored as a potential cancer therapy because telomerase, an enzyme that extends telomeres (protective caps on chromosomes), is often overexpressed in cancer cells, allowing them to replicate indefinitely. Inhibiting telomerase can potentially disrupt this immortality, leading to cancer cell death or enhanced sensitivity to other treatments. Telomerase inhibitors are being investigated for their potential to treat a variety of cancers, particularly those where telomerase expression is high. These include blood cancers like myelofibrosis and essential thrombocythemia, as well as certain solid tumors such as breast, prostate, ovarian, lung, pancreatic, liver, cervix, melanoma, and colorectal cancers.

Drugs: Rytelo.

Plants: Chanca piedra, espinheira santa, pau d'arco, and vassourinha.

c-Met Inhibitors

c-Met is a receptor tyrosine kinase that plays a significant role in cancer development and progression. It is often overexpressed or mutated in various cancers, driving processes like tumor growth, invasion, and metastasis. Aberrant c-Met signaling can also contribute to drug resistance. The types of cancer that benefit from c-Met inhibitors include non–small cell lung cancer, liver cancer, gastric cancer, pancreatic cancer, melanoma, and some breast and colorectal cancers.

Drugs: Capmatinib, tepotinib, and telisotuzumab vedotin-tllv.

Plants: Bitter melon and graviola.

Notch Signaling Inhibitors

The Notch pathway powerfully influences stem cell maintenance, development, and cell fate; it is increasingly recognized for the key roles it plays in cancer. Notch promotes cell survival, angiogenesis, and treatment resistance in numerous cancers, making it a promising target for cancer therapy. It also crosstalks with other critical cancer genes, providing a means to affect numerous signaling pathways with one intervention. Notch signaling inhibitors show promise in treating a variety of cancers, particularly those with aberrant Notch activation. These include certain types of breast cancer, lung cancer (especially non–small cell lung cancer), T-cell acute lymphoblastic leukemia, and diffuse large B-cell lymphoma. Additionally, they are being explored for use in ovarian, pancreatic, and colon cancers, as well as glioblastoma.

Drugs: One drug has been approved (nirogacestat), and several others are in development.

Plants: Anamu, bitter melon, chanca piedra, espinheira santa, graviola, guacatonga, and picão preto have been shown to affect Notch signaling in various beneficial ways. See Part 3 for more information.

β-Glucuronidase Inhibitors

These inhibitors may increase the safety and tolerability of anti-cancer agents and chemotherapy drugs. For example, research suggests that inhibiting gut bacterial β-glucuronidase enzymes can reduce the gastrointestinal toxicity caused by irinotecan, a cancer drug that treats colorectal and pancreatic cancers. β-Glucuronidase (βG) inhibitors show promise in the treatment of several cancers, primarily by mitigating chemotherapy-induced side effects and potentially enhancing treatment efficacy. Specifically, these inhibitors have shown benefit or potential benefit in breast, colorectal, pancreatic, prostate, and non–small cell and small cell lung cancers.

Drugs: While no β-glucuronidase-inhibitor drugs are specifically FDA approved solely for cancer treatment, some existing drugs with other primary indications are being explored for potential cancer-related applications, including amoxapine, nialamide, and isocarboxazid.

Plants: In research, vassourinha demonstrated βG-inhibitor actions.

Hsp90 Inhibitors

Heat shock proteins (Hsp) are critical for cell survival and protection from stressful stimuli, including oxidative stress. Hsp90 inhibitors are a type of targeted cancer therapy that works by blocking the Hsp90 protein. By inhibiting Hsp90, these drugs can force cancer cells to degrade and die. Hsp90 inhibitors have shown potential in treating various cancers, particularly those where specific proteins (client proteins) are heavily reliant on Hsp90 for stability and function. Examples include HER2-positive breast cancer, prostate cancer, some non–small cell lung cancers, and melanoma, leukemias, and multiple myeloma.

Drugs: Ganetespib has shown synergy with chemotherapy drugs like doxorubicin and etoposide in preclinical studies but has not been approved to treat cancer yet.

Plants: Anamu and espinheira santa can inhibit Hsp90.

NQO1 Inhibitors

NAD(P)H:quinone oxidoreductase 1 (NQO1) inhibitors are a new molecular target for new chemotherapy drugs since NQO1 protects cancer cells from the oxidative stress that would normally instigate apoptosis. NQO1 is upregulated in many human cancers including breast cancer, colorectal cancer, lung cancer, pancreatic cancer, uterine cancer, cervical cancer, and melanoma.

Drugs: There are no FDA-approved drugs available yet; however, several plant-based chemicals have been approved as small-molecule drugs for research, including one found in pau d'arco, beta lapachone, which is in human clinical trials.

Plants: Pau d'arco.

NADH Oxidase Inhibitors

The plasma membrane in some cancers can promote too much of an enzyme (NADH oxidase), which contributes to uncontrolled cell proliferation. These include some breast cancers, gastric cancer, chronic myelogenous leukemia, acute myelogenous leukemia, chronic myeloid leukemia, and colorectal, bile duct, cervix, and anal cancers. This makes its inhibition a potential therapeutic strategy for cancer that uses the enzyme to enhance proliferation.

Drugs: Several new drugs are in clinical trials, but none have been approved yet.

Plants: Graviola and simarouba.

COL1A1 Inhibitors

This type of collagen gene is implicated in cancer, particularly in its progression, metastasis, drug resistance, and prognosis. Cancer can significantly affect COL1A1 expression and function. Some cancers significantly increase the expression of this gene, including breast, colorectal, and liver cancers.

Drugs: There are no approved cancer drugs that inhibit COL1A1.

Plants: Mullaca was shown to inhibit COL1A1.

PI3K/AKT/mTOR Inhibitors

This pathway is a signaling network in cells that regulates cell growth, survival, and the cell cycle. It's involved in many normal cellular functions, including protein synthesis, energy balance and nutrition, and controlling growth. Cancers with alterations in this pathway that benefit from this type of inhibitor include hormone receptor-positive breast cancer, HER2-negative advanced breast cancer, triple negative breast cancer, melanoma, and ovarian, prostate, colon, gastric, pancreatic, and thyroid cancers.

Drugs: Alpelisib, copanlisib, idelalisib, duvelisib, and umbralisib.

Plants: Anamu, espinheira santa, chanca piedra, graviola, mullaca, and vassourinha.

mTOR Inhibitors

mTOR inhibitors are a class of drugs used in cancer treatment that target the mTOR signaling pathway, a key pathway involved in cell growth and proliferation. By inhibiting mTOR, these drugs can help slow down or stop the growth of cancer cells. mTOR inhibitors have been approved for the treatment of certain types of cancer, including renal cell carcinoma and breast cancer. In many cancers, the mTOR pathway is abnormally activated, leading to uncontrolled cell growth and tumor development. mTOR also plays a role in the formation of new blood vessels (angiogenesis) that tumors need to grow. Inhibiting mTOR can help prevent the development of new blood vessels, thus limiting tumor growth. mTOR inhibitors are used to treat several types of cancer, including renal cell carcinoma, breast cancer, and neuroendocrine tumors. They have also shown promise in treating other cancers like lung cancer, gastric carcinoma, colorectal cancer, and prostate cancer.

Drugs: Approved mTOR-inhibitor drugs for cancer include sirolimus, everolimus, and temsirolimus.

Plants: Graviola and vassourinha are reported to inhibit mTOR.

Inhibition of the Wnt/β-catenin Signaling Pathway

Wnt/β-catenin signaling is a highly conserved pathway that regulates cell proliferation, differentiation, apoptosis, stem cell self-renewal, tissue homeostasis, and wound healing. Several cancers exhibit dysregulation of Wnt signaling pathways, including breast cancer, colorectal cancer, endometrial cancer, lung cancer, gastric cancer, and melanoma. Inhibition of the Wnt/β-catenin pathway is also being explored as a strategy to overcome drug resistance in cancer and target cancer stem cells. Several cancers are known to benefit from therapies targeting the Wnt/β-catenin pathway including melanoma and colorectal, pancreatic, gastric, lung, renal, and liver cancers.

Drugs: While no drugs are specifically FDA approved solely for inhibiting the Wnt/β-catenin pathway in cancer, several existing drugs and compounds show potential as Wnt pathway inhibitors and are being investigated for their anti-cancer properties. Some of these include the anti-parasite drugs niclosamide, ivermectin, mebendazole, albendazole, pyrvinium, and guanabenz, as well as the anticoccidial agent salinomycin.

Plants: Bitter melon, cat's claw, chanca piedra, picão preto, simarouba, and vassourinha.

Inhibition of TGF-β-Associated EMT Progression

TGF-β (Transforming Growth Factor beta) is an important protein that helps control a process called Epithelial-Mesenchymal Transition (EMT), which is involved in cancer spread. During EMT, cancer cells change shape, lose their ability to stick together, and become more mobile and invasive. TGF-β helps drive this change, making it easier for cancer to spread and harder to treat. Inhibiting this process has become a new target in cancer research to reduce invasiveness and metastasis of various cancers. Cancers that are known to benefit from EMT inhibitors include head and neck squamous cell carcinoma and breast, pancreatic, lung, bladder, and ovarian cancers. These cancers are often associated with increased invasiveness and resistance to therapy due to the EMT process.

Drugs: Existing EMT inhibitors are largely still in research and development phases, with a few clinical trials under way focused on targeting EMT in cancer. None have been FDA approved for cancer treatment as of the current date. While several TGF-β inhibitors are in clinical trials, either alone or in combination with other therapies, none have received full FDA approval for cancer.

Plants: Bitter melon juice, espinheira santa, picão preto, simarouba, and vassourinha have demonstrated in cancer research to be able to inhibit EMT.

RSK1 Inhibitors

RSK1, a member of the RSK (ribosomal protein S6 kinase) family, is implicated in both promoting and suppressing tumor growth, depending on the specific cancer type. These inhibitors are being researched as potential anti-cancer agents due to the role of RSK1 in cell growth, survival, and motility, which are all important processes in cancer development. Studies have shown that RSK1 inhibitors have shown potential in treating a variety of cancers, including lung adenocarcinoma, leukemia, colorectal cancer, renal cancer, ovarian cancer, and glioma. Specifically, they have demonstrated efficacy in preclinical models of breast cancer and have entered clinical trials for metastatic breast cancer.

Drugs: There are no FDA-approved drugs that specifically target RSK1 for cancer treatment. While RSK1 is a validated target for cancer therapy, and some RSK inhibitors are in development, including those for breast cancer, none have received FDA approval yet.

Plants: Anamu has shown the ability to inhibit RSK1.

MMP Inhibitors

Matrix metalloproteinases (MMPs) are enzymes that break down the outer layer of cells (the extracellular matrix), and they are linked to occurrence and promotion of tumor invasion, metastasis, and angiogenesis. Because of this, blocking MMPs and stopping the breakdown of the extracellular matrix has become a new focus in cancer treatment. MMP inhibitors have shown promise in preclinical studies for treating various cancers, including melanoma and breast, colon, prostate, pancreatic, and lung cancers.

Drugs: MMP inhibitors have been studied as potential anti-cancer drugs, but early initial clinical trials were not successful due to lack of specificity and unforeseen side effects. Doxycycline is the only FDA-approved MMP inhibitor (approved for periodontal disease). Newer drugs have been developed that have better specificity and fewer side effects; these are in clinical trials currently, including one being tested in gastric cancer patients.

Plants: Bitter melon, chanca piedra, espinheira santa, graviola, mullaca, pau d'arco, and vassourinha have MMP-inhibitor properties as follows:

- Studies have shown that ethanol extracts from bitter melon leaves can reduce the movement and invasion of prostate cancer cells in lab tests by reducing the release of MMP-2 and MMP-9.

- Chanca piedra suppressed breast carcinoma metastasis and proliferation by suppressing matrix metalloprotein 2 and 9 expression via inhibition of the extracellular signal-related kinase (ERK) pathway. It also inhibited tumor metastasis and angiogenesis through the suppression of 4 MMP (matrix metalloproteinase) enzymes in prostate and melanoma cancers. In osteosarcoma cells, a main active chemical (geraniin) reduced the expression of MMP-9 through the PI3K/Akt and ERK1/2 signaling pathways.

- Espinheira santa causes a loss of mitochondrial membrane potential and decreased the expression of MMPs. MMP2 and MMP9 were decreased by espinheira santa in esophageal cancer cells.
- Graviola reduced MMP expression via upregulation of Bax and downregulation of Bcl-2 at the gene expression level, accompanied by cytochrome c release to the cytosol.
- Mullaca was reported to inhibit cancer cell proliferation, migration, and angiogenesis through reducing MMP activity and vascular endothelial growth factor (VEGF) expression, which results in antimetastatic properties.
- A pau d'arco chemical (lapachol) was reported to inhibit MMPs.
- Vassourinha inhibits metastasis by decreasing NF-κB/MMP-2 signaling.

P-glycoprotein (ABCB1) Inhibitors

P-glycoprotein (P-gp), also known as ABCB1, is a transmembrane protein that can actively export many foreign substances, including various chemotherapeutic drugs, out of cells. P-glycoprotein acts as an energy-dependent efflux pump, meaning it uses ATP energy to pump substances (like chemo drugs) out of the cells. This process of drug efflux can lead to multidrug resistance (MDR), where cancer cells become resistant to multiple types of chemotherapy drugs. Cancers where ABCB1 overexpression is a significant factor in resistance, such as leukemia and certain breast, lung, ovarian, colorectal, and prostate cancers, may benefit from the use of ABCB1 inhibitors in combination with chemotherapy.

Drugs: Several antibiotics and heart drugs inhibit ABCB1, but they haven't been approved for cancer. Several new cancer ABCB1-inhibitor drugs are in human clinical trials with mixed results.

Plants: Cancer research on bitter melon fruit and leaf, chanca piedra, graviola, and simarouba has demonstrated ABCB1-inhibitor actions.

Mucin Inhibitors

Mucins are a family of heavily glycosylated proteins that play a role in various cellular processes, including cell signaling, cell adhesion, and protection of mucosal surfaces. In cancer, mucins can be overexpressed and contribute to tumor growth, metastasis, and resistance to therapy. For example, MUC4 plays an important role in the etiology of many different types of cancer, including pancreatic cancer, ovarian cancers, and head and neck cancers. MUC4 suppresses apoptosis and induces resistance to several chemotherapeutic agents by modulating STAT and the PI-3K, Ras/RAF/extracellular signal-regulated kinase (ERK1/2) signaling pathways through physical interaction and stabilization of the ErbB family of growth factor RTKs.

Drugs: No mucin inhibitors are currently FDA approved specifically for cancer treatment yet. Several are under development, and at least two approved mucin-inhibitor drugs for other diseases are under research to repurpose for cancer.

Plants: Graviola, mullaca, and picão preto can inhibit MUC4.

IFN-γ Stimulant

IFN-γ is a protein secreted by immune cells that is crucial for activating cellular immunity, boosting antitumor responses, and modulating immune responses, including inflammation and autoimmunity.

Drugs: None.

Plants: Picão preto and suma were capable of stimulating IFN-γ in clinical research.

THE AUTOPHAGY PATHWAY

Autophagy is like a cleanup process for your cells. When a cell is damaged or has parts it doesn't need, it breaks them down and recycles them to keep the cell healthy. This helps the cell get rid of waste, stay balanced, and even provide energy when it's under stress. Autophagy in cancer biology serves a dual function, encompassing both tumor promotion and inhibition. The induction of autophagy in response to diverse cellular stressors plays a crucial role in regulating cell death, therefore offering a promising avenue for developing novel anti-cancer therapeutics. In addition, autophagy regulates the properties of cancer stem cells by contributing to the maintenance of stemness, the induction of recurrence, and the development of resistance to anti-cancer reagents. Although some autophagy modulators, such as rapamycin and chloroquine, are used to regulate autophagy in anti-cancer therapy, since this process also plays roles in both tumor suppression and promotion, the precise mechanism of autophagy in cancer requires further study.

Molecular targets being researched in this pathway include mTOR, PI3K, ULK1, VPS34, ATG4B, Beclin 1, and LC3.

TREATING CANCER THROUGH THE MAIN CANCER PATHWAYS

Plants: The rainforest plants that have been reported to kill cancer cells through triggering autophagy include bitter melon, chanca piedra, espinheira santa, mullaca, picão preto, and vassourinha.

Summary

As you can see, quite a few molecular targets have been identified in all the new cancer research that started with the Human Genome Project. We are in a much better position to finally counteract the many changes that cancer can make, which is the only way we will ever win the war on cancer. Remember, however, the average time from discovery to a new approved cancer drug is 30–50 years, and we are, at best, 10–20 years into that long process on many of the drugs discussed in this chapter.

Our conventional health care system is still hampered by the single molecule drug approval process, when it's clear that multiple chemicals are required to address multiple targets simultaneously, if a cure is possible. Chemically rich medicinal plants, as well as combination formulas combining multiple plants together may well be the only approach that works.

For example, let's look at one plant, anamu (see page 198), that is beneficial for breast cancer. One single chemical in anamu (diallyl trisulfide) affected 22 signaling pathways and/or molecular targets within those pathways to fight breast cancer alone. The effects were reported to inhibit proliferation, ROS formation, AhR expression, cell migration, cell proliferation, cancer stem cell characteristics, cell invasion, cell viabilities, metastasis, and cell progression. In addition, it can induce cell death and apoptosis, arrest the cell cycle, and increase sensitivity to chemotherapy drugs.

One chemical had 14 different beneficial effects against one type of cancer. The plant has shown similar benefits for 16 different types of cancers, using even more signaling pathways and molecular targets. So, multiply that by 16. Anamu has more than 100 different active chemicals, so multiply by 100. The plant was delivered in a natural remedy containing anamu and seven other plants with a similar amount of signaling pathways, molecular targets, and benefits.

How likely is it that cancer can mutate fast enough to defend against so many different chemicals working together simultaneously? In Part 2, we will look at natural cancer remedies in this manner and discuss how to combine these chemically rich rainforest plants using these new molecular targets to increase the efficacy of the natural remedy.

PART 2

Harnessing the Power of the Plants

Now that you've learned more about the new methods to treat cancer and how these rainforest plants can react with cancer on a molecular level, it's time to apply that knowledge to help you fight cancer with it. Let's review what we've already learned that will help in the process.

SINGLE-CHEMICAL DRUGS VERSUS MULTIPLE-CHEMICAL PLANTS

With cancer being a multifaceted and complex disease, the old paradigm of one magic bullet for one cancer is simply not going to work. We've proven that quite well over the last 50 years. Cancer can change too many genes, molecules, and signaling pathways, and multiple moving targets will have to be addressed to ever hope to have a cure. A medicinal plant, like those found in this book, with 300–400 plant chemicals that we now know can hit multiple targets at once has a much better chance than any single molecule drug. But even that is not enough!

WHY YOU CAN'T IGNORE CANCER'S DEFENSIVE AND RECURRENCE MECHANISMS

Cancer seems to have an enormous will to survive and has spent many years creatively devising ways to survive and thrive—and it gets complicated quickly. For example, cancer uses a strategy called angiogenesis to create new blood vessels to bring additional nutrients to a tumor, which it needs to divide and grow at a much faster rate than normal cells. We have known this for many years and have developed angiogenesis inhibitor drugs to combat this strategy. The problem is that cancer has developed more than one strategy to achieve angiogenesis, and it can quickly change strategies when one is blocked by a drug or even a plant chemical. Just for angiogenesis alone, scientists have (so far) discovered six different genes with at least a dozen different molecules in each one of those genetic pathways, which cancer can use to trigger and achieve angiogenesis. Today, oncologists are prescribing at least two—and sometimes three—anti-angiogenetic drugs to combat this, while just hoping they can kill enough cancer cells using other methods to be effective. And angiogenesis is just one process cancer has to thrive and survive, out of at least 100 or more. There's a lot going on, and all at the same time!

SMALL-MOLECULE PLANT DRUGS GO MAINSTREAM

In chapters 3 and 5, you also learned about a new type of drug that came out of the new methods to treat cancer called "targeted therapies" and "small-molecule drugs." Targeted therapies are a type of cancer treatment that uses drugs or other substances to identify and attack specific molecules in cancer cells, disrupting their growth and spread while minimizing damage to healthy cells. Unlike traditional chemotherapy, which affects all rapidly dividing cells, targeted therapies aim for specific molecules that are crucial for cancer cell survival.

These targeted therapies can also target specific molecules (usually proteins and enzymes) in a signaling pathway that a cancer created or changed. This precision approach can lead to more effective treatments with fewer side effects by selectively changing something that is only found in cancer's defensive and recurrence pathways and has no effect on healthy cells' normal pathways.

The majority of the targeted therapies developed so far involve a newer small-molecule drug. A small-molecule drug is an organic compound, typically a plant chemical, that can be chemically synthesized in a laboratory. The molecules in these drugs are small in size and can easily penetrate cell membranes and interact with specific targets within cells, like proteins or enzymes, to produce a therapeutic effect. Many plant chemicals from rainforest plants, including those found in this book, have been used to create small-molecule drugs and are being studied for cancer. Some are an exact copy of the plant chemical, while others have been changed slightly, but enough to be patented as a new molecule. You'll learn about the small-molecule drugs in more detail reading about each rainforest plant in Part 3.

The problem is mainstream medicine is still stuck in the one magic bullet–one target paradigm. Their single-chemical small-molecule drug doesn't have the diversity of actions necessary to address the multiple pathways cancer uses, and oftentimes a single medicinal plant may not either. That's where multi-plant natural remedies may hold the key.

Harnessing the Power of the Plants Means Effective Multi-Plant Remedies

The combination of medicinal plants is of great importance because additive or synergistic interactions can enhance their biological activity. Multiple plants can affect multiple targets more efficiently and quickly. Resistance to treatment is less likely to occur when active compounds derived from different plants are used in combination than when they are used individually because they can act on multiple molecular targets and pathways simultaneously.

Part 2 of the book is about the anti-cancer natural remedies I have created over the years using rainforest plants, and how to use them today to fight cancer. And while these remedies are now in the public domain, and I make nothing on their sales, they are available to purchase. In fact, because they are so effective, they have been sold and used for almost 25 years. Writing this book has given me the opportunity to review all the new research on the plants used for these remedies (and there has been a lot), as well as all the new research and information on how cancer is working on a molecular level, to understand why these remedies are so effective and how to make them better.

Part 2 is divided into three chapters. Chapter 6 provides information on the history and use of three anti-cancer natural remedies, and in general, how to use them. Included is where to source the products, dosages to use, possible contraindication, drug interactions, practitioners' observations, and how to combine them with conventional cancer treatments, when appropriate. The chapter also provides additional information on how to support immune function and offers helpful advice on dietary and lifestyle choices.

Chapter 7 provides a specific cancer plan by cancer type detailing which natural remedies to use, with the assumption that readers will be purchasing the manufactured natural remedies discussed that are available from various natural product manufacturers. It provides the protocols as well as new information on other plant products to add to the cancer plan to address specific defense and recurrence mechanisms that each cancer type employs. This information is based on thousands of research studies on the plants and the cancers published over the last 10 years. The chapter also offers specific dosages and instructions.

Chapter 8 supplies similar information, but with the assumption that readers, trained practitioners, and/or compounding pharmacies may want to make their own natural cancer remedies. It provides the recipes to make the original three N-Tense formulas, as well as specific instruction on how to make capsules, infusions, tinctures, and glycerin extract remedies with the combination of plants. It then provides a recipe for each cancer type on the best way to combine the ingredients in N-Tense necessary for that particular cancer, with new additional plants needed to help with defense and recurrence mechanisms.

In both chapters 7 and 8, cancer plans are included for bladder, bone, brain, breast, cervical, colorectal, endometrial, esophageal, gastric, kidney, and laryngeal cancers; leukemias; liver and lung cancers; lymphomas, melanoma, and multiple myeloma; and nasopharyngeal, ovarian, pancreatic, prostate, skin, testicular, and thyroid cancers.

6

A NATUROPATHIC APPROACH TO NATURAL ANTI-CANCER REMEDIES

As you may have seen in Part 1, my being a naturopath and herbalist has allowed me to view healing in a different light. There is no question that modern medicine has allowed us to cure many terrible diseases and helped extend life, but it also has a number of shortcomings. Sometimes it can be limited in its views, evolve too slowly, or be too motivated by money. On the other hand, allowing yourself to understand healing from a different perspective can open many doors. Having traveled to the Amazon rainforest over the years, I had come to meet many Indigenous people—individuals whose only link to health was their "medicine men." I saw firsthand the power of rainforest plants used to heal the sick. I clearly understood that the chemicals found in these plants actually worked against a variety of serious health disorders. This was the beginning of my journey.

As a naturopath, I took it upon myself to learn as much as I could about these many medicinal plants. Based on my research, I put together many remedy-specific formulas, which were only sold to practitioners. It was cancer, however, that got my attention: first on a personal level and then on a professional one. Over the past 25 years, I have worked with many health care professionals who have used these formulas successfully that I had developed. Although the process took some time, it ultimately led to the development of three basic formulas—N-Tense, NTense-2, and N-Tense Topical—which will be discussed in Part 2. What I have also found is that the new research on the rainforest plants over the past decade have only added to the power of these three formulas.

The N-Tense Formulas

The first formula was called **N-Tense**, and it was created as a natural remedy for solid tumors. It is a combination of graviola, mullaca, guacatonga, espinheira santa, bitter melon, vassourinha, mutamba, and cat's claw. When it moved to the retail line, the label only said: "N-TENSE combines the rainforest's most potent and powerful plants into one intensive formula" without any other indication of its uses.

The second formula was called **NTense-2** (now renamed by other manufacturers to N-Tense 2), and it was created as a natural remedy for blood cancers such as leukemias, lymphomas, and multiple myeloma. When it was moved to the retail product line, the label read "An intensive combination of mullaca and anamu with 6 other rainforest plants." Again, without ever saying what to take it for, it is a combination of mullaca, anamu, vassourinha, simarouba, picão preto, suma, cat's claw, and espinheira santa.

The third formula was called **N-Tense Topical**, which was created as a natural remedy for skin cancers (basal and squamous cell) and meant to be used topically on the skin. It is a combination of sangre de grado, copaiba, graviola, espinheira santa, suma, pau d'arco, mullaca, vassourinha, and mutamba.

Sourcing Products

Even though Raintree Nutrition is long gone, many of its effective natural remedies are still available to purchase from other manufacturers, including the three N-Tense products and many of the practitioner formulas (called *Amazon Support*). When I closed my company, I posted all of the formulas of my proprietary and practitioner products on the rain-tree.com website so any company could re-create them. And some did! See the "Resources" section (page 327) or do an internet search using the keywords *N-Tense Herbal Supplement* to find them.

If you want to make any of the N-Tense formulas yourself, just go to chapter 8 to find the recipes and instructions on how to do it. While it can save money over purchasing manufactured products, it does take more time to find, order, and receive the bulk plants. And then you'll need additional time to put them into capsules or prepare extracts with the combined plants.

Dosages

Dosages for N-Tense and NTense-2 are 2–3 grams, three times daily. The difference between 2 and 3 grams is based on your cancer stage or grade rather than body weight. If you are dealing with a stage 1 cancer, use 2 grams. If you have stage 2, 3, or 4, use 3 grams. If your cancer is considered low grade, use the 2-gram dosage, and if it's considered a high-grade cancer, use 3 grams. If you are dealing with a metastatic or a recurring cancer, always choose the higher 3-gram dosage.

The N-Tense formulas are offered by several manufacturers; some sell them in 700 mg capsules and some in 500 mg capsules. For 2 grams, you would take three 700 mg capsules or four 500 mg capsules. For 3 grams, you'd take four 700 mg capsules (even though it's a tad short at 2,800 mg), or six 500 mg capsules.

Adjusting dosages for animals is done by body weight. For dogs weighing 75 pounds and more, use 2 grams twice daily. For dogs weighing 45–74 pounds, use 1 gram twice daily. For animals under 45 pounds, use one 500 mg capsule twice daily. Veterinarians have used N-Tense in dogs with good results for osteosarcomas and melanomas and NTense-2 in dogs with mast cell tumors and lymphomas.

Maintenance Dosages

As you'll learn in chapters 7 and 8, the majority of cancers have a chance to recur after successful treatment/remission; some have a very high rate of recurrence. Special types of cells called *cancer stem cells* can hide from the immune system (as well as drug and/or traditional medicine treatments) because they are much slower growing than regular cancer cells (most cancer therapies target fast-growing cells) or they employ other unique defense mechanisms that only stem cells use. These stem cells can start dividing and multiplying to form a new tumor, months to even years later. For that reason, the original instructions, as well as the new instructions for these cancer remedies herein, recommend a maintenance dosage to help lower recurrence rates. Most of the extra remedies in the plans are to specifically target these types of cancer stem cells and other mechanisms regular cancer cells use to recur.

The length of time you need to take the remedies will vary based on the cancer type, stage at diagnosis, types of treatments employed, and how your body and your cancer respond to the remedies. The remedies listed in the cancer plans herein should be taken for as long as it takes to achieve remission or "disease stabilization" (see below). This is usually confirmed initially with a simple blood test if your type of cancer has standard tumor markers that can be tested. Then it is usually confirmed with imaging tests (CT scan, PET scan, MRI, etc.). Those cancer types without tumor markers usually rely solely on imaging tests. Most users of the formulas waited until they had taken the remedies for four months before checking on the status of their cancer by testing. It depends, however, on how they were feeling. If cancer symptoms were getting better or worse, some tested sooner or later based on how they were feeling.

Remember, these remedies won't work for everyone. Unfortunately, sometimes they don't work at all. Taking them for at least four months will give you a good idea if they'll work or not. As you'll read in the following cancer plans, I've tried to provide information on what my personal experiences are to help with expectations. You'll see that in some particular types of cancer, patients responded, but it was with an anti-proliferative response (meaning the tumors just stopped growing and didn't metastasize, but they didn't disappear) instead of a full remission response. Once they've stopped growing for usually six months or longer, it is usually called "disease stabilization." Most of these responses required the patient to keep taking the remedies long term to stay stabilized, and when they discontinued the remedies, the tumor would begin growing again.

Once you've confirmed you're in remission, the cancer plan will instruct you to take the remedies for one or two months more. Take them at the same dosages to help clean up any microscopic cells or hidden stem cells that may be hanging around that may take longer to find and kill. Some types of cancers have much higher recurrence rates (or employ multiple mechanisms to recur) and you'll take the remedies for two more months; those with lower recurrence rates will take them for one more month. You'll find this information in the cancer plans in the next chapter.

Then the maintenance dosage schedule begins: After the one- or two-month cleanup period, discontinue the use of the remedies for three months. Begin taking the remedies again at the same original dosage for 30 days; then discontinue use again for three months. You will repeat this schedule two more times. So the schedule, after your cleanup period of one or two months, is this: three months off the remedies; one month on the remedies;

three months off; one month on; three months off; one month on. Most were done at this point. Some practitioners, however, recommended to patients with metastatic cancers, and cancers with very high recurrence rates (brain, lung, pancreatic, ovarian, etc.), to take the remedies for 30 days, twice annually thereafter and long term.

Possible Contraindications and Side Effects Using N-Tense
Contraindications:

- This formula is not to be used during pregnancy or while breastfeeding.
- Several ingredients in this formula have demonstrated hypotensive, vasodilator, and cardiac depressant activities in animal studies. People with low blood pressure should monitor their blood pressure for this possible effect.

Drug Interactions: Although not confirmed in humans, this product may enhance or increase the effect of high blood pressure drugs.

Other Practitioner Observations:

- Several ingredients in this formula have demonstrated significant *in vitro* antimicrobial properties. Supplementing the diet with probiotic supplements (or regularly consuming live-cultured yogurt) is advisable when this product is used for longer than 30 days.
- Taking CoQ10 and other supplements that increase cellular ATP might reduce the effects of N-Tense.

Possible Contraindications and Side Effects Using NTense-2
Contraindications:

- This formula is not to be used during pregnancy or while breastfeeding.
- Several plants in this formula have demonstrated immunostimulant effects; therefore, this formula is contraindicated before or following any organ or bone marrow transplant or skin graft.

Drug Interactions: None reported.

Possible Contraindications and Side Effects Using N-Tense Topical

Because this product was not taken orally but, rather, applied topically, there were never any contraindications or drug interactions. There is a warning that the product will stain the skin temporarily and other surfaces (like clothing, countertops, and flooring) permanently a reddish brown color. This was mostly due to the blood-red sangre de drago resin in the formula. If you unintentionally spill any of it, clean it up immediately with a heavy-duty cleanser (preferably containing bleach) to avoid permanent stains.

Combining with Conventional Therapies

Raintree's practitioners who used the remedy-specific product line were MDs with integrative practices (combining conventional medicine and alternative medicine), naturopathic doctors and naturopaths, DOs (doctors of osteopathic medicine), chiropractors, and others. From the first day the N-Tense formulas were made available, they were used in conjunction with both radiation and chemotherapy by the practitioners. Over the years, the N-Tense formulas were combined with just about every standard first-line chemotherapy drug on the market. In my personal knowledge, it was even used with some experimental drugs in clinical trials.

There were no serious complications, contraindications, side effects, or drug reactions reported by the practitioners who were using these formulas in combination with radiation and chemotherapy. In fact, many reported that there were fewer standard chemotherapy side effects noted. There was one issue, however, that was reported in about 25% of users. When the N-Tense formula was used in combination with chemotherapy drugs, it increased the amount of dead cancer cells the body needed to clean up and eliminate. In some instances, the lymphatic system got sluggish with all the dead and dying cancer cells. Many of the alternative practitioners recommended their patients stay well hydrated and increase water intake as well as prepare a Lemon Lymph Flush drink (see recipe on page 330) to help stimulate lymphatic flow. This seemed to be effective for the majority and became a part of the protocols used.

Supporting Immune Function

Cancer has evolved over the years, learning new defense mechanisms to survive. One of these mechanisms was learning how to hide from the immune system and immune cells that were meant to monitor foreign harmful cells and eliminate them. Now there are more than a dozen ways that cancer can choose to escape detection or change immune cells to evade them. Some of the most promising new cancer drugs are those called *immunotherapies*, which were designed to counteract some of these mechanisms.

Our natural remedy protocol usually recommended taking a single plant or multi-plant formula to support and increase immune function. This was always true when the patient was using immunosuppressive chemotherapy drugs. The single plant used was cat's claw (page 217), and the multi-plant formula used was called Amazon Immune Support. See the "Resources" section (page 327) for more information on this formula. To learn more, see the information in Part 3 (page 217) on how cat's claw was turned into an adjunctive herbal drug for cancer patients more than 20 years ago to keep the immune system intact while taking chemotherapy drugs.

While cat's claw is important, as with natural remedies, a multi-plant formula usually works better than single plants, especially when there are multiple targets and pathways that need to be addressed. I still recommend the Immune Support formula, and it is usually available from the manufacturers that currently offer the N-Tense formulas.

Dietary and Lifestyle Choices

So, let's face it—if we ended up with cancer, for the most part, our bodies weren't doing the job they were supposed to do, to keep us healthy. Maybe our built-in antioxidant system was overwhelmed by our bad dietary choices, and the resulting chronic oxidative stress was the catalyst that caused the cancer to form. Maybe our lifestyle choices like smoking, drinking too much, or living a sedentary lifestyle helped it along or impaired our built-in immune systems designed to protect us (and kill cancer cells as they are formed). Whatever it was, now is the time to fix it, if you want to survive.

It doesn't make much sense to try and fight cancer with natural remedies like those in this book if our bodies are still continuously producing more cancer cells based on all these detrimental dietary and lifestyle choices. So, if you smoke, stop. Yes, it's hard. Do it anyway. Your life depends on it now. Buy a good book on cancer diets and read it. You'll probably figure out pretty quickly what went wrong with your dietary choices, and how to fix it now. Yes, changing dietary habits is really hard. But it's really important to do it, if you want to survive. Think of it as your "wake-up call." Cancer has changed your life. Now it's time for *you* to change your life to fight it. These choices are now life and death choices.

In the meantime, remember, fresh fruits and vegetables are full of beneficial anti-cancer polyphenols that will help you fight cancer. Highly processed foods and fast foods with tons of human-made chemicals promote chronic oxidative damage linked to healthy cells mutating into cancerous cells. Sugar in the diet is one of the main ingredients cancer cells need to make more energy to fuel their rapid growth. Reducing or eliminating sugar in your diet has the potential to slow down or stop the growth of your cancer. You can do this. I've been there and know it's hard. You just need to choose to do it, then make those same choices daily. Take it day by day.

Summary

It's quite remarkable how much we've learned in the last 20 years about cancer—how it works on a genetic and molecular level to promote its growth and survival. If the drug approval process wasn't so long, arduous, and expensive, I'm sure we'd have many more new cancer drugs available today—effective drugs that are much less toxic with much fewer toxic side effects. While new drugs may be many years off, these rainforest plants, where the original novel molecules came from, are available now. It also proves a point I've known for many years—nature is a much better chemist than humankind who can only hope to copy it. Using the whole plant that nature provides gives us the multiple chemicals necessary to address the many chemical targets it uses to survive.

As I organized all the research on the plants in each of the cancer formulas I used, it gave me a much better understanding of why my original formulas were so effective and why it worked on so many different types of cancer. Every plant has multiple actions against multiple cancers. The average number of actions is 23 different mechanisms of action. Not only that, but every single plant also addresses multiple defense and/or recurrence mechanisms that multiple cancer types use. So while we didn't know yet about all these underlying molecular targets and how these plants were fighting cancer on a molecular level 20-plus years ago, the combinations of plants for these formulas had what they needed for the majority of cancers.

For example, cancer stem cells survive many types of chemotherapy drugs and are a leading cause of why cancer recurs after treatment. One of the main ways to kill cancer stem cells is to disrupt their mitochondrial function/metabolism. Graviola alone can disrupt mitochondrial function in four different ways, and the other seven ingredients in N-Tense provide five other ways to disrupt it. Twenty-five years ago, when I first developed N-Tense, we didn't know much about cancer stem cells, but its ability to avoid recurrences in many cancers was probably due to these mitochondrial-disrupting ingredients and active chemicals.

Just as important, I was able to learn which mechanisms each cancer was using that the plant ingredients did not affect. This also helped explain why the products worked much better on some types of cancers than others. That made it much easier to add those plants with those actions needed to these new cancer plans you'll find in the next chapter. These additional plants can affect any missing defense and recurrence mechanisms to achieve better results. I am even more excited to share this new and important information in the cancer plans, which you'll find by turning the page.

7

CANCER PLANS BY CANCER TYPE

This chapter describes cancer protocols that I have used for many years, which have now been updated to include all the new information and research on how these rainforest plants are working on a molecular level. It can be complicated because each type of cancer can employ different ways to turn on or off particular genes. These changes can affect particular chemicals in the genes' signaling pathways and other complicated molecular changes within the cancer cell to create defense mechanisms and recurrence strategies for it to thrive and survive. In addition, each plant can affect different molecules and pathways based on what type of cancer one has.

For that reason, the information in this chapter is organized by cancer type and provides a "cancer plan" specifically for each type of cancer. The types of cancer included are bladder, bone, brain, breast, cervical, colorectal, endometrial, esophageal, gastric, kidney, laryngeal, leukemia, liver, lung, lymphoma, melanoma, multiple myeloma, nasopharyngeal, ovarian, pancreatic, prostate, skin, testicular, and thyroid.

For each cancer plan, you will find a short description of the cancer, including survival rates and recurrence rates using conventional cancer therapies. Regarding survival rates, the phrase "the five-year survival rate is 51%," for example, means that, at the end of five years, 51% (or 51 people out of 100) will still be alive. Following that are the natural remedies I have used for that particular cancer, and new remedies recommended based on new research, and why. Finally, you will be provided with dosage information and instructions on how to take them.

These plans start with one of the N-Tense formulas. Side effects and contraindications for these products are shown in chapter 6 (see page 84). Please refer to the plant detail information in Part 3 (see page 192) for other possible side effects and contraindications on each of the plants added to the plan.

THE CANCER PLANS

BLADDER/KIDNEY CANCER

Bladder cancer occurs when abnormal cells grow uncontrollably in the bladder lining. It is the seventh most diagnosed cancer in the United States and the third most common in men. Most bladder cancers are called urothelial carcinomas or transitional cell carcinomas. Cancers confined to the inner lining of the bladder are called "superficial" or "stage 1" and comprise 70–80% of all bladder cancers diagnosed. Cancers that have spread into the bladder wall are called "deep" bladder cancers or "stage 2," and those that have spread to lymph nodes and/or distantly to the lungs, liver, or other organs are referred to as "metastatic" or "stage 3 or 4" depending on where the cancer spread. Common treatments include surgery, radiation therapy, chemotherapy, immunotherapy, and targeted therapy. In many cases, a combination of these treatments is used. The recurrence rate for this cancer is 6–10% for stages 1 and 2 (and 30–60% within five years for stages 3 and 4), depending on which treatments were used.

Kidney Cancer

Kidney cancer, also known as renal cancer, occurs when cells in the kidneys grow out of control, forming a tumor, and are staged much like bladder cancer. The most common type (90% of cases) is renal cell carcinoma (RCC), which starts in the lining of the kidney's tubules. It is treated much like bladder cancer. Transitional cell carcinoma (TCC) can develop in the renal pelvis or ureter; it is often treated like bladder cancer as well. Kidney cancer recurrence rates vary, but approximately 20–30% of patients with localized kidney cancer experience a recurrence after surgery (kidney removal). Most recurrences happen within the first five years after surgery, with a significant portion occurring within the first two years.

CANCER PLANS BY CANCER TYPE

Natural Remedies for Bladder and Kidney Cancer

N-Tense has a long history of being effectively used for these types of cancer by addressing the initial tumor(s), and quickly, especially stage 1 tumors. Several patients reported starting N-Tense shortly after the first diagnostic biopsy and the surgeon not finding any tumor to remove only 30–45 days later during surgery. A well-known defense mechanism is used by these cancers to escape detection from the immune system. Several chemicals in N-Tense disable this mechanism.

Adding chanca piedra and picão preto to the N-Tense capsules can help direct the plants specifically to the bladder and kidneys, reduce symptoms (bladder and kidney irritation, inflammation, pain, urinary urgency), and address three other defense mechanisms these cancers use to recur. Both plants have their own anti-cancer/antitumor actions as well. In addition, both plants may help reduce common side effects of chemotherapy drugs for those taking them. See the information on these two plants in Part 3 for more information on these defense mechanisms.

THE BLADDER AND KIDNEY CANCER PLAN

Dosage

N-Tense capsules: 2–3 g, three times daily, based on cancer stage/grade (see page 82).

Chanca piedra: 1 g in capsules or 2 ml of a glycerin liquid extract, three times daily.

Picão preto: 1 g in capsules or 2 ml of a tincture extract, three times daily.

Instructions

- Take all natural remedies together (for synergistic/additive effects), three times daily.
- They can be taken either with or between meals.
- When/if you achieve remission, continue taking the remedies for two months longer.
- Discontinue use for three months; then follow the instructions for the maintenance dosage and schedule provided on page 82.

BONE CANCERS/SARCOMAS

There are several different types of primary bone cancers including osteosarcoma (20–40%), Ewing sarcoma (10–15%), and chondrosarcoma (20–30%). Osteosarcoma begins in the cells that form bones, most often in the long bones of the legs and sometimes the arms. Osteosarcoma tends to happen most often in teenagers and young adults; however, it can occur at any age. Osteosarcoma can occur in soft tissue outside the bone, but it is rare. An osteosarcoma that has not responded to treatment or has returned after an initial response to treatment is considered recurrent. Recurrent osteosarcoma occurs in 30–50% of patients with initial localized disease and 80% of patients presenting with metastatic disease.

Ewing sarcoma is a type of bone cancer that begins in the bones and the soft tissue around the bones. It most often begins in the leg bones and in the pelvis, but it can happen in any bone. This cancer occurs mostly in children and young adults, although it can happen at any age. Approximately 30–40% of patients with non-metastatic Ewing sarcoma will experience a recurrence after achieving remission. The recurrence can be either local (at the original tumor site) or metastatic (spreading to other parts of the body). Most recurrences happen within the first two years after diagnosis, but late relapses can occur. Patients with recurrence have a reported five-year survival rate of 13% with conventional standard therapies.

Chondrosarcoma is a type of bone cancer that usually begins in the bones, but it can sometimes occur in the soft tissue. Chondrosarcoma happens most often in the pelvis, hip, and shoulder. It occurs most often in middle-aged and older adults. Those with a low-grade chondrosarcoma tumor have an 83% five-year survival rate. Intermediate-grade (grade 2) drops to 53% and for high-grade (grade 3) tumors, the five-year survival rate is around 29%.

Chondrosarcoma recurrence rates vary based on factors like grade, location, and treatment but generally range from 15–58%. Lower-grade chondrosarcomas (grade 1 and 2) tend to have a lower recurrence rate compared to higher-grade tumors (grade 3 and 4).

Conventional treatment of these bone cancers typically involves a combination of surgery, chemotherapy, and radiation therapy.

Natural Remedies for Bone Cancer

N-Tense had quite a reputation for osteosarcomas with Raintree's practitioners, including veterinarians. Many types of large-breed dogs have a higher risk of developing osteosarcomas. When a handful of vets found that N-Tense could eliminate them in 30–60 days, word got out pretty quickly. It worked almost as quickly in people with osteosarcomas and chondrosarcomas. The natural remedy plan is to use N-Tense to fight the bone tumors, while also providing two mechanisms of action, which prevents drug resistance and reduces recurrences, and adding chanca piedra to the plan.

Five newer studies describe how two main active plant chemicals in chanca piedra have a direct toxic effect to osteosarcoma cancer cells as well as demonstrating it may prevent drug resistance and migration/metastasis. Adding chanca piedra to the plan may reduce rates of recurrence by combating defense mechanisms. See the plant information for chanca piedra (page 226) for more on these defense mechanisms.

THE BONE CANCER PLAN

Dosage

N-Tense: 2–3 g in capsules, three times daily, based on stage/grade (see page 82).

Chanca piedra: 1 g in capsules or 2 ml glycerin extract, three times daily.

Instructions

- Take both remedies together at the same time (for synergistic/additive effects), three times daily.
- They can be taken either with or between meals.
- When/if you achieve remission, take the remedies for two months longer.
- Discontinue use for three months; then follow the instructions for the maintenance dosage and schedule provided on page 82.

BRAIN CANCERS

There are more than 120 different types of brain tumors, lesions, and cysts, which are differentiated by where they occur and what kinds of cells that compose them. Brain tumors can be classified as either primary (originating in the brain) or secondary (metastatic, spreading from other parts of the body). Primary tumors are further categorized as glial (arising from glial cells like astrocytomas, oligodendrogliomas, and glioblastomas) or non-glial (like meningiomas, medulloblastomas, and pituitary adenomas). Metastatic tumors are cancerous growths that have spread to the brain from other areas of the body, most commonly lung, breast, or melanoma.

The most common type of malignant brain tumors are glioblastomas and medulloblastomas. Glioblastomas are the most common and aggressive type of glioma in adults, characterized by rapid growth and poor prognosis. This type of brain tumor is currently not curable using conventional therapy, even if caught early. While treatment can extend life and improve quality of life, glioblastoma is known for its rapid growth and recurrence, making it difficult to eradicate completely. The standard treatment involves surgery, radiation, and chemotherapy, but these are typically not curative. While not a cure, advancements in treatment have led to improved survival rates, with some patients living longer than the average 15–18 months after diagnosis. Glioblastomas almost always recur (90%), even after initial treatment, usually within 6–12 months after initial treatment.

Medulloblastoma is a type of cancerous brain tumor that originates in the cerebellum, the part of the brain responsible for balance and coordination. It is the most common malignant brain tumor in children, though it can also occur in adults. Medulloblastomas can spread to other parts of the brain and spinal cord but rarely metastasize outside the central nervous system. Survival rates for medulloblastoma have improved significantly over the past 20 years. While the tumor is considered high grade and can spread, many children are cured with current treatment approaches. Medulloblastoma can come back after treatment, however. It can recur in up to 30% of children. Recurrent medulloblastoma is often difficult to treat and can significantly reduce survival rates.

Natural Remedies for Brain Cancers

N-Tense has a long history of use as a natural remedy for glioblastomas; however, I am unaware of any person who was actually cured. While most plant chemicals are considered small molecules, most are not small enough to pass the blood-brain barrier to get to a tumor in the brain to have a positive effect. About 30–40% of users experienced a stabilization of their tumors (they stopped growing), and some reduced in size, but none disappeared completely. It widely varied how long this stabilization lasted. In two people I worked with personally in Austin, Texas, they achieved stable disease for quite a few years (6 years and 10 years). They were still taking the formula when I moved from Austin to Nevada, and I lost touch with them about a year later. These two ladies, however, were very committed to making the dietary and lifestyle changes that contributed to their cancers and were no longer creating higher risks of making more cells to mutate into cancerous cells. These two were the exception, however. In more than half the people with glioblastoma, the N-Tense had no appreciable effect. To my knowledge, N-Tense wasn't used in children with medulloblastomas due to their inability to swallow capsules and the objectionable taste of extracts. It is rare in adults, but one practitioner did report disease stabilization in one patient.

Simarouba has been used for brain tumors, and several studies confirm that it has anti-cancer actions against four different types of brain cancer. See the plant information on simarouba (page 304) for more.

The Brain Cancer Plan

Dosage

N-Tense capsules: 2–3 g in capsules, three times daily, based on stage/grade (see page 82).

Simarouba: 1.5 g in capsules or 3 ml tincture (very bitter taste), three times daily.

Instructions

- Take both remedies together at the same time (for synergistic/additive effects), three times daily.
- They can be taken either with or between meals.
- When/if you achieve remission, take the remedies for two months longer.
- Discontinue use for three months; then follow the instructions for the maintenance dosage and schedule provided on page 82.

BREAST CANCER (HORMONE-POSITIVE)

Hormone receptor-positive (HR+) breast cancer is a type of breast cancer where the cancer cells have receptors that interact with hormones like estrogen and progesterone. These hormones essentially fuel the growth of the cancer cells, causing them to divide and the tumor to enlarge. HR+ breast cancer can have receptors for estrogen (ER+), progesterone (PR+), or both (ER/PR+). Treatment often involves surgery as well as hormone therapy, which works to block the effects of these hormones, slowing or stopping the growth of the cancer. HR+ breast cancer is the most common form, making up about 70% of all breast cancer cases. It tends to grow more slowly than hormone receptor-negative cancers. The five-year survival rate for hormone receptor-positive breast cancer is generally very high, often exceeding 90%. Although HR+ cancers often have a favorable short-term prognosis, there is still a risk of recurrence that may persist for many years.

Recurrence rates largely depend on tumor size, stage, and whether lymph nodes were involved at the time of diagnosis. Generally, if caught at an early stage and without lymph node involvement, the recurrence rate is only 6%. If the cancer had spread to nearby lymph nodes, recurrence increased to 25%; however, when radiation was used to treat it, the recurrence rate dropped back to 6%.

Natural Remedies for Hormone-Positive Breast Cancer

N-Tense has been used for more than 20 years with good results as a natural remedy for breast cancer. The protocols always added extra cat's claw to the N-Tense for hormone-positive cancers. One study compared the actions of cat's claw to Tamoxifen (a drug used for estrogen positive cancers to block estrogen receptors) and reported that cat's claw provided similar results.

If your cancer has BRCA mutations, newer research indicates adding pau d'arco would be beneficial. Only buy a product that extracts pau d'arco in alcohol (a tincture), however. The beneficial chemicals needed are not water soluble. See the plant information in Part 3 (page 284) for more.

The Hormone-Positive Breast Cancer Plan
Dosage

N-Tense: 2–3 g in capsules, three times daily, based on stage/grade (see page 82).

Cat's claw: 1.5 g in capsules, three times daily.

If necessary for BRCA mutations add:

Pau d'arco alcohol tincture: 2 ml, three times daily.

Instructions

• Take the remedies together at the same time (for synergistic/additive effects), three times daily.

• They can be taken either with or between meals.

• When/if you achieve remission, take the remedies for two months longer.

• Discontinue use for three months; then follow the instructions for the maintenance dosage and schedule provided on page 82.

BREAST CANCER (HORMONE-NEGATIVE)

Hormone receptor-negative breast cancer means the cancer cells do not have receptors for estrogen and progesterone, meaning they do not respond to hormone therapy. It is important to note that about 25–30% of breast cancers are hormone receptor-negative. Other treatments like surgery, radiation therapy, and chemotherapy are used to treat hormone receptor-negative breast cancer. Hormone-negative cancers tend to grow and spread more quickly than hormone receptor-positive cancers and tend to have a less favorable prognosis.

The five-year survival rate for localized disease is 91%. If the cancer has spread to nearby lymph nodes (regional), the rate drops to 66%. If the cancer has metastasized to distant parts of the body, the rate is only 12%. Approximately 50% of patients with earlier-stage hormone-negative cancer (stages 1–3) experience a recurrence after standard treatment, often within the first two to three years after diagnosis.

Natural Remedies for Hormone-Negative Breast Cancer

N-Tense has been used for more than 20 years with good results as a natural remedy for breast cancer. Based on newer research adding chanca piedra to target and kill cancer stem cells and primary breast cancer cells may be beneficial. For triple negative breast cancer, which grows and spreads much faster, a more aggressive approach is advised. For this type of cancer, adding anamu and a concentrated bitter melon fruit extract to the plan is beneficial. Additionally, if your cancer has BRCA mutations, newer research indicates adding pau d'arco would be beneficial. Only buy a product that extracts pau d'arco in alcohol (a tincture), however. The beneficial chemicals needed are not water soluble and need extracting in alcohol. There are numerous bitter melon concentrated fruit extracts in capsules available to choose from. See the plant information in Part 3 (page 207) for more.

THE HORMONE-NEGATIVE BREAST CANCER PLAN

Dosage

N-Tense: 2–3 g in capsules, three times daily, based on stage/grade (see page 82).

Chanca piedra: 1 g in capsules, three times daily.

For Triple Negative cancers add:

Anamu: 1.5 g in capsules, three times daily.

Bitter melon concentrated fruit extract in capsules: 1 g, three times daily, or follow labeled dosages.

If necessary for BRCA mutations add:

Pau d'arco tincture: 2 ml, three times daily.

Instructions

- Take all remedies together at the same time (for synergistic/additive effects), three times daily.
- They can be taken either with or between meals.
- When/if you achieve remission, take the remedies for two months longer.
- Discontinue use for three months; then follow the instructions for the maintenance dosage and schedule provided on page 82.

BREAST CANCER (HER2-POSITIVE)

About one in five women with breast cancer has a type called HER2-positive and can include both hormone positive and negative cancer types. HER2 stands for human epidermal growth factor receptor 2. This means that the cancer cells have a gene that makes HER2 protein. This protein causes cancer cells to grow and spread quickly. HER2+ cancers are usually considered more aggressive (they grow more quickly) and more invasive (they spread to other sites more easily). Treatments for HER2-positive breast cancer target the cells that make the protein. This helps slow the cancer's growth and stop it from spreading. Recurrence rates vary depending on factors like tumor stage and treatment but generally range from 15% to 30% within 10 years after treatment.

Natural Remedies for HER2-Positive Breast Cancer

N-Tense has been used for more than 20 years with good results as a natural remedy for breast cancer. Based on newer research adding anamu and picão preto to the plan will help address HER2-positive cancers. Both plants have a direct toxic action as well as address stem cells and defense mechanisms of HER2-positive breast cancer.

Additionally, if your cancer has BRCA mutations, newer research indicates adding pau d'arco would be beneficial. Only buy a product that extracts pau d'arco in alcohol (a tincture), however. The beneficial chemicals needed are not water soluble and need extracting in alcohol. See the plant information in Part 3 (page 284) for more on these defense mechanisms.

THE HER2-POSITIVE BREAST CANCER PLAN

Dosage

N-Tense: 2–3 g in capsules, three times daily, based on stage/grade (see page 82).

Anamu: 1.5 g in capsules, three times daily.

Picão preto: 1.5 g in capsules, three times daily.

If necessary for BRCA mutations add:

Pau d'arco tincture: 2 ml, three times daily.

Instructions

- Take all remedies together at the same time (for synergistic/additive effects), three times daily.
- They can be taken either with or between meals.
- When/if you achieve remission, take the remedies for two months longer.
- Discontinue use for three months; then follow the instructions for the maintenance dosage and schedule provided on page 82.

CERVICAL CANCER

Cervical cancer is a type of cancer that develops in the cervix, the lower part of the uterus that connects to the vagina. It is usually caused by persistent infection with human papillomavirus (HPV). Early stages may have no noticeable symptoms, which is why routine cervical cancer screening (Pap and/or HPV tests), are recommended for all sexually active women. Cervical cancer is highly treatable in its early stages but gets more difficult in higher stages since it can spread to other sites in the body. Treatment options depend on the cancer stage and type and may include surgery, radiation therapy, chemotherapy, targeted therapy, and immunotherapy.

For early-stage (localized) cervical cancer, the five-year relative survival rate is around 91%. If the cancer has spread to nearby tissues or lymph nodes, the rate is about 60%. If the cancer has spread to distant parts of the body, the rate is approximately 19%. Recurrence rates for stage 1 and 2 cancers are 11–22%, while more advanced stages (stages 3 and 4) have a higher recurrence rate of 28–64%.

Natural Remedies for Cervical Cancer

N-Tense has long been used for cervical cancer. If caught at an early stage, all that is needed is just N-Tense capsules. Research indicates that many of the N-Tense ingredients address cervical cancer's defense mechanisms and have a direct anti-cancer action. For late stage or recurrent cervical cancer, add pau d'arco and picão preto. Only use an alcohol tincture of pau d'arco as the beneficial plant chemicals are not water soluble and require extraction in alcohol.

The Cervical Cancer Plan

Dosage

N-Tense capsules: 2–3 g in capsules, three times daily, based on stage/grade (see page 82).

If necessary (for late stage) add:

Picão preto: 1 g (two 500 mg capsules) or 2 ml tincture, three times daily.

Pau d'arco tincture: 2 ml extract, three times daily.

Instructions

- Take all remedies together at the same time (for synergistic/additive effects), three times daily.
- They can be taken either with or between meals.
- When/if you achieve remission, take the remedies for one month longer.
- Discontinue use for three months; then follow the instructions for the maintenance dosage and schedule provided on page 82.

COLORECTAL CANCER

Colorectal cancer (also known as colon cancer or rectal cancer) is a cancer that starts in the large intestine (colon) or rectum. It is primarily an adenocarcinoma, a cancer of the mucus-secreting cells lining the colon and rectum (although other rarer types exist). It often develops from pre-cancerous polyps, which are abnormal growths in the colon or rectum. Colorectal cancer is one of the most common cancers and is the third leading cause of cancer death in both men and women in the United States. It mostly occurs in people who are 45 years and older.

Early detection through screening is crucial, as it can often be treated more effectively when found early. Currently, only one in three cases are diagnosed at stage 1 or 2. A total of 35–50% of patients present with distant metastasis at diagnosis, and this confers a five-year survival rate of less than 10%. The age you should start screening really depends on your risk factors. Risk factors include age, family history, and inflammatory bowel disease;

lifestyle factors like diet, obesity, smoking, and lack of physical activity; and inherited genetic disorders.

The overall five-year survival rate for colorectal cancer is around 65%. This rate varies significantly, however, depending on the stage of the cancer at diagnosis. Early-stage (stage 1) colorectal cancer has a very high five-year survival rate, often exceeding 90%, while late-stage (stage 4) cancer has a much lower rate, around 10–17%.

Colorectal cancer recurrence rates vary based on several factors, including cancer stage, but generally, around 20–30% of patients experience recurrence within five years of initial treatment, with most happening within the first two years. The longer you go without a recurrence, the lower your chances are of having the cancer return. This is why follow-up screening for the first two years is very important.

Natural Remedies for Colorectal Cancer

N-Tense capsules have had good results with colorectal cancer (CRC) in all stages. It was often combined with another Raintree formula called Amazon Bowel Support, especially if the patient was doing conventional chemotherapy/radiation and/or had stage 3 or 4 CRC. (See page 330 for more information about this product.) Some of the plants in this formula have direct anti-cancer actions against CRC. Others protect against chemo and radiation side effects, and some have immune system benefits while mitigating CRC defense mechanisms.

THE COLORECTAL CANCER PLAN

Dosage

N-Tense capsules: 2–3 g in capsules, three times daily, based on stage/grade (see page 82).

If necessary (for late stage) add:

Amazon Bowel Support: 1.5 g in capsules, three times daily. (See page 330 for more information about this product.)

Instructions

- Take both remedies together (if using Bowel Support) at the same time (for synergistic/additive effects), three times daily.

- They can be taken either with or between meals.
- When/if you achieve remission, take the remedies for one month longer.
- Discontinue use for three months; then follow the instructions for the maintenance dosage and schedule provided on page 82.

ENDOMETRIAL CANCER

Endometrial cancer is a type of cancer that develops in the lining of the uterus (the endometrium). It is the most common type of gynecologic cancer in women and is also referred to as uterine cancer. The average age at diagnosis for endometrial cancer is 60; it is rare among those younger than 45. It is the fourth most common cancer among women in the United States and the sixth leading cause of cancer-related deaths among women. Approximately 70% of women are diagnosed at stage 1, when the cancer is easiest to treat. Initially, it may spread to nearby organs like the ovaries, fallopian tubes, or cervix (stage 3). It can also spread through lymphatic or blood vessels to distant organs such as the lungs, liver, bones, and brain (stage 4). The lungs are the most common site for distant spread.

Survival rates vary, but overall, the five-year survival rate is high, especially for early-stage localized disease (95%). In stage 2 and 3 where the cancer has spread in the same region, rates drop to 70%. In later stages, when the cancer has spread to distant sites, the five-year survival rate drops to around 18%.

Approximately 15–20% of endometrial cancer patients experience a recurrence after initial treatment, with the majority occurring within the first two to three years. Factors like stage, grade, and lymph node involvement influence the risk of recurrence. Even when the uterus is surgically removed to treat the cancer, there is a chance of recurrence in other areas (most commonly found in the vagina and pelvis). Endometrial cancer can also recur in the ovaries, fallopian tubes, or cervix; this is why radical hysterectomies (which remove all these organs/tissues along with the uterus) are part of the standard level of care for most.

Natural Remedies for Endometrial Cancer

Most of the ingredients in N-Tense have some kind of research indicating that it is toxic to endometrial cancer. In addition, several of the plants in the formula address several main defense mechanisms this cancer uses to become drug resistant, and recur.

Anamu is also toxic to endometrial cancer and addresses another defense mechanism the cancer uses to hide from the immune system as well as recur. It relieves pain as well as reduces inflammation (which has anti-cancer benefits as well). See the plant information for anamu (page 198) for more on these defense mechanisms.

THE ENDOMETRIAL CANCER PLAN

Dosage

N-Tense capsules: 2–3 g in capsules, three times daily, based on stage/grade (see page 82).

Anamu: 1 g in capsules or 1 ml tincture, three times daily.

Instructions

- Take both remedies together at the same time (for synergistic/additive effects), three times daily.
- They can be taken either with or between meals.
- When/if you achieve remission, take the remedies for two months longer.
- Discontinue use for three months; then follow the instructions for the maintenance dosage and schedule provided on page 82.

ESOPHAGEAL CANCER

Esophageal cancer develops in the esophagus, the tube connecting the throat to the stomach. It is often diagnosed at later stages due to a lack of early symptoms, but early detection and treatment are crucial for a better prognosis. The two main types of esophageal cancer are squamous cell carcinoma and adenocarcinoma. Squamous cell carcinoma (the most prevalent type) develops in the flat, thin cells lining the esophagus, while adenocarcinoma arises in the glandular cells that produce mucus and other fluids.

Esophageal squamous cell carcinoma (ESCC) is an aggressive form of esophageal cancer that is often diagnosed only after the cancer has already spread. This means survival rates for ESCC are much lower than some other cancers. It ranks seventh in incidence and sixth in mortality among all malignancies worldwide. ESCC is primarily caused by tobacco use (including smokeless/vapes) and excessive alcohol consumption. Additionally, other factors like poor diets (low in fruits and vegetables, high in processed meats), drinking very hot beverages, some vitamin deficiencies (beta-carotene, vitamin E, selenium, or iron), and infection with human papillomavirus increase risks.

Esophageal adenocarcinoma (EA) is primarily linked to chronic irritation and changes in the esophageal lining, particularly in the lower esophagus. Key risk factors include gastroesophageal reflux disease (GERD), Barrett's esophagus, obesity, and tobacco use. It has a better prognosis, mainly because it is discovered sooner and at an earlier stage. Doctors usually regularly screen their GERD and Barrett's patients for this cancer and find it in early stages in highly developed countries like the United States.

When treated conventionally with concurrent chemotherapy and radiation, five-year survival rates for esophageal cancers are 48% for stage 1, 20–30% for stages 2 and 3, and 5% for stage 4. Roughly half of patients experience recurrence after treatment, with a significant proportion occurring within the first two years. Recurrences can be local (at the original tumor site), regional (in nearby lymph nodes), or distant (in other organs). Distant metastases are the most common type of recurrence, most commonly in the lungs, liver, and bones.

Natural Remedies for Esophageal Cancer

N-Tense capsules have been used for esophageal cancer for many years. It is one of the cancers that provided rather dramatic results—usually a noticeable and significant reduction in tumor size in as little as two weeks. Oftentimes, as with conventional therapy, many patients were in late stages and had large tumors that prevented swallowing much besides liquids when they started taking N-Tense.

The advice was (and is) to open the capsules and place the powder in a teacup and pour 6 ounces of boiling water into the cup. Cover and let soak until lukewarm (about 15 minutes), stirring once after about 5–7 minutes. Then drink slowly (even though it tastes dreadful). The ground plants will settle to the bottom of the cup so you can drink the tea off the top, or run through a strainer or coffee filter. Avoid drinking or eating for at least one hour afterward. Because the tea, full of anti-cancerous plant chemicals, is coming into direct contact with the cancer in the esophagus, the results are pretty rapid. Many switched over to swallowing the capsules after they were eating food again, but if you can tolerate the taste, it will be more effective and work faster taking it as a tea. Quite a few patients were cancer free in two to three months or less, but we did see some recurrences (including some who didn't change their diet/lifestyle to lower their risks).

With all the new research on defense mechanisms and cancer stem cells (which increase the risk of recurrences), we've learned that adding pau d'arco and picão preto to the cancer plan may help lower the risk of specific defense mechanisms this cancer employs and may help kill stem cells to help avoid recurrences. See the plant information in Part 3 (pages 284 and 294) for more information on the other plants in the plan. Pau d'arco requires alcohol to extract the active chemicals needed so only purchase a tincture (widely available). Adding it to the tea with the boiling water will evaporate off the alcohol content to avoid throat irritation. The picão preto is available to purchase as a powder or in capsules and can be added to the same teacup.

Adding a tea bag or teaspoon of loose green tea to the N-Tense tea may be beneficial. Green tea contains an abundance of a polyphenol chemical called EGCG. Compelling research reports that EGCG can prevent the self-renewal ability of esophageal squamous carcinoma stem cells and reduce recurrence rates. Adding a cup or glass of green tea as a beverage you drink daily as a lifestyle change may be very beneficial as well; just avoid really hot beverages in general and let them cool to lukewarm or drink them iced.

The Esophageal Cancer Plan

Dosage

N-Tense capsules: 3 g in capsules, three times daily (see page 81). Open capsules and prepare into a tea as described earlier.

Pau d'arco tincture: 2 ml, three times daily, and added to the N-Tense tea while still hot.

Picão preto: 1 g in powder or capsules (opened), three times daily, and added to the N-Tense tea while still hot.

Instructions

- Drink the tea 3 times daily with or between meals.
- When/if you achieve remission, take the remedy twice daily for three months longer.
- Discontinue use for three months; then follow the instructions for the maintenance dosage and schedule provided on page 82.

GASTRIC CANCER

Gastric cancer, also known as stomach cancer, develops in the stomach lining. There are several types with adenocarcinoma being the most common type (accounting for 90–95% of all stomach cancers), arising from the stomach's glandular cells that line the stomach. While it can occur in anyone, certain factors like age, gender, and lifestyle choices can increase the risk. Other types of gastric cancer include gastrointestinal stromal tumors (GISTs), neuroendocrine tumors (including carcinoid tumors), and lymphomas. These cancers are classified based on the type of cells where the cancer originates and are considered rare.

Overall, gastric cancer incidence rates have decreased over time in the United States and are much lower in highly developed nations like the United States. This is probably due to our regularly and effectively treating one of the main causes of gastric cancer before it causes cancer: *H. pylori* bacterial infections (also one of the leading causes of gastric ulcers).

For localized stomach cancer, the five-year survival rate is approximately 71%, while for regional cancer it drops to 33%, and for distant (metastatic) cancer, it is around 6%. Gastric cancer recurrence rates vary widely, ranging from 14–60%, with higher tumor stages (3 and 4) associated with higher recurrence rates.

Natural Remedies for Gastric Cancer

N-Tense has long been used for gastric cancer; however, the number of patients were much lower than other types of cancer. We seem to be doing a pretty good job here in the United States either preventing it or catching this cancer early. The average time it took for those taking N-Tense was two months. Again, like esophageal cancer, if you can get all the anti-cancer chemicals from the N-Tense ingredients in direct contact with the cancer cells in the stomach, the efficacy and speed increases.

Based on more recent research, adding anamu and picão preto to the plan might address all of the defense mechanisms this cancer uses to recur. Both plants also have shown to have direct toxic actions to gastric cancer cells. See the plant information in Part 3 (pages 198 and 294) for more on these defense mechanisms. It is recommended to add these two plants if the cancer has already spread to the local lymph nodes and beyond (stage 2, 3, or 4).

The Gastric Cancer Plan

Dosage

N-Tense capsules: 2–3 g in capsules, three times daily, based on stage/grade (see page 82).

Anamu: 1 g in capsules, three times daily, or 2 ml of a tincture, three times daily.

Picão preto: 1.5 g in capsules or 3 ml of a tincture, three times daily.

Instructions

- Take all remedies together at the same time (for synergistic/additive effects), three times daily.
- They can be taken either with or between meals.
- When/if you achieve remission, take the remedies for two months longer.
- Discontinue use for three months; then follow the instructions for the maintenance dosage and schedule provided on page 82.

KIDNEY/RENAL CANCER—see BLADDER CANCER

LARYNGEAL AND NASOPHARYNGEAL CANCERS

Laryngeal cancer, also known as larynx cancer, is a type of cancer that develops in the tissues of the larynx (voice box). It is a type of head and neck cancer and is more common in men over 60. The larynx plays a vital role in breathing, speaking, and swallowing. The primary type of laryngeal cancer is squamous cell carcinoma, which originates in the thin, flat cells lining the larynx (voice box). Rarer types include adenocarcinoma (originating in mucus-producing cells), sarcomas (cancers of connective tissues), and lymphomas (cancers of lymphatic tissue). The overall five-year survival rate for laryngeal cancer is approximately 77% and 84%, respectively, for stages 1 and 2 and dropping to 46% and 30%, respectively, for stages 3 and 4. Recurrence rates for stage 1 cancers are 5–13%, 25–30% for stage 2, 30% for stage 3, and 50% for stage 4. Different treatment modalities (surgery, radiation, chemotherapy) can affect recurrence rates.

Nasopharyngeal cancer is a less common cancer that develops in the nasopharynx, the upper part of the throat behind the nose. It is more common in certain parts of the world, particularly Southeast Asia. Risk factors include Epstein-Barr virus (EBV) infection and genetic predisposition. It is also known as nasopharyngeal carcinoma (NPC) and has three subtypes (types 1, 2, and 3). It originates from the epithelial cells lining the nasopharynx and is classified as a squamous cell cancer, like laryngeal cancer, and treated in a similar fashion. The overall five-year survival rate for nasopharyngeal cancer is approximately 82% for stage 1 and dropping to 48% at stage 4. The recurrence rate for NPC after initial treatment, which usually involves radiotherapy with or without chemotherapy, ranges from 15–58% depending on the stage at diagnosis and lifestyle/dietary habits.

Natural Remedies for Laryngeal and Nasopharyngeal Cancers

Laryngeal and nasopharyngeal cancers always had a very good response rate to N-Tense. For laryngeal cancer, it was generally recommended to brew a tea with the N-Tense capsules (see instructions on page 140) so that the active chemicals in the formula could come into direct contact with the cancer to provide results more quickly. Nasopharyngeal cancer patients can just use the capsules to take by mouth.

With all the new research on defense mechanisms and cancer stem cells, which we now know increase the risk of recurrences, we've learned that adding pau d'arco and picão preto to the cancer plan may help lower the risk of specific defense mechanisms this cancer employs and may help kill cancer stem cells to help avoid recurrences. See the plant information in Part 3 (pages 284 and 294) for more on these defense mechanisms. Pau d'arco needs alcohol to extract the active chemicals needed so only purchase a tincture (widely available). If you're brewing a tea, put the tincture in the cup with the other plant powders before pouring in the boiling water to help evaporate off the alcohol in the tincture. Picão preto can be purchased in tinctures, capsules, and powder and can also be added directly into the teacup with the other products (opening the capsules) in the same manner.

The Laryngeal and Nasopharyngeal Cancer Plan
Dosage

N-Tense capsules: 2–3 g in capsules, three times daily, based on stage/grade (see page 82).

Pau d'arco tincture: 2 ml, three times daily.

Picão preto: 1 g in powder or capsules or 2 ml of a tincture, three times daily.

Instructions
- Take all remedies together at the same time (for synergistic/additive effects), three times daily.
- They can be taken either with or between meals.
- When/if you achieve remission, take the remedies for two months longer.
- Discontinue use for three months; then follow the instructions for the maintenance dosage and schedule provided on page 82.

LEUKEMIA

Leukemia is a type of cancer that affects the blood and bone marrow, where blood cells are produced. It's characterized by the uncontrolled production of abnormal white blood cells that don't function properly. These abnormal cells can crowd out healthy blood cells, leading to various complications. Leukemia is classified based on how quickly it progresses (acute or chronic) and the type of white blood cell affected (lymphoid or myeloid). Leukemia can affect both children and adults, with some types being more common in certain age groups. Acute lymphocytic leukemia (ALL) and acute myeloid leukemia (AML) are the acute types, while chronic lymphocytic leukemia (CLL) and chronic myeloid leukemia (CML) are the chronic types.

There are a few more rare types of leukemia, but we'll focus on the common types herein. The acute leukemias are more deadly because they grow more rapidly. The five-year survival rate for AML (most common in adults) is 31.9%, and the rate is 72% for ALL (most common in children). The five-year survival rate for CLL is 88.5% and 70% for CML. Leukemia recurrence rates vary significantly depending on the type of leukemia, with some forms having a higher likelihood of returning than others. For example, in ALL, relapse rates can be around 10–15% in children, while for adults, it can be closer to 50%. About 50% of AML patients will experience a relapse. While most leukemia relapses occur within the first few years, late relapses (several years after initial remission) can occur, though they are less common.

Natural Remedies for Leukemia

NTense-2 was created specifically with plant ingredients that had demonstrated anti-leukemic actions. It has been sold for approximately 24 years, becoming a natural herbal remedy for both leukemias and lymphomas. For the chronic leukemias (CLL and CML), generally all that was recommended was the NTense-2 capsules. With all the newer research on defense mechanisms and how this cancer can recur on a molecular level, I would add two other plants to the cancer plan for the acute leukemias (AML and ALL): graviola and chanca piedra. Between these two plants, stem cells can be targeted, and five defense mechanisms that leukemia uses to recur can be addressed. See Part 3 (pages 226 and 252) for more information on these two plants.

THE LEUKEMIA CANCER PLAN

Remedies for CLL and CML

NTense-2 capsules: 2–3 g in capsules, three times daily, based on stage/grade (see page 82).

Remedies for AML and ALL

NTense-2 capsules: 3 g in capsules, three times daily.

Chanca piedra: 1.5 g in capsules or 3 ml of a glycerin extract, three times daily.

Graviola: 1.5 g in capsules or 3 ml of a tincture, three times daily.

Instructions

• Take all remedies together at the same time (for synergistic/additive effects), three times daily.

• They can be taken either with or between meals.

• When/if you achieve remission, take the remedies for two months longer.

• Discontinue use for three months; then follow the instructions for the maintenance dosage and schedule provided on page 82.

LIVER CANCER

Liver cancer is a disease in which cancerous cells form in the tissues of the liver. It can be primary, meaning it originates in the liver, or secondary, meaning it has spread from another part of the body. The most common type of primary liver cancer is hepatocellular carcinoma (HCC), which develops in the main liver cells called hepatocytes. Risk factors for getting liver cancer include chronic Hepatitis B and C infections, cirrhosis (scarring of the liver, often caused by chronic hepatitis or excessive alcohol consumption), excessive alcohol consumption, aflatoxins, and nonalcoholic steatohepatitis, a type of fatty liver disease that can lead to cirrhosis.

Liver cancer is often diagnosed at a later stage because symptoms are typically absent in the early stages. This means that by the time symptoms appear, the cancer may have already progressed to an advanced stage. For localized liver cancer, meaning the cancer hasn't spread beyond the liver, the five-year survival rate is 31%. If the cancer has spread to nearby organs or lymph nodes, however, the rate drops to 13%, and if it has spread to distant parts of the body, the rate is only 3%.

The recurrence rate of liver cancer, specifically HCC, after surgery to remove the tumor is high, with estimates ranging from 50–70% at five years. Recurrence can happen early (within weeks or months) or late (up to 10 years) after treatment. Several factors influence the risk of recurrence, including tumor size, presence of microvascular invasion, and underlying liver conditions like cirrhosis.

Natural Remedies for Liver Cancer

N-Tense had some great results with liver cancer; however, it was almost always combined with another Raintree formula called Amazon Liver

Support. The second formula was especially important for patients with hepatitis infections and damage to the liver from cirrhosis and fatty liver as well as late-stage cancers. Several of the plant ingredients in Liver Support have toxic actions against liver cancer cells, while others have healing, repairing, and protective effects to the liver. (See page 330 for more information about these products.)

The Liver Cancer Plan
Dosage
N-Tense capsules: 2–3 g in capsules, three times daily, based on stage/grade (see page 82).

Amazon Liver Support: 1.5 g in capsules, three times daily. (See page 330 for more information about this product.)

Instructions
- Take both remedies together at the same time (for synergistic/additive effects), three times daily.
- They can be taken either with or between meals.
- When/if you achieve remission, take the remedies for two months longer.
- Discontinue use for three months; then follow the instructions for the maintenance dosage and schedule provided on page 82.

LUNG CANCER (SMALL CELL)

Small cell lung cancer (SCLC) represents between 13 and 15% of all new cases of lung cancers. It is a highly aggressive form of lung cancer that originates from neuroendocrine cells in the lungs and is considered a neuroendocrine tumor. A neuroendocrine tumor (NET) is a rare type of cancer that develops from neuroendocrine cells, which are cells that have characteristics of both nerve cells and hormone-producing cells. These cells and resulting tumors are found in various parts of the body, including in or on the outside of the lungs/bronchus. SCLC is known for its rapid growth and tendency to spread to other parts of the body easily. Luckily, SCLC readily responds to chemotherapy and/or radiation as well as plant-based therapies, oftentimes reducing or eliminating initial tumors rather quickly. The reason it has such a poor prognosis is because this cancer can regularly return a few months to a year later to form new tumors. These tumors are drug resistant and grow even more quickly. NET tumors have several different and highly effective defense mechanisms that allow them to hide from detection.

The estimated five-year overall survival rate is 42.9% with chemo/radiation followed by immunotherapy. The five-year survival rate for limited-stage small cell lung cancer (LS-SCLC) without it is typically around 25–30%. Unfortunately, approximately 70% of new SCLC diagnoses are extensive-stage (the cancer has already spread outside the lungs), which has a survival rate without treatment of 2–4 months and 7–11 months with standard chemo/radiation treatment. Immunotherapy has increased the five-year survival rate from 1–2% to around 12% in extensive late-stage SCLC.

Natural Remedies for Small Cell Lung Cancer

The natural remedy plan is to use the plants in the N-Tense formula to fight the tumor(s) (including previously treated and drug-resistant tumors) and to add plants that will target the specific mechanisms that this cancer uses to return and to become drug resistant. The graviola in the N-Tense formula can address one defense mechanism and one type of drug resistance, and adding more espinheira santa (already in N-Tense) can better address a third defense mechanism. Importantly, adding picão preto and pau d'arco can help the N-Tense ingredients target and/or kill cancer stem cells and another defensive molecule in two different ways (the fourth and strongest mechanism that enables the cancer to return). See the plant information in Part 3 (pages 284 and 294) for more on these defense mechanisms. Only purchase an alcohol tincture of pau d'arco as the active plant chemicals needed are not water soluble and must be extracted in alcohol.

THE SMALL CELL LUNG CANCER PLAN

Dosage

N-Tense Capsules: 3 g in capsules, three times daily.

Picão preto: 1.5 g in capsules or 3 ml of a tincture, three times daily.

Espinheira santa: 1 g in capsules, three times daily.

Pau d'arco tincture: 2 ml, three times daily.

CANCER PLANS BY CANCER TYPE

Instructions
- Take all remedies together at the same time (for synergistic/additive effects), three times daily.
- They can be taken either with or between meals.
- When/if you achieve remission, take the remedies for two months longer.
- Discontinue use for three months; then follow the instructions for the maintenance dosage and schedule provided on page 82.

LUNG CANCER (NON-SMALL CELL)

Non–small cell lung cancer (NSCLC) is a type of lung cancer that includes several subtypes, the most common being adenocarcinoma, squamous cell carcinoma, and large cell carcinoma. It is the most prevalent form of lung cancer, accounting for roughly 85% of cases. NSCLC is characterized by uncontrolled growth of epithelial cells in the lungs. NSCLC is categorized into three main subtypes: adenocarcinoma, squamous cell carcinoma, and large cell carcinoma. Smoking is the leading risk factor, but NSCLC can also occur in nonsmokers. Treatment options vary based on the stage and subtype of NSCLC, and it may include surgery, chemotherapy, radiation therapy, and targeted therapy. Advances in treatment, including targeted therapies and immunotherapies, have improved survival rates, especially for certain subtypes and stages of NSCLC. Adenocarcinomas have a better prognosis than squamous cell carcinomas.

Around 65% of patients with localized NSCLC (cancer confined to the lung) survive five years or longer. The survival rate decreases to about 37% for stages 2 and 3 and drops to 6% at stage 4. Early-stage NSCLC (stage 1) can have recurrence rates between 5% and 19% and between 11% and 27% for stage 2. Advanced stages may experience recurrence in 24–40% of cases in stage 3 and around 66% for stage 4.

Natural Remedies for Non–Small Cell Lung Cancer
N-Tense had a very good response to NSCLC and has been used for more than 20 years as a natural remedy for this cancer. Newer research indicates that adding anamu and chanca piedra to the plan might help reduce recurrences and address specific defense mechanisms that this cancer uses to become drug resistant, proliferate, and metastasize.

The Non–Small Cell Lung Cancer Plan

Dosage

N-Tense capsules: 2–3 g in capsules, three times daily, based on stage/grade (see page 82).

Anamu: 2 g in capsules or 2 ml of a tincture, three times daily.

Chanca piedra: 2 g in capsules or 2 ml of a glycerin extract, three times daily.

Instructions

- Take all remedies together at the same time (for synergistic/additive effects), three times daily.
- They can be taken either with or between meals.
- When/if you achieve remission, take the remedies for two months longer.
- Discontinue use for three months; then follow the instructions for the maintenance dosage and schedule provided on page 82.

LYMPHOMA

Lymphoma is a cancer that originates in the lymphatic system, a part of the body's immune system, and specifically affects lymphocytes, a type of white blood cell. It's characterized by the abnormal growth and multiplication of lymphocytes, which can lead to the formation of tumors in lymph nodes and other parts of the body. There are more than 20 different types of lymphoma with the two main types being Hodgkin lymphoma (HL) and non-Hodgkin lymphoma (NHL). In the United States, NHL is one of the most common cancers, accounting for about 4% of all cancers.

Aggressive lymphomas are fast-growing types of NHL that require prompt treatment. Common aggressive NHL subtypes include diffuse large B-cell lymphoma, Burkitt lymphoma, mantle cell lymphoma, peripheral T-cell lymphoma, and lymphoblastic lymphoma. B-cell lymphomas account for the vast majority (85%) of all NHL cases and are formed in a type of white blood cell called a B-cell.

The lymphatic system includes lymph nodes, lymphatic vessels, and other tissues that help fight infections. Lymphoma disrupts the normal function of this system. It is classified as a "hematological" or blood cancer. NHL is more common in men, individuals over 65, and those with autoimmune diseases or family history of blood cancers. HL often affects young adults (20–34 age group) and older adults (55+). HL is more common in males and individuals with a history of certain infections (like Epstein-Barr virus) or autoimmune diseases.

Lymphoma treatment varies based on the specific type and stage of the cancer, but common approaches include chemotherapy, radiation therapy, immunotherapy, targeted therapy, and stem cell transplantation (bone marrow transplant). For certain lymphomas, particularly early-stage or slow-growing types, watchful waiting or active surveillance may be appropriate. Treatment for lymphoma, particularly with chemotherapy and radiation, can increase the risk of developing a second cancer later in life (especially leukemia).

The five-year survival rate for HL is generally very high, often around 90%, while the five-year survival rate for NHL is around 74%. These are general statistics, however, and the actual survival rate can vary significantly based on several factors, including the specific type of lymphoma, the stage at diagnosis, the patient's age and overall health, and how well the lymphoma responds to treatment. HL has a recurrence rate of around 5% (early stage) to 30% (late stage). The recurrence rate of lymphoma also varies significantly based on several factors, including the specific type of lymphoma, the stage at diagnosis, and the type of initial treatment received.

Natural Remedies for Lymphoma

NTense-2 was designed specifically for blood cancers such as lymphomas and leukemias. It has long been used as a natural remedy for most of the common lymphomas for many years with good results. The plan then and now is to add graviola to this formula. Graviola has specific ways it can find the lymphoma cells and kill them; it also shuts down defense mechanisms that allow the cells to become drug resistant and metastasize.

THE LYMPHOMA CANCER PLAN

Dosage

NTense-2: 2–3 g in capsules, three times daily, based on stage/grade (see page 82).

Graviola: 1 g in capsules or 2 ml of a tincture, three times daily.

Instructions

- Take both remedies together at the same time (for synergistic/additive effects), three times daily.
- They can be taken either with or between meals.
- When/if you achieve remission, take the remedies for two months longer.
- Discontinue use for three months; then follow the instructions for the maintenance dosage and schedule provided on page 82.

MELANOMA

Melanoma is a type of skin cancer that develops in melanocytes, the cells that produce melanin (the pigment that gives skin its color). Melanoma is the most serious type of skin cancer, but it is highly curable if detected and treated early. Regular skin self-exams and sun protection measures are essential for early detection and prevention. While melanoma is less frequent than other types of skin cancers, it is responsible for the majority of skin cancer–related deaths. Rates of melanoma are rising rapidly, especially in younger people. In fact, cases of melanoma have tripled in the last 30 years, at a time when cancer rates for other common cancers have declined. Melanoma can be broadly categorized into cutaneous (on the skin), mucosal (in mucus membranes), and ocular melanoma (in the eye). Cutaneous melanoma, the most common type, is further classified into subtypes like superficial spreading, nodular, lentigo maligna, and acral lentiginous melanoma.

The five-year survival rate for melanoma varies significantly based on stage at diagnosis. When detected and treated early (stages 0, 1, 2), the survival rate is very high, often exceeding 99%. When melanoma has spread to nearby lymph nodes (stage 3), the five-year survival rate is around 66% and when it has spread to distant sites, the survival rate drops to 15–50%. Overall, 2–5% of melanomas are estimated to recur, but this can be higher for advanced stages. Higher-stage melanomas (thicker, with ulceration, or involving lymph nodes) have a higher risk of recurrence and tend to recur faster. While many recurrences happen within two to three years, some can occur much later—even more than 10 years after the initial diagnosis. Recurrences can happen in the same skin area or in distant sites (lungs, liver, brain, or other organs).

Natural Remedies for Melanoma

N-Tense capsules have been used as a natural remedy for melanoma for more than 20 years. Results have varied with about 50% seeing benefits. Based on all the new research on chanca piedra, I would try adding it to the cancer plan to see if better results are achieved. Newer research reports that chanca piedra has six different ways to kill melanoma cancer cells, and it prevents several defense mechanisms.

THE MELANOMA CANCER PLAN

Dosage

N-Tense capsules: 2–3 g in capsules, three times daily, based on stage/grade (see page 82).

Chanca piedra: 1 g in capsules, three times daily.

Instructions

- Take both remedies together at the same time (for synergistic/additive effects), three times daily.
- They can be taken either with or between meals.
- When/if you achieve remission, take the remedies for one month longer.
- Discontinue use for three months; then follow the instructions for the maintenance dosage and schedule provided on page 82.

MULTIPLE MYELOMA

Multiple myeloma (MM) is a cancer that develops from plasma cells, a type of white blood cell in the bone marrow. MM is classified as a blood cancer. These cancerous plasma cells, called myeloma cells, multiply uncontrollably and produce abnormal antibodies. The abnormal antibodies can lead to various complications like bone damage, kidney problems, and immune system issues. Multiple myeloma is considered treatable but is generally not curable. Treatments can induce remission and manage symptoms. Many people with multiple myeloma live for many years with treatment and support. Survival rates vary depending on factors like the stage of the disease, age, and overall health. Early-stage multiple myeloma has a higher five-year survival rate (around 82% for stage 1 and 69% for stage 2) than later stages (around 60% for stage 3 and 40% for stage 4).

Multiple myeloma is known to relapse, and the rate can vary based on factors like the initial stage and individual patient characteristics. Most people with multiple myeloma will experience periods of remission and relapse throughout the course of their disease. While some patients may experience remission for several years, others may relapse sooner, even within the first year. Unlike many other cancers, MM doesn't have as many defense mechanisms to become drug resistant. If a patient relapses, doctors will often consider reusing the same therapy that induced the initial remission, as it may still be effective, especially if the remission lasted for a year or longer.

Natural Remedies for Multiple Myeloma

NTense-2 capsules were specially designed for blood cancers like multiple myeloma and have been used as a natural remedy for blood cancers for more than 20 years with good results. Adding a pau d'arco alcohol tincture to the plan should help avoid relapse because it disables most of the defense mechanisms this cancer uses as well as targets cancer stem cells. The beneficial plant chemicals in pau d'arco must be extracted from the bark in alcohol, so avoid buying capsules and instead buy an alcohol tincture.

THE MULTIPLE MYELOMA CANCER PLAN

Dosage

NTense-2 capsules: 2–3 g, three times daily, based on stage/grade (see page 82).

Pau d'arco tincture: 2 ml, three times daily.

Instructions

- Take both remedies together at the same time (for synergistic/additive effects), three times daily.
- They can be taken either with or between meals.
- When/if you achieve remission, take the remedies for one month longer.
- Discontinue use for three months; then follow the instructions for the maintenance dosage and schedule provided on page 82.

NASOPHARYNGEAL CANCER—see LARYNGEAL CANCER

ORAL CANCER

Oral cancer is a malignant tumor that can develop on the lips, tongue, gums, floor of the mouth, and other areas of the mouth and throat. Early detection is crucial for successful treatment, so regular dental checkups are recommended. The most common type is squamous cell carcinoma (about 90% of oral cancers), which originates in the thin, flat squamous cells lining the mouth and throat. Risk factors include tobacco use, excessive alcohol consumption, and HPV infection. Other types of oral cancers include verrucous carcinoma, salivary gland cancers, lymphomas (which can occur in the tonsils or base of the tongue), and melanomas (which occur in the gums or roof of the mouth).

If the cancer is found and treated before it spreads (stage 1), the five-year survival rate can be as high as 80–90%. The survival rate drops to around 60–70% for cancers that have spread to nearby areas or nearby lymph nodes in the neck (stage 2 and 3). If the cancer has spread to distant parts of the body, survival rates drop to around 30–40%. Approximately 20–47% of patients experience recurrence after initial treatment, depending on the stage at diagnosis and initial treatment. Recurrence can manifest as local recurrence in the same area, second primary tumors, or metastases to lymph nodes or distant sites like the lungs or bones.

Natural Remedies for Oral Cancer
N-Tense has been used for many years as a natural remedy for oral cancers. It is best to open the capsules and prepare a tea with the plant powder inside. This increases efficacy and speed by getting the anti-cancerous plant chemicals in direct contact with the cancer. It really is worth it, despite the bad taste of the tea. Open the capsules and place the contents in a teacup and pour 6 ounces of boiling water into the cup. Cover and let soak until lukewarm (about 15 minutes), stirring once after about 5–7 minutes. The plant powder will settle to the bottom of the cup so you can drink the tea off the top, or pour the tea through a fine strainer or coffee filter. Then drink slowly, swishing around in the mouth before swallowing. Avoid drinking or eating for at least one hour afterward.

Adding chanca piedra to the tea will be very beneficial as it addresses several of the defense mechanisms this cancer uses to become drug resistant and recur. Chanca piedra capsules are now widely available and are inexpensive. Just open the capsules and put the powder in the cup with the N-Tense powder.

For oral lymphomas, see the cancer plan and instructions in the "Lymphoma" section.

For oral melanomas, see the cancer plan and instructions in the "Melanoma" section.

The Oral Cancer Plan

Dosage

N-Tense capsules: 2–3 g, three times daily, based on stage/grade (see page 82).

Chanca piedra: 1–2 g, three times daily, based on stage/grade.

Instructions

- Open the capsules and prepare a tea/infusion with the powder inside as described earlier.
- Drink the tea three times daily.
- It can be taken either with or between meals.
- When/if you achieve remission, drink the remedy twice daily for one month longer.
- Discontinue use for three months; then follow the instructions for the maintenance dosage and schedule provided on page 82.

OVARIAN CANCER

Ovarian cancer is a disease where cancerous cells form in the ovaries, the female reproductive organs that produce eggs. It is often called a "silent disease" because symptoms may not appear until later stages. Most ovarian cancers are epithelial ovarian carcinomas, which originate in the cells covering the ovaries. Other types include germ cell tumors and stromal cell tumors. Ovarian cancer ranks as the eighth most common cancer among women globally. While not the most common cancer, it is the deadliest gynecologic cancer.

The five-year survival rate for ovarian cancer varies significantly based on the stage at diagnosis. If the cancer is found early (localized to the ovary), the five-year survival rate can be as high as 90–92%. For advanced stages, the five-year survival rate is much lower, around 30%. Ovarian cancer grows quickly and can progress from early stages to an advanced stage within a year. Most patients are diagnosed after the cancer has spread (metastasized) from the ovaries to other areas of the body (stages 3 and 4). This is because early-stage ovarian cancer often has vague or no symptoms. The large majority of ovarian cancer cases are diagnosed in postmenopausal women, with 63 being the average age at diagnosis.

About 10–20% of women with early-stage ovarian cancer will experience a recurrence (stages 1 and 2). Recurrence rates for advanced-stage ovarian cancer (stages 3 and 4) are 70% and 95%, respectively.

Natural Remedies for Ovarian Cancer

N-Tense has long been used as a natural remedy for ovarian cancer with mixed results. This particular cancer is hard to treat conventionally as well as naturally. In my personal experience, it benefited about 45–50% who took it. Those benefits, however, were mostly disease stabilization (the tumor reduced in size and then stopped growing but didn't disappear) in late-stage cancers. Or, in earlier stages, the cancer disappeared but then recurred in a year or two. It seemed that as long as they continued to take the N-Tense, their results were sustained, with several patients I knew personally remaining stable for longer than five years. The progression of the disease, however, was pretty rapid when they stopped taking it.

With all the new information on how cancer behaves on a molecular and genetic level and what signaling pathways they use to thrive and survive, when I started really looking at the new research, I quickly understood why this particular cancer was so hard to treat. Researchers have discovered (to date) at least 32 different mechanisms that ovarian cancer uses to avoid death, recur, and metastasize in 22 different signaling pathways. And it's likely to be much more than that—researchers just haven't found them all. It has 12 different mechanisms to choose from just to become drug resistant (which it does quite well).

Based on all the new research, I would have to add four more plants to the cancer plan to hope to address the majority of the defense mechanisms this cancer uses. These plants include chanca piedra, picão preto, anamu, and pau d'arco. These plants are available in capsules; however, only purchase an alcohol tincture of pau d'arco. The beneficial plant chemicals in the plant aren't water soluble and need alcohol to extract them.

The Ovarian Cancer Plan

Dosage

N-Tense capsules: 3 g, three times daily.

Chanca piedra: 1.5 g in capsules, three times daily.

Anamu: 1 g in capsules, three times daily.

Picão preto: 1.5 g in capsules or 3 ml of a tincture, three times daily.

Pau d'arco tincture: 2 ml, three times daily.

Instructions

- Take all remedies together at the same time (for synergistic/additive effects), three times daily.

- They can be taken either with or between meals.

- When/if you achieve remission, take the remedies for two months longer.

- Discontinue use for three months; then follow the instructions for the maintenance dosage and schedule provided on page 82.

PANCREATIC CANCER

Pancreatic cancer is a disease where cancer cells form in the tissues of the pancreas, a gland located behind the stomach. It's often difficult to detect early, and the prognosis is generally poor, though survival rates vary depending on the stage at diagnosis. Pancreatic cancer is primarily categorized into exocrine and neuroendocrine tumors, with exocrine being more common and neuroendocrine harder to treat. The most prevalent type is adenocarcinoma, originating in the cells lining the pancreatic ducts. Neuroendocrine tumors develop from hormone-producing cells in the pancreas and are less frequent.

In the United States, pancreatic cancer rates are rising (probably due to an aging population and rising rates of type 2 diabetes that increases risk), and the disease has a high mortality rate. This is because it often doesn't cause noticeable symptoms in the early stages. Many patients are diagnosed after the cancer has already spread to the liver, lungs, or other locations (stage 4). It is the third leading cause of cancer-related death and is expected to be the second leading cause by 2030. While it can take a decade or more for the initial cancer cell to develop into a detectable tumor, the transition from an early stage to a more advanced and inoperable stage can be rapid (a little over a year).

The life expectancy for pancreatic cancer varies significantly based on stage at diagnosis. Early-stage pancreatic cancer (stage 1 and 2) has a five-year survival rate of around 44%, while stage 3 pancreatic cancer has a survival rate of 13%. In advanced cancers (stage 4), survival rate drops to just 3%. Pancreatic cancer recurrence is unfortunately common, with up to 80% of patients experiencing it after potentially curative surgery (usually stages 1 and 2 before the cancer spreads outside of the pancreas). Many recurrences happen within the first two years following surgery. A small percentage (around 10%) of patients, however, can achieve long-term disease-free survival after surgery. Recurrences can be local (within the pancreas or surrounding tissues), distant (in other organs like the liver or lungs), or a combination of both. Recurrent tumors are usually drug resistant and grow quickly.

Natural Remedies for Pancreatic Cancer

N-Tense has long been used as a natural remedy for pancreatic cancer with mixed results. This particular cancer (like ovarian cancer) is particularly hard to treat conventionally as well as naturally. In my personal experience, it benefited about 40–50% who took it. Those benefits, however, were mostly disease stabilization (the tumor reduced in size and then stopped growing but didn't disappear) in late-stage cancers. Or, in earlier stages, the cancer disappeared but then recurred in a year or two. It seemed as long as they continued to take the N-Tense, their results were sustained, with several I knew personally remaining stable for longer than five years.

Based on all the new research, I would have to add several more plants to the cancer plan to address the majority of the defense mechanisms this cancer uses. This is an aggressive cancer needing an aggressive approach. First, add pau d'arco. A natural pau d'arco chemical is a new small-molecule drug in human trials showing it seeks out and selectively kills pancreatic cancer cells in a novel manner. Other chemicals directly kill the cancer, as well as stem cells, in several different ways. Only purchase an alcohol tincture of pau d'arco since this chemical is not water soluble and needs alcohol to extract it.

Bitter melon juice provides six different mechanisms of action against pancreatic cancer; however, there is not enough of this ingredient in N-Tense to replicate the compelling newer research on it targeting and killing cancer stem cells to avoid relapse. Therefore, I'm adding a concentrated spray-dried or freeze-dried extract of bitter melon juice. Quite a few of these products are available in capsules and are the easiest to take (many find the concentrated juice has an unpleasant bitter taste and avoid liquid extracts).

Finally, I would add an anamu capsule product. Based on earlier test-tube and animal studies, a new anamu herbal drug was created and is now in human Phase II clinical trials for pancreatic and gastric cancers in Colombia. Other research shows anamu can kill pancreatic cancer in at least five different ways, including stem cells.

The Pancreatic Cancer Plan

Dosage

N-Tense capsules: 3 g, three times daily.

Pau d'arco tincture: 2 ml, three times daily.

Bitter melon fruit juice extract (freeze-dried or spray-dried) capsules: 1 g, three times daily.

Anamu: 1.5 g in capsules, three times daily.

Instructions

- Take all remedies together at the same time (for synergistic/additive effects), three times daily.
- They can be taken either with or between meals.
- When/if you achieve remission, take the remedies for two months longer.
- Discontinue use for three months; then follow the instructions for the maintenance dosage and schedule provided on page 82.

PROSTATE CANCER

Prostate cancer is a type of cancer that develops in the prostate gland, a small gland in males that produces seminal fluid. It's one of the most common cancers in men, and while it often grows slowly and can be successfully treated, some types can be more aggressive and spread to other parts of the body. Prostate cancer is a significant health concern, being the second leading cause of cancer death in American men. Prostate cancer is primarily classified into types based on cell origin. The most common type is adenocarcinoma, which develops from the gland cells of the prostate. Other, less common types include small cell carcinoma, neuroendocrine tumors, transitional cell carcinoma, and sarcomas.

The Gleason score, along with Grade Groups, helps doctors assess the aggressiveness of prostate cancer. The Gleason score is a system used to grade prostate cancer based on how abnormal the cancer cells look under a microscope. It ranges from 2 to 10, with lower scores indicating less aggressive cancer. Nonaggressive prostate cancer, also known as low-grade (grade 1), is a type of prostate cancer that is characterized by its slow progression and low risk of spreading (Gleason score of 6 or less). Many men with this type of cancer may not require immediate treatment and can be managed with active surveillance (monitoring the cancer's progression). A Gleason score of 7 in prostate cancer indicates intermediate-grade cancer, with a higher likelihood of tumor growth. A score of 8, 9, or 10 represents high-grade tumors that are likely to grow and spread quickly and are treated more aggressively.

The five-year survival rate for prostate cancer in the United States is generally very high but varies significantly based on the stage of the cancer at diagnosis. For localized and regional prostate cancer (cancer contained within the prostate or surrounding areas), the five-year survival rate is nearly 100%. When the cancer has spread to distant parts of the body (distant stage), the five-year survival rate drops to around 37%. Approximately 20–30% of men treated for prostate cancer will experience a recurrence, even after initial successful treatment like surgery or radiation. The risk of recurrence varies based on factors like the initial cancer's stage, grade, and individual patient characteristics.

Natural Remedies for Prostate Cancer
Raintree probably helped more men with prostate cancer than any other type of cancer because it is so common. Word-of-mouth referrals reporting how

well it worked is what fueled the sale of N-Tense capsules as an effective natural remedy for prostate cancer. It was routinely combined with another Raintree formula called Amazon Prostate Support. This formula helped direct the anti-cancer plants to the prostate more efficiently, reduced inflammation, and relieved some of the symptoms of prostate cancer. Some of the ingredients of Prostate Support are also the subject of research for prostate cancer as well. This combination of products always worked faster and more efficiently than N-Tense alone. (See page 330 for more information on Amazon Prostate Support.)

The Prostate Cancer Plan

Dosage

N-Tense capsules: 2–3 g, three times daily, based on stage/grade (see page 82).

Amazon Prostate Support capsules: 1.5 g in capsules, three times daily (see page 82 for more information about this product).

Instructions

- Take both remedies together at the same time (for synergistic/additive effects), three times daily.
- They can be taken either with or between meals.
- When/if you achieve remission, take the remedies for two months longer.
- Discontinue use for three months; then follow the instructions for the maintenance dosage and schedule provided on page 82.

SARCOMAS—*see* BONE CANCERS

SKIN CANCER

Skin cancer is an abnormal growth of skin cells, often caused by sun exposure. The main types are basal cell carcinoma, squamous cell carcinoma, and melanoma. See the separate "Melanoma" section. The type of skin cancer a person gets is determined by where the cancer begins. If the cancer begins in skin cells called basal cells, the person has basal cell skin cancer (BCC). BCCs often look like a flesh-colored round growth, pearl-like bump, or a pinkish patch of skin. They usually develop after years of frequent sun exposure or indoor tanning and are common on the head, neck, and arms; however, they can form anywhere.

Squamous cell carcinoma (SCC) of the skin is the second most common type of skin cancer. Squamous cells are located in the upper layers of the skin, near the surface. People who have light skin are most likely to develop SCC. It often looks like a red firm bump, scaly patch, or a sore that heals and then reopens. While generally treatable, it can be more likely to grow deeper and spread than BCC.

The five-year relative survival rate for skin cancer is generally excellent, with 100% for BCC and 95% for SCC, when detected early. Approximately 20% of patients with skin cancer will experience a recurrence at some point, especially if the BCC or SCC was large, deeply invasive, or not completely removed.

Natural Remedies for Skin Cancer

After many practitioner requests, I developed an N-Tense formula that could be used topically on standard skin cancers such as basal cell and squamous cell carcinomas. It had a huge following and worked well. If it doesn't react at all to the extract, it's probably a non-cancerous spot on the skin. Depending on the size of the cancer, it can take as little as a week and up to a month or a little longer to disappear. If the spot reacted to the topical extract but still isn't healed completely after a month, schedule an appointment with your dermatologist. The spot may be a melanoma and needs to be biopsied (see the information in the "Melanoma" section).

Please note, this product will temporarily stain the skin and may permanently stain other surfaces and clothing reddish-brown. Also note this product is unlike other skin cancer products on the market called "black salves" or "drawing salves" that are corrosive to the skin, leave scars, and/or remove flesh. This product leaves no scars, and the "reaction" seen looks like a minor irritation with a tad of inflammation, not the corrosive damage the black salves create.

The Skin Cancer Plan

Dosage

N-Tense Topical extract: Apply 3–4 drops on affected area, twice daily.

Instructions

- Soak the affected area with a wet, warm wash rag or paper towel to gently remove any scab.

- Place several drops of the extract on the affected area to cover completely and let dry completely.

- Apply in this manner twice daily. It will actually look a bit worse before it gets better as the anti-cancer plants go to work to remove the cancer.

- One ingredient (sangre de drago) promotes wound healing and scabbing, which is normal. Always gently remove the scab before reapplying.

TESTICULAR CANCER

Testicular cancer is a disease where cancerous cells form in one or both testicles. It's the most common cancer in young and middle-aged men, typically diagnosed between the ages of 20 and 34. While rare overall, it's highly treatable and often curable, especially when detected early. The majority of testicular cancers are called germ cell tumors, which originate from cells that produce sperm. There are two main types of germ cell tumors: seminomas and non-seminomas. Seminomas tend to grow slower and respond well to radiation and chemotherapy. Non-seminomas are more common in younger men and tend to grow faster.

Testicular cancer generally has a very high survival rate, with most patients experiencing a normal life expectancy after treatment. More than 95% of men diagnosed with testicular cancer survive at least five years, and the cure rate can be as high as 90%. Localized testicular cancer (confined to the testicle) has a 99% five-year survival rate, while even regional cancer (spread to nearby lymph nodes) has a 96% five-year survival rate. Treatment typically involves surgery (removing the cancerous testicle), and sometimes chemotherapy or radiation therapy, and is often successful in curing the cancer. The overall crude relapse rate is 8–19.3%, with most relapses occurring in the first two years.

Natural Remedies for Testicular Cancer

N-Tense has been used as a natural remedy for testicular cancer with good results for numerous years. It worked well on its own and with a low relapse rate. There wasn't a need to add anything else. Most of the N-Tense ingredients addressed the defense mechanisms this cancer uses. If you are dealing with a recurrence of testicular cancer, or worry about a relapse based on the type of testicular cancer you have, you can add a concentrated spray-dried or freeze-dried extract of bitter melon juice.

Research reports that in dosages higher than what N-Tense provides, this juice can selectively target testicular cancer stem cells and kill them in various ways. These concentrated fruit extracts of bitter melon are available from several larger manufacturers and are sold as dry extract powders in capsules or bulk. Capsules are typically preferred because, as the name indicates, the juice tastes bitter. See the plant information in Part 3 (page 207) for more on the new research.

THE TESTICULAR CANCER PLAN

Dosage
N-Tense capsules: 2–3 g, three times daily, based on stage/grade (see page 82).

If needed/desired:
Bitter melon fruit extract capsules: 1 g, three times daily.

Instructions
• Take both remedies together at the same time (for synergistic/additive effects), three times daily.

• They can be taken either with or between meals.

• When/if you achieve remission, take the remedies for one month longer.

• Discontinue use for three months; then follow the instructions for the maintenance dosage and schedule provided on page 82.

THYROID CANCER

Thyroid cancer is a disease where malignant (cancerous) cells form in the tissues of the thyroid gland. The thyroid, a butterfly-shaped gland at the base of the neck, produces hormones that regulate the body's energy use. There are multiple types of thyroid cancer, including papillary, follicular, medullary, anaplastic, and Hurthle cell thyroid cancers. Papillary thyroid cancer is the most common type, which is often slow growing and typically affects one lobe of the thyroid. Anaplastic thyroid cancer is the deadliest; average median survival is generally four to five months after diagnosis. All anaplastic thyroid cancers are considered stage 4 at diagnosis because they are aggressive and can spread quickly.

Women are three times more likely to get thyroid cancer than men. In the United States, thyroid cancer is relatively common. While it's not one of the most prevalent cancers overall, it's the 13th most commonly diagnosed cancer and the sixth most common in women. Although it can occur at any age, it generally affects people ages 30 to 50. The incidence of thyroid cancer has been increasing, particularly in women, though mortality rates remain low.

The overall five-year survival rate for thyroid cancer is very high, around 98%. Survival rates vary significantly, however, depending on the stage and type of cancer. For example, localized (early stage) papillary and follicular thyroid cancers have survival rates near 100%. Papillary and follicular thyroid cancer recurrence rates vary depending on several factors, but generally, it's considered to have a high survival rate with a lower recurrence risk (2–20%).

Natural Remedies for Thyroid Cancer

N-Tense has long been used as a natural remedy for thyroid cancer with good results. It worked well on its own and with a low relapse rate, there wasn't a need to add anything else. Most of the N-Tense ingredients address the defense mechanisms this cancer uses. If you are dealing with a recurrence of thyroid cancer, or worry about a relapse based on the type of cancer you have, you can add chanca piedra to the cancer plan. Research reports that it can selectively target cancer stem cells and kill them in various ways. See the plant information in Part 3 (page 226) for more.

The Thyroid Cancer Plan

Dosage

N-Tense capsules: 2–3 g, three times daily, based on stage/grade (see page 82).

If needed/desired:

Chanca piedra capsules: 1 g, three times daily.

Instructions

- Take both remedies together at the same time (for synergistic/additive effects), three times daily.
- They can be taken either with or between meals.
- When/if you achieve remission, take the remedies for two months longer.
- Discontinue use for three months; then follow the instructions for the maintenance dosage and schedule provided on page 82.

UTERINE CANCER—see ENDOMETRIAL CANCER

Summary

When I started compiling all the new research describing how cancer acts on a molecular level, as well as how plants and their large complement of active chemicals can address those actions, I began to understand that natural remedies might be the only thing that has a real chance to address so many defense mechanisms simultaneously to actually cure cancer. We know how incredibly complicated cancer is and how complex cancer cells' innate survival instincts are to create so many defense mechanisms to avoid death and to continue to grow and spread. When a single-chemical drug or even a single-plant chemical thwarts one of their defense mechanisms, they simply mutate against it, or choose a new pathway and a new chemical to use in the complicated chain reaction of cascading molecular reactions to achieve the same outcome.

The research shows that all of the active chemicals in a multi-plant formula like N-Tense have the potential to affect hundreds of different molecules and pathways all at once. We will never know everything the plant chemicals (and all the new chemicals they make binding with one another or by reacting in the body during metabolism) might be doing in all of these complicated signaling pathways. But do we really have to? If it works, it works. What it showed me was a peek inside why these formulas worked so well for so many years, for so many different types of cancer, and how I might make them better. That's good enough for me.

8

HOW TO PREPARE YOUR OWN NATURAL ANTI-CANCER REMEDIES

While it is a bit more trouble and time consuming, making your own natural remedies is usually much more economical than purchasing manufactured products. These savings, however, are seen only after a much higher initial investment to purchase all the plant powders and whatever equipment you might need. Some of the plants can only be purchased by the pound or the kilogram and can cost as much as $20–$30 per pound or more.

In this chapter, you will find everything you need to know about making the N-Tense formulas into teas, capsules, and extracts, as well as how to customize the recipes to help fight the particular cancer you may be fighting.

Buying Plant-Based Products

While you may not be familiar with purchasing plant-based products, there are two important factors to consider. The first is the form these plants come in. You will want to use a form that works best for you. The second has to do with the storage of these plant products. There are a number of important factors to think about when storing plants in your home. The following section will provide you with some key facts that deal with the types of products available and the storage of these products.

Sourcing Products

The first step in preparing these remedies is sourcing good raw plant materials. Most coming from South America and the Amazon (featured in this book) will only be available in a dried state and are either a tea-cut herb or a ground powder form. Find a reputable supplier who exports regularly from the region, and please, ask questions about their harvesting practices. Many South American plants are harvested unsustainably—causing more rainforest destruction, rather than helping to preserve it. Again, do the research required to find a good supplier, ask questions, and make sure that you are obtaining the correct species of plant (using the Latin botanical name), that it is fresh, and that it has been sustainably harvested. See the "Resources" section on page 327 for companies that sell bulk rainforest plants by the ounce, pound, or kilogram (2.2 pounds).

Tea-Cut Plants versus Powders

While all the plants (and recipes) in this book can be found to purchase retail in powder form, some may not be available in tea-cut form. It is not always necessary to find a tea-cut plant to prepare a tea or extract; ground powders can be used to make teas, tinctures, and extracts just as well. Since the plant is finely ground, it usually makes a stronger remedy as more surface area of the plant is available to extract in the liquid. Many herbalists prefer working with powders instead of bulky cut herbs since they make stronger teas and extracts. Others use plants cut into pieces (tea-cut) because it's easier to strain out the plants before storing the remedy. You can also combine tea-cut plants with powdered plants when extracting them.

It is recommended that you use distilled or purified water when extracting medicinal plants. Regular tap water can contain chlorine, fluoride, and other chemicals that might have an interaction or chain reaction with one or more of the many chemicals found in plants.

Storing Bulk Plants

If you don't plan on using all of the plant(s) immediately, it's best to keep them unopened, in their original packaging, and away from direct sunlight (just put them in a closed cupboard/cabinet or drawer). Many plants will absorb moisture and humidity from the air, so if they are opened, reseal them tightly or put them into glass jars with a tight-fitting lid (avoid metal containers). Most will never require refrigeration or freezing—just keep them at average room temperature (70–80 degrees). Generally, the "shelf-life" for optimum freshness will be about a year for dried leaves, and two years for dried barks and roots if stored properly. If you live in a warm, high humidity area, it may be impossible to keep moisture out of regularly opened and closed glass containers, and the plants may become moldy. If this happens, discard them and purchase fresh ones.

You can also consider storing the leaves in a larger container, taking out some leaves to place into a smaller container that can be used on a more regular basis. In addition, try storing them in paper lunch bags, so they can "breathe" (although this will reduce the shelf life significantly).

When the combined plant formula is stored and handled properly, its shelf life is one to two years (depending on humidity levels). If you are opening a jar with the formula in it three times a day to brew tea every day, and you live in a humid climate, plan on a one-year shelf life or less.

The N-Tense Formulas

There are three N-Tense recipes: N-Tense used for solid tumors, NTense-2 used for blood-based cancers, and N-Tense Topical used for skin cancers. The following is a breakdown of the plants each formula contains. Throughout chapter 7 and this chapter, the amount of plants suggested for use are described as "parts." This is a general term. A part can be a tablespoon, an ounce, a cup, or a pound, or any measurement you'd like. The important thing to remember is that when putting a formula together, all the parts are measured in the same quantity. Therefore, when measuring in ounces, 10 parts graviola is equal to 10 ounces of graviola, while 1 part bitter melon is equal to 1 ounce of bitter melon, and so on.

The N-Tense Product Recipes

N-Tense for Solid Tumors:

10 parts graviola	1 part bitter melon
2 parts mullaca	2 parts vassourinha
2 parts guacatonga	1 part cat's claw
2 parts espinheira santa	

To make a smaller amount, 1 part could be a tablespoon (you'd have 20 tablespoons of the blended herbal formula).

NTense-2 for Blood Cancers (Leukemia, Lymphoma, Myeloma, etc.):

1 part mullaca	1 part picão preto
1 part anamu	1 part suma
1 part vassourinha	1 part cat's claw
1 part simarouba	1 part espinheira santa

To make a small amount, 1 part could be a tablespoon (you'd have 8 tablespoons of the blended formula).

Instructions

- Combine all the plants together well in a glass, a plastic bowl, or jar. Avoid metals.

- The formula can then be put into capsules (see instructions on page 140) or brewed into tea/infusions (see instructions on page 140); used to prepare alcohol tinctures or glycerin extracts (see instructions on pages 141 and 142); stirred into juice or other liquid; or taken however you'd like.

- Store the combined plant formula at room temperature, in the dark, and in a tightly closed glass or plastic container that will keep humidity out.

N-Tense Topical for Skin Cancers:

1 part sangre de grado	1 part pau d'arco
1 part copaiba	1 part mullaca
1 part graviola	1 part vassourinha
1 part espinheira santa	1 part mutamba extracted in
1 part suma	distilled water and alcohol

To make a small amount, 1 part could be a tablespoon (you'd have 7 tablespoons of the blended formula). For larger amounts 1 part could be 1 ounce, or 1 cup, or 1 pound.

HOW TO PREPARE YOUR OWN NATURAL ANTI-CANCER REMEDIES

Instructions

- To prepare this, combine equal parts of graviola, espinheira santa, suma, pau d'arco, mullaca, vassourinha, and mutamba.
- To make a tincture, follow the instructions on page 141.
- Once the tincture is finished, measure it. For every four parts of the finished tincture, add one part sangre de grado resin and one part copaiba oil. Mix together and bottle it in a dark glass bottle; it will naturally separate, so just shake well before using.
- Store at room temperature, away from light, for up to a year.

Choose the Type of Remedy You Want

In traditional medicine systems, natural remedies are prepared in several rather standardized ways, which usually vary based upon the plant utilized and, sometimes, what condition is being treated. You have several options on how to prepare the N-Tense formula once you've combined the plants. The best method is one that results in a product that is the easiest for you to take. These methods include capsules, infusions (hot teas), tinctures (alcohol and water extracts), and non-alcohol extracts (made with vegetable glycerin).

Swallowing capsules is probably the easiest, and you don't have to worry about the objectionable taste of the plants. The easiest, physically, is to just prepare a cup of tea (infusion) by stirring the powder into almost boiling water. Many people, however, find the taste to be too unpleasant to put up with three times a day, day after day. Tinctures and extracts can also have an objectionable taste, but you have swallowed much less of it than a 6-to-8-ounce cup of tea. A good idea is to first make a cup of tea with the plant powder and see how it tastes to you before you commit to which method to use. Some find it worse than others, especially those already struggling with nausea issues if they're taking the formula along with standard chemotherapy drugs that cause nausea.

These formulas can be prepared using different methods. The most common are preparing capsules, infusion/teas, tinctures, and glycerin extracts, and as you will read, they can also be customized to meet your specific situation. The following section will provide a more specific explanation of each of these methods.

Capsules

Capsules are not all that hard to make if you use a specialized manual capsule filler. There are several available to purchase that make 24 or 100 capsules at a time and cost around $20–$40. Once you get the hang of it; you can make 100 capsules in about 10 minutes. See page 329 in the "Resources" section for links to purchase one. Purchasing empty capsules is easy; Amazon.com has some of the best prices. They are also sold by larger natural product or bulk herb suppliers such as Swansons (who sell empty capsules and capsule fillers). Standard gelatin capsules and vegetable-base capsules are available (around $7–$8 for 250 capsules). Again, see page 329 in the "Resources" section for more information.

The important thing to remember is that there are different capsule sizes, and the size of the capsule needs to be the same as the size of capsule filler (which also comes in three standard sizes) you purchase. Capsules (and fillers) are sold by the "aught," single 0, double 00, and triple 000. A single 0 capsule will hold approximately 500–570 mgs of plant powder depending on how well you pack the powder into the capsules. A double 00 capsule will hold between 750 and 800 mgs. The traditional remedies shown in this book are stated in grams; usually 2–3 grams, three times daily for the N-Tense formulas. One gram is the equivalent of 1,000 mgs. Therefore, four capsules would equal 2 grams if using 0 (500 mg) capsules; 750 mgs is 1.5 grams, and four capsules would equal 3 grams if using 00 capsules.

To make the capsules, just follow the directions that come with the capsule filler machine. It is pretty straightforward. There are also demonstrations on how it can be used to fill capsules on YouTube.com. See the "Resources" section for more information and links.

Store the filled capsules in glass or plastic jars with a tight lid at room temperature and away from the direct light (inside a dark cabinet or drawer). Shelf life for capsules is approximately two years if stored properly.

Infusions/Teas

Preparing an infusion is much like making a cup of tea. Water is brought to a boil and then poured over the N-Tense combination of plants. It is covered and allowed to sit/steep for 15 minutes. It can be prepared in the drinking cup (by just pouring the heated water over the plant formula in the cup) or by dropping the plant formula into the same pot you used to heat the water.

Empty gauze teabags are even available on Amazon; these can be filled with herbs and then sealed with an iron. (See the "Resources" section.) If an infusion is prepared in the heating pan/pot, it's best to use a ceramic pot with a lid (avoid metal pots). Stirring it a few times while steeping (especially with tea-cut herbs) is helpful. Keeping the infusion covered while steeping is generally recommended as well (place a saucer on top of the cup, or a lid on top of the pot).

Dosage: Use 1 rounded teaspoon of the powdered plant formula or 2 rounded teaspoons of tea-cut plant formula in a 6-to-8-ounce cup of water and taken three times daily. If using powdered plants, stir once halfway through the seeping time and let the powder settle to the bottom of the cup; then drink the infusion off the top (leaving the sediment in the bottom of the cup). If using a cut herb, strain the infusion with a tea-strainer after seeping. Infusions are best prepared as needed and taken the same day it is prepared. It can be taken hot, warm, or cold. If desired, the entire day's dosage can be prepared in the morning (3 cups at one time), and the remainder refrigerated until ready to use.

Tinctures

A tincture is an alcohol and water extract used when plants have active chemicals that are not very soluble in water, and/or when a larger quantity is prepared for convenience with longer-term storage. Many properly prepared plant tinctures can last several years or more without losing potency. The percentage of alcohol usually helps determine its shelf life: the more alcohol used, the longer the shelf life. The type of alcohol can vary from vodka, rum, or 90–180 proof grain alcohol (sold as "everclear" in liquor stores and oftentimes cheaper than vodka). Vodka is fine. But remember, if it says 80 proof, it is 40% alcohol and the rest is water.

To prepare a tincture with a shelf life of at least one to two years, plan on using a minimum of 40% alcohol (so you can extract an herb in a bottle of 80 proof vodka or rum without adding any water). Use a clean glass bottle or jar with a tight-fitting lid or cork. Use a dark-colored bottle (like a recycled green/amber wine bottle) or plan on storing the bottle out of the sunlight inside a dark cabinet.

When working with dried plants, use 2 ounces of plant material (cut or powder) for every 8 ounces (1 cup) of liquid. Since many cut herbs can be bulky compared to much denser powders, measure the amount of cut herb by weight and not volume. Most cooks would tell you that 2 tablespoons of butter is 1 ounce; however, a lightweight bulky leaf is not as heavy as butter in the same volume or by the tablespoon. A "standard 4:1 tincture" means 4 parts liquid to 1 part plant (or as above, 4 ounces of liquid to 1 ounce plant).

To prepare approximately 1 cup of tincture (some of the liquid will be absorbed by the dry plant material), place 2 ounces of the herb (cut up or powdered) into your clean glass container. Pour ½ cup (4 ounces) of distilled water and a ½ cup (4 ounces) of 180 proof alcohol into the container (or just use 1 cup of straight 80 proof vodka and no water). Seal the container and store at room temperature away from direct sunlight. Shake the bottle/jar at least once daily while allowing it to soak/extract for at least two weeks for powders (tea-cut plant pieces should soak for four weeks). At the end of the soaking time, filter the tincture through a strainer to remove the plant parts (pressing hard on the plant material to get as much liquid out as possible), pour into a fresh, clean glass container, and seal. Some like to pour it through a cheesecloth and then use the cheesecloth to more easily wring out the liquid from the plant material.

Since this method uses a higher ratio of plant to liquid and helps concentrate the chemicals through the use of alcohol, dosages needed for tinctures are usually much less than infusions. Dosages for the N-Tense tincture is 5 milliliters (or about 1 teaspoon), three times daily. The tincture can be placed directly in the mouth for immediate absorption, or placed in a small amount of water or juice. If you dislike the alcohol content (or want to give the remedy to a child), place the dosage in about 1–2 ounces of very hot water and most of the alcohol will be evaporated in the hot water in a minute or two. (Let it cool before taking.) Store the tincture at room temperature and away from direct sunlight. A properly prepared 4:1 standard tincture, has a shelf life of three years or more.

Glycerin Extracts

Basically, preparing this type of extract is similar to a tincture but 75% vegetable glycerin, and 25% distilled water is used instead of the ratios of water and alcohol. Fill a clean jar half full with the ground plant powder. In a separate same-sized jar, combine 3 parts vegetable glycerin with 1 part distilled water. This is a 3:1 ratio. Cap the jar and shake to thoroughly combine. Pour the liquid mixture over the powdered plants in the jar to within 1 inch of the top to completely cover the plant material. Stir well with a long, clean spoon or knife to release any air bubbles. Add more glycerin/water mixture as necessary to bring liquid back up to 1 inch from the top of the jar to completely cover plant material and stir again.

Cap the jar tightly and set aside away from sunlight at room temperature to soak for four weeks. Shake daily to mix. After four weeks, strain through three to four layers of cheesecloth to remove all plant material. Be sure to squeeze the cheesecloth to get every last drop of extract. Bottle in a clean amber or cobalt glass bottle or jar with an airtight lid. Label with ingredients, ratios, and date strained. Store in a cool, dark area.

Vegetable glycerin is available from Amazon.com and also found in some retail stores like Walmart and Michaels, some grocery stores and pharmacies, and some larger suppliers that sell herbs in bulk. Look for "USP Grade" or "Food Grade" vegetable glycerin. See the "Resources" section for more information.

CUSTOMIZING THE FORMULAS BASED ON CANCER TYPE

Once again, like the previous chapter, the last section of this chapter provides information and a cancer plan for each type of cancer. Since you are planning on preparing the natural remedy yourself, however, the section that follows will give you a new recipe for N-Tense or NTense-2 that incorporates the new plants to address defense and recurrence mechanisms into one complete formula (with a few exceptions). Just follow the instructions in this chapter to use these new recipes that follow to prepare teas, capsules, or extracts as described herein. Some new ingredients replace old ingredients (which may not have been effective for a particular cancer), and ratios/parts of some plant ingredients have changed based on efficacy/research. When the N-Tense formulas were first created, they were formulated as broad-spectrum formulas that would hit a large number of different cancer types. Creating a recipe for each cancer type allows for better customization of which plants work the best for each unique cancer type.

THE CANCER PLANS

BLADDER/KIDNEY CANCER

Bladder cancer occurs when abnormal cells grow uncontrollably in the bladder lining. It is the seventh most diagnosed cancer in the United States and the third most common in men. Most bladder cancers are called urothelial carcinomas or transitional cell carcinomas. Cancers confined to the inner lining of the bladder are called "superficial" or "stage 1" and comprise 70–80% of all bladder cancers diagnosed. Cancers that have spread into the bladder wall are called "deep" bladder cancers or "stage 2," and those that have spread to lymph nodes and/or distantly to the lungs, liver, or other organs are referred to as "metastatic" or "stage 3 or 4" depending on where the cancer spread. Common treatments include surgery, radiation therapy, chemotherapy, immunotherapy, and targeted therapy. In many cases, a combination of these treatments is used. The recurrence rates for this cancer are 6–10% for stages 1 and 2 (and 30–60% within five years for stages 3 and 4), depending on which treatments were used.

Kidney Cancer

Kidney cancer, also known as renal cancer, occurs when cells in the kidneys grow out of control, forming a tumor, and are staged much like bladder cancer. The most common type (90% of cases) is renal cell carcinoma (RCC), which starts in the lining of the kidney's tubules. It is treated much like bladder cancer. Transitional cell carcinoma (TCC) can develop in the renal pelvis or ureter; it is often treated like bladder cancer as well. Kidney cancer recurrence rates vary, but approximately 20–30% of patients with localized kidney cancer experience a recurrence after surgery (kidney removal). Most recurrences happen within the first five years after surgery, with a significant portion occurring within the first two years.

Natural Remedies for Bladder and Kidney Cancer

N-Tense has a long history of being effectively used for these types of cancer by addressing the initial tumor(s), and quickly, especially stage 1 tumors. Several patients reported starting N-Tense shortly after the first diagnostic biopsy and the surgeon not finding any tumor to remove only 30–45 days later during surgery. A well-known defense mechanism is used by these cancers to escape detection from the immune system. Several chemicals in N-Tense disable this mechanism.

Adding chanca piedra and picão preto to the N-Tense capsules can help direct the plants specifically to the bladder and kidneys, reduce symptoms (bladder and kidney irritation, inflammation, pain, urinary urgency), and address three other defense mechanisms these cancers use to recur. Both plants have their own anti-cancer/antitumor actions as well. In addition, both plants may help reduce common side effects of chemotherapy drugs for those taking them. See the information on these two plants in Part 3 for more information on these defense mechanisms.

THE BLADDER AND KIDNEY CANCER PLAN

Recipe

10 parts graviola

2 parts espinheira santa

2 parts chanca piedra

1 part mullaca

1 part guacatonga

1 part bitter melon fruit extract

1 part vassourinha

1 picão preto

1 part cat's claw

Dosages

Capsules: 2–3 g in capsules, three times daily, based on stage/grade (see page 82); *or*

Tincture or glycerin extract: 1 teaspoon, three times daily; *or*

Infusion/tea: 1 cup, three times daily.

Instructions

- This natural remedy can be taken either with or between meals.
- When/if you achieve remission, take the remedy for two months longer.
- Discontinue use for three months; then follow the instructions for the maintenance dosage and schedule provided on page 82.

BONE CANCERS/SARCOMAS

There are several different types of primary bone cancers including osteosarcoma (20–40%), Ewing sarcoma (10–15%), and chondrosarcoma (20–30%). Osteosarcoma begins in the cells that form bones, most often in the long bones of the legs and sometimes the arms. Osteosarcoma tends to happen most often in teenagers and young adults; however, it can occur at any age.

Osteosarcoma can occur in soft tissue outside the bone, but it is rare. An osteosarcoma that has not responded to treatment or has returned after an initial response to treatment is considered recurrent. Recurrent osteosarcoma occurs in 30–50% of patients with initial localized disease and 80% of patients presenting with metastatic disease.

Ewing sarcoma is a type of bone cancer that begins in the bones and the soft tissue around the bones. It most often begins in the leg bones and in the pelvis, but it can happen in any bone. This cancer occurs mostly in children and young adults, although it can happen at any age. Approximately 30–40% of patients with non-metastatic Ewing sarcoma will experience a recurrence after achieving remission. The recurrence can be either local (at the original tumor site) or metastatic (spreading to other parts of the body). Most recurrences happen within the first two years after diagnosis, but late relapses can occur. Patients with recurrence have a reported five-year survival rate of 13% with conventional standard therapies.

Chondrosarcoma is a type of bone cancer that usually begins in the bones, but it can sometimes occur in the soft tissue. Chondrosarcoma happens most often in the pelvis, hip, and shoulder. It occurs most often in middle-aged and older adults. Chondrosarcoma recurrence rates vary based on factors like grade, location, and treatment, but these generally range from 15% to 58%. Low-grade chondrosarcomas (grades 1 and 2) tend to have a lower recurrence rate compared to higher-grade tumors (grades 3 and 4).

Conventional treatment of these bone cancers typically involves a combination of surgery, chemotherapy, and radiation therapy.

Natural Remedies for Bone Cancer

N-Tense had quite a reputation for osteosarcomas with Raintree's practitioners, including veterinarians. Many types of large-breed dogs have a higher risk of developing osteosarcomas. When a handful of vets found that N-Tense could eliminate them in 30–60 days, word got out pretty quickly. It worked almost as quickly in people with osteosarcomas and chondrosarcomas. The natural remedy plan is to use N-Tense to fight the bone tumors, while also providing two mechanisms of action that prevent drug resistance and reduce recurrences, and by adding chanca piedra to the plan.

Five newer studies describe how two main active plant chemicals in chanca piedra have a direct toxic effect to osteosarcoma cancer cells as well as demonstrating it may prevent drug resistance and migration/metastasis. Adding chanca piedra to the plan may reduce rates of recurrence by combating defense mechanisms. (See the plant information for chanca piedra in Part 3, page 226, for more on these defense mechanisms.)

The Bone Cancer Plan

Recipe

10 parts graviola

2 parts mullaca

2 parts chanca piedra

2 parts espinheira santa

1 part guacatonga

1 part bitter melon fruit extract

1 part vassourinha

1 part cat's claw

Dosages

Capsules: 2–3 g in capsules, three times daily, based on stage/grade (see page 82); *or*

Tincture or glycerin extract: 1 teaspoon, three times daily; *or*

Infusion/tea: 1 cup, three times daily.

Instructions

- This natural remedy can be taken either with or between meals.
- When/if you achieve remission, take the remedy for two months longer.
- Discontinue use for three months; then follow the instructions for the maintenance dosage and schedule provided on page 82.

BRAIN CANCERS

There are more than 120 different types of brain tumors, lesions, and cysts, which are differentiated by where they occur and what kinds of cells that compose them. Brain tumors can be classified as either primary (originating in the brain) or secondary (metastatic, spreading from other parts of the body). Primary tumors are further categorized as glial (arising from glial cells like astrocytomas, oligodendrogliomas, and glioblastomas) or non-glial (like meningiomas, medulloblastomas, and pituitary adenomas). Metastatic tumors are cancerous growths that have spread to the brain from other areas of the body, most commonly lung, breast, or melanoma.

The most common type of malignant brain tumors are glioblastomas and medulloblastomas. Glioblastomas are the most common and aggressive type of glioma in adults, characterized by rapid growth and poor prognosis. This type of brain tumor is currently not curable using conventional therapy, even if caught early. While treatment can extend life and improve quality of life, glioblastoma is known for its rapid growth and recurrence, making it difficult to eradicate completely. The standard treatment involves surgery, radiation, and chemotherapy, but these are typically not curative. While not a cure, advancements in treatment have led to improved survival rates, with some patients living longer than the average 15–18 months after diagnosis. Glioblastomas almost always recur (90%), even after initial treatment, usually within 6–12 months after initial treatment.

Medulloblastoma is a type of cancerous brain tumor that originates in the cerebellum, the part of the brain responsible for balance and coordination. It is the most common malignant brain tumor in children, though it can also occur in adults. Medulloblastomas can spread to other parts of the brain and spinal cord but rarely metastasize outside the central nervous system. Survival rates for medulloblastoma have improved significantly over the past 20 years. While the tumor is considered high grade and can spread, many children are cured with current treatment approaches. Medulloblastoma can come back after treatment, however. It can recur in up to 30% of children. Recurrent medulloblastoma is often difficult to treat and can significantly reduce survival rates.

Natural Remedies for Brain Cancers

N-Tense has a long history of use as a natural remedy for glioblastomas; however, I am unaware of any person who was actually cured. While most plant chemicals are considered small molecules, most are not small enough to pass the blood-brain barrier to get to a tumor in the brain to have a positive effect. About 30–40% of users experienced a stabilization of their tumors (they stopped growing), and some reduced in size, but none disappeared completely. It widely varied how long this stabilization lasted. In two people I worked with personally in Austin, Texas, they achieved stable disease for quite a few years (6 years and 10 years). They were still taking the formula when I moved from Austin to Nevada, and I lost touch with them about a year later. These two ladies, however, were very committed to making the dietary and lifestyle changes that contributed to their cancers and were no longer creating higher risks of making more cells to mutate into cancerous cells. These two were the exception, however. In more than half the people with glioblastoma, the N-Tense had no appreciable effect. To my knowledge, N-Tense wasn't used in children with medulloblastomas due to their inability to swallow capsules and the objectionable taste of extracts. It is rare in adults, but one practitioner did report disease stabilization in one patient.

Simarouba has been used for brain tumors, and several studies confirm that is has anti-cancer actions against four different types of brain cancer. See the plant information in Part 3 (page 304) for more.

The Brain Cancer Plan

Recipe

10 parts graviola	1 part bitter melon fruit extract
4 parts simarouba	1 part vassourinha
2 parts espinheira santa	1 part guacatonga
1 part mullaca	1 part cat's claw

Dosages

Capsules: 2–3 g in capsules, three times daily, based on stage/grade (see page 82); *or*

Tincture or glycerin extract: 1 teaspoon, three times daily; *or*

Infusion/tea: 1 cup, three times daily.

Instructions

- This natural remedy can be taken either with or between meals.
- When/if you achieve remission, take the remedy for two months longer.
- Discontinue use for three months; then follow the instructions for the maintenance dosage and schedule provided on page 82.

BREAST CANCER (HORMONE-POSITIVE)

Hormone receptor-positive (HR+) breast cancer is a type of breast cancer where the cancer cells have receptors that interact with hormones like estrogen and progesterone. These hormones essentially fuel the growth of the cancer cells, causing them to divide and the tumor to enlarge. HR+ breast cancer can have receptors for estrogen (ER+), progesterone (PR+), or both (ER/PR+). Treatment often involves surgery as well as hormone therapy, which works to block the effects of these hormones, slowing or stopping the growth of the cancer. HR+ breast cancer is the most common form, making up about 70% of all breast cancer cases. It tends to grow more slowly than hormone receptor-negative cancers. The five-year survival rate for hormone receptor-positive breast cancer is generally very high, often exceeding 90%. Although HR+ cancers often have a favorable short-term prognosis, there is still a risk of recurrence that may persist for many years.

Recurrence rates largely depend on tumor size, stage, and whether lymph nodes were involved at the time of diagnosis. Generally, if caught at an early stage and without lymph node involvement, the recurrence rate is only 6%. If the cancer had spread to nearby lymph nodes, recurrence increased to 25%; however, when radiation was used to treat it, the recurrence rate dropped back to 6%.

Natural Remedies for Hormone-Positive Breast Cancer

N-Tense has been used for more than 20 years with good results as a natural remedy for breast cancer. The protocols always added extra cat's claw to the N-Tense for hormone-positive cancers. One study compared the actions of cat's claw to Tamoxifen (a drug used for estrogen positive cancers to block estrogen receptors) and reported that cat's claw provided similar results.

If your cancer has BRCA mutations, newer research indicates adding pau d'arco would be beneficial. Only buy a product that extracts pau d'arco in alcohol (a tincture), however. The beneficial chemicals needed are not water soluble. See the plant information for each plant in Part 3 (pages 217 and 284) for more.

The Hormone-Positive Breast Cancer Plan
Recipe

10 parts graviola

4 parts cat's claw

2 parts espinheira santa

1 part bitter melon fruit extract

1 part mullaca

1 part guacatonga

1 part vassourinha

Dosages

Capsules: 2–3 g in capsules, three times daily, based on stage/grade (see page 82); *or*

Tincture or glycerin extract: 1 teaspoon, three times daily; *or*

Infusion/tea: 1 cup, three times daily.

If necessary for BRCA mutations add:

Pau d'arco tincture: 2 ml, three times daily.

Instructions

- Take both remedies together at the same time (for synergistic/additive effects), three times daily.
- This natural remedy can be taken either with or between meals.
- When/if your tumors disappear, take the remedies for two months longer.
- Discontinue use for three months; then follow the instructions for the maintenance dosage and schedule provided on page 82.

BREAST CANCER (HORMONE-NEGATIVE)

Hormone receptor-negative breast cancer means the cancer cells do not have receptors for estrogen and progesterone, meaning they do not respond to hormone therapy. It is important to note that about 25–30% of breast cancers are hormone receptor-negative. Other treatments like surgery, radiation therapy, and chemotherapy are used to treat hormone receptor-negative breast cancer. Hormone negative cancers tend to grow and spread more quickly than hormone receptor-positive cancers and tend to have a less favorable prognosis.

The five-year survival rate for localized disease is 91%. If the cancer has spread to nearby lymph nodes (regional), the rate drops to 66%. If the cancer has metastasized to distant parts of the body, the rate is only 12%. Approximately 50% of patients with earlier-stage hormone negative cancer (stages 1–3) experience a recurrence after standard treatment, often within the first two to three years after diagnosis.

Natural Remedies for Hormone-Negative Breast Cancer

N-Tense has been used for more than 20 years with good results as a natural remedy for breast cancer. Based on newer research adding chanca piedra to target and kill cancer stem cells and primary breast cancer cells may be beneficial. For triple negative breast cancer, which grows and spreads much faster, a more aggressive approach is advised. For this type of cancer, adding anamu and a concentrated bitter melon fruit extract to the plan is beneficial. Additionally, if your cancer has BRCA mutations, newer research indicates adding pau d'arco would be beneficial. Only buy a product that extracts pau d'arco in alcohol (a tincture), however. The beneficial chemicals needed are not water soluble and need extracting in alcohol. There are numerous bitter melon concentrated fruit extracts in capsules available to choose from. See the plant information in Part 3 (pages 198, 207, 226, and 284) for more.

THE HORMONE-NEGATIVE BREAST CANCER PLAN

Recipe

10 parts graviola	2 parts bitter melon fruit extract
2 parts mullaca	1 part guacatonga
2 parts chanca piedra	1 part vassourinha
2 parts espinheira santa	1 part cat's claw

Dosages

Capsules: 2–3 g in capsules, three times daily, based on stage/grade (see page 82); *or*

Tincture or glycerin extract: 1 teaspoon, three times daily; *or*

Infusion/tea: 1 cup, three times daily.

For Triple Negative cancers add:

Anamu: 1.5 g in capsules, three times daily.

If necessary for BRCA mutations add:

Pau d'arco alcohol tincture: 2 ml, three times daily.

Instructions

- Take all remedies together at the same time (for synergistic/additive effects), three times daily.
- They can be taken either with or between meals.
- When/if you achieve remission, take the remedies for two months longer.
- As a maintenance dose, take the remedies for one month, wait for three months, and then take again for one month. Repeat one more time.

BREAST CANCER (HER2-POSITIVE)

About one in five women with breast cancer has a type called HER2-positive and can include both hormone positive and negative cancer types. HER2 stands for human epidermal growth factor receptor 2. This means that the cancer cells have a gene that makes HER2 protein. This protein causes cancer cells to grow and spread quickly. HER2-positive cancers are usually considered more aggressive (they grow more quickly) and more invasive (they spread to other sites more easily). Treatments for HER2-positive breast cancer target the cells that make the protein. This helps to slow the cancer's growth and stop it from spreading. Recurrence rates vary depending on factors like tumor stage and treatment but generally range from 15% to 30% within 10 years after treatment.

Natural Remedies for HER2-Positive Breast Cancer

N-Tense has been used for more than 20 years with good results as a natural remedy for breast cancer. Based on newer research adding anamu and picão preto to the plan will help address HER2-positive cancers. Both plants have a direct toxic action as well as address stem cells and defense mechanisms of HER2-positive breast cancer.

Additionally, if your cancer has BRCA mutations, newer research indicates adding pau d'arco would be beneficial. Only buy a product that extracts pau d'arco in alcohol (a tincture). The beneficial chemicals needed are not water soluble and need extracting in alcohol. See the plant information in Part 3 (pages 198, 284, and 294) for more on these defense mechanisms.

The HER2-Positive Breast Cancer Plan

Recipe

10 parts graviola	1 part bitter melon fruit extract
2 parts anamu	1 part mullaca
2 parts espinheira santa	1 part guacatonga
2 parts picão preto	1 part vassourinha

Dosages

Capsules: 2–3 g in capsules, three times daily, based on stage/grade (see page 82); *or*

Tincture or glycerin extract: 1 teaspoon, three times daily; *or*

Infusion/tea: 1 cup, three times daily.

If necessary for BRCA mutations add:

Pau d'arco tincture: 2 ml, three times daily.

Instructions

- This natural remedy can be taken either with or between meals.
- When/if you achieve remission, take the remedy(s) for two months longer.
- Discontinue use for three months; then follow the instructions for the maintenance dosage and schedule provided on page 82.

CERVICAL CANCER

Cervical cancer is a type of cancer that develops in the cervix, the lower part of the uterus that connects to the vagina. It is usually caused by persistent infection with human papillomavirus (HPV). Early stages may have no noticeable symptoms, which is why routine cervical cancer screening (Pap and/or HPV tests) are recommended for all sexually active women. Cervical cancer is highly treatable in its early stages but gets more difficult in higher stages since it can spread to other sites in the body. Treatment options depend on the cancer stage and type and may include surgery, radiation therapy, chemotherapy, targeted therapy, and immunotherapy.

For early-stage (localized) cervical cancer, the five-year relative survival rate is around 91%. If the cancer has spread to nearby tissues or lymph nodes, the rate is about 60%. If the cancer has spread to distant parts of the body, the rate is approximately 19%. Recurrence rates for stage 1 and 2 cancers are 11–22%, while more advanced stages (stages 2b–4) have a higher recurrence rate of 28–64%.

Natural Remedies for Cervical Cancer

N-Tense has long been used for cervical cancer. If caught at an early stage, all that is needed is just N-Tense capsules. Research indicates that many of the N-Tense ingredients address cervical cancer's defense mechanisms and have a direct anti-cancer action. For late stage or recurrent cervical cancer add pau d'arco. Only use an alcohol tincture of pau d'arco as the beneficial plant chemicals are not water soluble and require extraction in alcohol.

THE CERVICAL CANCER PLAN

Recipe

10 parts graviola

2 parts mullaca

2 parts bitter melon fruit extract

2 parts espinheira santa

1 part guacatonga

1 part vassourinha

1 part picão preto

1 part cat's claw

Dosages

Capsules: 2–3 g in capsules, three times daily, based on stage/grade (see page 82); *or*

Tincture or glycerin extract: 1 teaspoon, three times daily; *or*

Infusion/tea: 1 cup, three times daily.

If necessary (for late stage):

Pau d'arco tincture: 2 ml, three times daily.

Instructions

- This natural remedy can be taken either with or between meals.
- When/if you achieve remission, take the remedy(s) for one month longer.
- Discontinue use for three months; then follow the instructions for the maintenance dosage and schedule provided on page 82.

COLORECTAL CANCER

Colorectal cancer (also known as colon cancer or rectal cancer) is a cancer that starts in the large intestine (colon) or rectum. It is primarily an adenocarcinoma, a cancer of the mucus-secreting cells lining the colon and rectum (although other rarer types exist). It often develops from pre-cancerous polyps, which are abnormal growths in the colon or rectum. Colorectal cancer is one of the most common cancers and is the third leading cause of cancer death in both men and women in the United States. It mostly occurs in people who are 45 years and older.

Early detection through screening is crucial, as it can often be treated more effectively when found early. Currently, only one in three cases are diagnosed at stage 1 or 2. A total of 35–50% of patients present with distant metastasis at diagnosis, and this confers a five-year survival rate of less than 10%. The age you should start screening really depends on your risk factors. Risk factors include age, family history, and inflammatory bowel disease; lifestyle factors like diet, obesity, smoking, and lack of physical activity; and inherited genetic disorders.

The overall five-year survival rate for colorectal cancer is around 65%. This rate varies significantly, however, depending on the stage of the cancer at diagnosis. Early-stage (stage 1) colorectal cancer has a very high five-year survival rate, often exceeding 90%, while late-stage (stage 4) cancer has a much lower rate, around 10–17%.

Colorectal cancer recurrence rates vary based on several factors, including cancer stage, but generally, around 20–30% of patients experience recurrence within five years of initial treatment, with most happening within the first two years. The longer you go without a recurrence, the lower your chances are of having the cancer return. This is why follow-up screening for the first two years is very important.

Natural Remedies for Colorectal Cancer

N-Tense has had very good results with colorectal cancer (CRC) in all stages. It was often combined with another Raintree formula called Amazon Bowel Support, especially if the patient was doing conventional chemotherapy/radiation and/or had stage 3 or 4 CRC. (More information on this product can be found on page 330.) Some of the plants in this formula have direct anti-cancer actions against CRC; others protect against chemo and radiation side effects; and still others have immune system benefits while mitigating CRC defense mechanisms.

THE COLORECTAL CANCER PLAN

Recipe

10 parts graviola	1 part bitter melon fruit extract
2 parts mullaca	1 part vassourinha
2 parts guacatonga	1 part mutamba
2 parts espinheira santa	1 part cat's claw

Dosages

Capsules: 2–3 g, three times daily, based on stage/grade (see page 82); *or*

Tincture or glycerin extract: 1 teaspoon, three times daily; *or*

Infusion/tea: 1 cup, three times daily.

If necessary (for later stage):

Amazon Bowel Support: 1.5 g in capsules, three times daily. (See page 330 for more information about this product.)

Instructions

- Take both remedies at the same time (for synergistic/additive effects), three times daily.
- These natural remedies can be taken either with or between meals.
- When/if you achieve remission, take the remedies for one month longer.
- Discontinue use for three months; then follow the instructions for the maintenance dosage and schedule provided on page 82.

ENDOMETRIAL CANCER

Endometrial cancer is a type of cancer that develops in the lining of the uterus (the endometrium). It is the most common type of gynecologic cancer in women and is also referred to as uterine cancer. The average age at diagnosis for endometrial cancer is 60; it is rare among those younger than 45. It is the fourth most common cancer among women in the United States and the sixth leading cause of cancer-related deaths among women. Approximately 70% of women are diagnosed at stage 1, when the cancer is easiest to treat. Initially, it may spread to nearby organs like the ovaries, fallopian tubes, or cervix (stage 3). It can also spread through lymphatic or blood vessels to distant organs such as the lungs, liver, bones, and brain (stage 4). The lungs are the most common site for distant spread.

Survival rates vary, but overall, the five-year survival rate is high, especially for early-stage localized disease (95%). In stage 2 and 3 where the cancer has spread in the same region, rates drop to 70%. In later stages, when the cancer has spread to distant sites, the five-year survival rate drops to around 18%.

Approximately 15–20% of endometrial cancer patients experience a recurrence after initial treatment, with the majority occurring within the first two to three years. Factors like stage, grade, and lymph node involvement influence the risk of recurrence. Even when the uterus is surgically removed to treat the cancer, there is a chance of recurrence in other areas (most commonly found in the vagina and pelvis). Endometrial cancer can also recur in the ovaries, fallopian tubes, or cervix; this is why radical hysterectomies (which remove all these organs/tissues along with the uterus) are part of the standard level of care for most.

Natural Remedies for Endometrial Cancer

Most of the ingredients in N-Tense have some kind of research indicating that it is toxic to endometrial cancer. In addition, several of the plants in the formula address several main defense mechanisms this cancer uses to become drug resistant, and recur.

Anamu is also toxic to endometrial cancer and addresses another defense mechanism the cancer uses to hide from the immune system as well as recur. It relieves pain as well as reduces inflammation (which has anti-cancer benefits as well). See the plant information in Part 3 (page 198) for more on these defense mechanisms.

THE ENDOMETRIAL CANCER PLAN

Recipe

10 parts graviola	1 part bitter melon
2 parts mullaca	1 part guacatonga
2 parts anamu	1 part vassourinha
2 parts espinheira santa	1 part cat's claw

Dosages

Capsules: 2–3 g, three times daily, based on stage/grade (see page 82); *or*

Tincture or glycerin extract: 1 teaspoon, three times daily; *or*

Infusion/tea: 1 cup, three times daily.

Instructions

- This natural remedy can be taken either with or between meals.
- When/if you achieve remission, take the remedy for two months longer.
- Discontinue use for three months; then follow the instructions for the maintenance dosage and schedule provided on page 82.

ESOPHAGEAL CANCER

Esophageal cancer develops in the esophagus, the tube connecting the throat to the stomach. It is often diagnosed at later stages due to a lack of early symptoms, but early detection and treatment are crucial for a better prognosis. The two main types of esophageal cancer are squamous cell carcinoma and adenocarcinoma. Squamous cell carcinoma (the most prevalent type) develops in the flat, thin cells lining the esophagus, while adenocarcinoma arises in the glandular cells that produce mucus and other fluids.

Esophageal squamous cell carcinoma (ESCC) is an aggressive form of esophageal cancer that is often diagnosed only after the cancer has already spread. This means survival rates for ESCC are much lower than some other cancers. It ranks seventh in incidence and sixth in mortality among all malignancies worldwide. ESCC is primarily caused by tobacco use (including smokeless/vapes) and excessive alcohol consumption. Additionally, other factors like poor diets (low in fruits and vegetables, high in processed meats), drinking very hot beverages, some vitamin deficiencies (beta-carotene, vitamin E, selenium, or iron), and infection with human papillomavirus increases risks.

Esophageal adenocarcinoma (EA) is primarily linked to chronic irritation and changes in the esophageal lining, particularly in the lower esophagus. Key risk factors include gastroesophageal reflux disease (GERD), Barrett's esophagus, obesity, and tobacco use. It has a better prognosis, mainly because it is discovered sooner and at an earlier stage. Doctors usually regularly screen their GERD and Barrett's patients for this cancer and find it in early stages in highly developed countries like the United States.

When treated conventionally with concurrent chemotherapy and radiation, five-year survival rates for esophageal cancers are 48% for stage 1, 20–30% for stage 2 and 3, and 5% for stage 4. Roughly half of patients experience recurrence after treatment, with a significant proportion occurring within the first two years. Recurrences can be local (at the original tumor site), regional (in nearby lymph nodes), or distant (in other organs). Distant metastases are the most common type of recurrence, most commonly in the lungs, liver, and bones.

Natural Remedies for Esophageal Cancer

N-Tense capsules have been used for esophageal cancer for many years. It is one of the cancers that provided rather dramatic results—usually a noticeable and significant reduction in tumor size in as little as two weeks. Oftentimes, as with conventional therapy, many patients were in late stages, and had large tumors that prevented swallowing much besides liquids when they started taking N-Tense.

The advice was (and is) to prepare this remedy as a tea/infusion (see instructions on page 140). Allow the tea to cool to lukewarm and drink slowly. Avoid drinking or eating for at least one hour afterward. Because the tea, full of anti-cancerous plant chemicals, is coming into direct contact with the cancer in the esophagus, the results are pretty rapid. Many switched over to swallowing the capsules after they were eating food again, but if you can tolerate the taste, it will be more effective and work faster taking it as a tea. Quite a few patients were cancer free in two to three months or less, but we did see some recurrences (including some who didn't change their diet/lifestyle to lower their risks).

With all the new research on defense mechanisms and cancer stem cells (which increase the risk of recurrences), we've learned that adding pau d'arco and picão preto to the cancer plan may help lower the risk of specific defense mechanisms this cancer employs and may help kill stem cells to help avoid recurrences. See the plant information in Part 3 (pages 284 and 294) for more on these defense mechanisms. Pau d'arco needs alcohol to extract the active chemicals needed so only purchase a tincture (widely available) and add it to the tea while still very hot.

Adding a tea bag or teaspoon of loose green tea to the N-Tense tea may be beneficial. Green tea contains an abundance of a polyphenol chemical called EGCG. Compelling research reports that EGCG can prevent the self-renewal ability of esophageal squamous carcinoma stem cells and reduce recurrence rates. Alternatively, adding a cup or glass of green tea as a beverage you drink daily as a lifestyle change may be very beneficial as well; just avoid really hot beverages in general and let them cool to lukewarm or drink them iced.

The Esophageal Cancer Plan
Recipe

10 parts graviola	1 part bitter melon
2 parts mullaca	1 part vassourinha
2 parts picão preto	1 part guacatonga
2 parts espinheira santa	1 part cat's claw

Dosages

Capsules: 2–3 g, three times daily, based on stage/grade (see page 82); *or*

Tincture or glycerin extract: 1 teaspoon, three times daily; *or*

Infusion/tea: 1 cup, three times daily.

Pau d'arco alcohol tincture: 2 ml, three times daily, and added to the N-Tense tea while still hot.

Instructions

- These natural remedies can be taken either with or between meals.
- When/if you achieve remission, take the remedies twice daily for three months longer.
- Discontinue use for three months; then follow the instructions for the maintenance dosage and schedule provided on page 82.

GASTRIC CANCER

Gastric cancer, also known as stomach cancer, develops in the stomach lining. There are several types with adenocarcinoma being the most common type (accounting for 90–95% of all stomach cancers), arising from the stomach's glandular cells that line the stomach. While it can occur in anyone, certain factors like age, gender, and lifestyle choices can increase the risk. Other types of gastric cancer include gastrointestinal stromal tumors (GISTs), neuroendocrine tumors (including carcinoid tumors), and lymphomas. These cancers are classified based on the type of cells where the cancer originates and are considered rare.

Overall, gastric cancer incidence rates have decreased over time in the United States and are much lower in highly developed nations like the United States. This is probably due to our regularly and effectively treating one of the main causes of gastric cancer before it causes cancer: *H. pylori* bacterial infections (also one of the leading causes of gastric ulcers).

For localized stomach cancer, the five-year survival rate is approximately 71%, while for regional cancer it drops to 33%, and for distant (metastatic) cancer, it is around 6%. Gastric cancer recurrence rates vary widely, ranging from 14% to 60%, with higher tumor stages (3 and 4) associated with higher recurrence rates.

Natural Remedies for Gastric Cancer

N-Tense has long been used for gastric cancer; however, the number of patients were much lower than other types of cancer. We seem to be doing a pretty good job here in the United States either preventing it or catching this cancer early. The average time it took for those taking N-Tense was two months. Again, like esophageal cancer, if you can get all the anti-cancer chemicals from the N-Tense ingredients in direct contact with the cancer cells in the stomach, the efficacy and speed increases.

Based on more recent research, adding anamu and picão preto to the plan might address all of the defense mechanisms this cancer uses to recur. Both plants have also shown to have direct toxic actions to gastric cancer cells. See the plant information in Part 3 (pages 198 and 294) for more on these defense mechanisms. It is recommended to add these two plants if the cancer has already spread to the local lymph nodes and beyond (stage 2, 3, or 4).

THE GASTRIC CANCER PLAN

Recipe

10 parts graviola

2 parts mullaca

2 parts picão preto

2 parts espinheira santa

1 part melon fruit extract

1 part vassourinha

1 part anamu

1 part guacatonga

1 part cat's claw

Dosages

Capsules: 2–3 g, three times daily, based on stage/grade (see page 82); *or*

Tincture or glycerin extract: 1 teaspoon, three times daily; *or*

Infusion/tea: 1 cup, three times daily.

Instructions

- This natural remedy can be taken either with or between meals.
- When/if you achieve remission, take the remedy for two months longer.
- Discontinue use for three months; then follow the instructions for the maintenance dosage and schedule provided on page 82.

KIDNEY/RENAL CANCER—*see* BLADDER CANCER

LARYNGEAL AND NASOPHARYNGEAL CANCERS

Laryngeal cancer, also known as larynx cancer, is a type of cancer that develops in the tissues of the larynx (voice box). It is a type of head and neck cancer and is more common in men over 60. The larynx plays a vital role in breathing, speaking, and swallowing. The primary type of laryngeal cancer is squamous cell carcinoma, which originates in the thin, flat cells lining the larynx (voice box). Rarer types include adenocarcinoma (originating in mucus-producing cells), sarcomas (cancers of connective tissues), and lymphomas (cancers of lymphatic tissue). The overall five-year survival rate for laryngeal cancer is approximately 77% and 84%, respectively, for stages 1 and 2 and dropping to 46% and 30%, respectively, for stages 3 and 4. Recurrence rates for stage 1 cancers are 5–13%, 25–30% for stage 2, 30% for stage 3, and 50% for stage 4. Different treatment modalities (surgery, radiation, chemotherapy) can affect recurrence rates.

Nasopharyngeal cancer is a less common cancer that develops in the nasopharynx, the upper part of the throat behind the nose. It is more common in certain parts of the world, particularly Southeast Asia. Risk factors include Epstein-Barr virus (EBV) infection and genetic predisposition. It is also known as nasopharyngeal carcinoma (NPC) and has three subtypes (types 1, 2, and 3). It originates from the epithelial cells lining the nasopharynx and is classified as a squamous cell cancer, like laryngeal cancer, and treated in a similar fashion. The overall five-year survival rate for laryngeal cancer is approximately 82% for stage 1 and dropping to 48% at stage 4. The recurrence rate for NPC after initial treatment, which usually involves radiotherapy with or without chemotherapy, ranges from 15% to 58% depending on the stage at diagnosis and lifestyle/dietary habits.

Natural Remedies for Laryngeal and Nasopharyngeal Cancers
Laryngeal and nasopharyngeal cancers always had a very good response rate to N-Tense. For laryngeal cancer, it was recommended to brew a tea with the N-Tense capsules (see instructions on page 140) so that the active chemicals in the formula could come into direct contact with the cancer to provide results more quickly. People with nasopharyngeal cancer can use any type of natural remedy preparation method.

With all the new research on defense mechanisms and cancer stem cells, which we now know increase the risk of recurrences, we've learned that adding pau d'arco and picão preto to the cancer plan may help lower the risk of specific defense mechanisms this cancer employs and may help kill stem cells to help avoid recurrences. See the plant information in Part 3 (pages 284 and 294) for more on these defense mechanisms. Pau d'arco needs alcohol to extract the active chemicals needed so only purchase a tincture (widely available). If you're brewing a tea, put the tincture in the cup with the other herbs before pouring in the boiling water to help evaporate off the alcohol in the tincture.

The Laryngeal and Nasopharyngeal Cancer Plan
Recipe

10 parts graviola

2 parts mullaca

2 parts picão preto

2 parts espinheira santa

1 part bitter melon

1 part vassourinha

1 part guacatonga

1 part cat's claw

Dosages
Infusion/tea: 1 cup, three times daily; *or*

Capsules: 2–3 g, three times daily, based on stage/grade (see page 82); *or*

Tincture or glycerin extract: 1 teaspoon, three times daily.

Pau d'arco tincture: 2 ml, three times daily, and added to the N-Tense tea while still hot.

Instructions

- These natural remedies can be taken either with or between meals.
- When/if you achieve remission, take the remedies for three months longer.
- Discontinue use for three months; then follow the instructions for the maintenance dosage and schedule provided on page 82.

LEUKEMIA

Leukemia is a type of cancer that affects the blood and bone marrow, where blood cells are produced. It's characterized by the uncontrolled production of abnormal white blood cells that don't function properly. These abnormal cells can crowd out healthy blood cells, leading to various complications. Leukemia is classified based on how quickly it progresses (acute or chronic) and the type of white blood cell affected (lymphoid or myeloid). Leukemia can affect both children and adults, with some types being more common in certain age groups. Acute lymphocytic leukemia (ALL) and acute myeloid leukemia (AML) are the acute types, while chronic lymphocytic leukemia (CLL) and chronic myeloid leukemia (CML) are the chronic types.

There are a few more rare types of leukemia but we'll focus on the common types herein. The acute leukemias are more deadly because they grow more rapidly. The five-year survival rate for AML (most common in adults) is 31.9%, and the rate is 72% for ALL (most common in children). The five-year survival rate for CLL is 88.5%, and it is 70% for CML. Leukemia recurrence rates vary significantly depending on the type of leukemia, with some forms having a higher likelihood of returning than others. For example, in ALL, relapse rates can be around 10–15% in children, while for adults, it can be closer to 50%. About 50% of AML patients will experience a relapse. While most leukemia relapses occur within the first few years, late relapses (several years after initial remission) can occur, though they are less common.

Natural Remedies for Leukemia

NTense-2 was created specifically with plant ingredients that had demonstrated anti-leukemic actions. It has been sold for approximately 24 years, becoming a natural herbal remedy for both leukemias and lymphomas. For the chronic leukemias (CLL and CML), generally all that was recommended was the NTense-2 capsules. With all the newer research on defense mechanisms and how this cancer can recur on a molecular level, I would add two other plants to the cancer plan for the acute leukemias (AML and ALL): graviola and chanca piedra. Between these two plants, stem cells can be targeted and five defense mechanisms that leukemia uses to recur can be addressed. See the plant information in Part 3 (pages 226 and 252) for more.

THE LEUKEMIA CANCER PLAN

Recipe for CLL and CML

1 part mullaca	1 part picão preto
1 part anamu	1 part suma
1 part vassourinha	1 part cat's claw
1 part simarouba	1 part espinheira santa

Recipe for AML and ALL

1 part mullaca	1 part picão preto
1 part anamu	1 part chanca piedra
1 part graviola	1 part cat's claw
1 part vassourinha	1 part espinheira santa
1 part simarouba	

Dosages

Capsules: 2–3 g, three times daily, based on stage/grade (see page 82); *or*

Tincture or glycerin extract: 1 teaspoon, three times daily; *or*

Infusion/tea: 1 cup, three times daily.

Instructions

• This natural remedy can be taken either with or between meals.

• When/if you achieve remission, take the remedy for two months longer.

• Discontinue use for three months; then follow the instructions for the maintenance dosage and schedule provided on page 82.

LIVER CANCER

Liver cancer is a disease in which cancerous cells form in the tissues of the liver. It can be primary, meaning it originates in the liver, or secondary, meaning it has spread from another part of the body. The most common type of primary liver cancer is hepatocellular carcinoma (HCC), which develops in the main liver cells called hepatocytes. Risk factors for getting liver cancer includes chronic Hepatitis B and C infections, cirrhosis (scarring of the liver, often caused by chronic hepatitis or excessive alcohol consumption), excessive alcohol consumption, aflatoxins, and nonalcoholic steatohepatitis, a type of fatty liver disease that can lead to cirrhosis.

Liver cancer is often diagnosed at a later stage because symptoms are typically absent in the early stages. This means that by the time symptoms appear, the cancer may have already progressed to an advanced stage. For localized liver cancer, meaning the cancer hasn't spread beyond the liver, the five-year survival rate is 31%. If the cancer has spread to nearby organs or lymph nodes, however, the rate drops to 13%, and if it has spread to distant parts of the body, the rate is only 3%.

The recurrence rate of liver cancer, specifically hepatocellular carcinoma (HCC), after surgery to remove the tumor is high, with estimates ranging from 50% to 70% at five years. Recurrence can happen early (within weeks or months) or late (up to 10 years) after treatment. Several factors influence the risk of recurrence, including tumor size, presence of microvascular invasion, and underlying liver conditions like cirrhosis.

Natural Remedies for Liver Cancer

N-Tense had some great results with liver cancer; however, it was almost always combined with another Raintree formula called Amazon Liver Support. The second formula was especially important for patients with hepatitis infections and damage to the liver from cirrhosis and fatty liver as well as late-stage cancers. Several of the plant ingredients in Liver Support have toxic actions against liver cancer cells, while others have healing, repairing, and protective effects to the liver. (More information on the product can be found on page 330.)

The Liver Cancer Plan

Recipe

10 parts graviola

2 parts mullaca

2 parts guacatonga

2 parts espinheira santa

1 part bitter melon

1 part vassourinha

1 part mutamba

1 part cat's claw

Dosages

Capsules: 2–3 g, three times daily, based on stage/grade (see page 82); *or*

Tincture or glycerin extract: 1 teaspoon, three times daily; *or*

Infusion/tea: 1 cup, three times daily.

Amazon Liver Support: 2 g in capsules, three times daily. (See page 330 for more information about this product.)

Instructions
- Take both remedies together at the same time (for synergistic/additive effects), three times daily.
- They can be taken either with or between meals.
- When/if you achieve remission, take the remedies for two months longer.
- Discontinue use for three months; then follow the instructions for the maintenance dosage and schedule provided on page 82.

LUNG CANCER (SMALL CELL)

Small cell lung cancer (SCLC) represents between 13% and 15% of all new cases of lung cancers. It is a highly aggressive form of lung cancer that originates from neuroendocrine cells in the lungs and is considered a neuroendocrine tumor. A neuroendocrine tumor (NET) is a rare type of cancer that develops from neuroendocrine cells, which are cells that have characteristics of both nerve cells and hormone-producing cells. These cells and resulting tumors are found in various parts of the body, including in or on the outside of the lungs/bronchus. SCLC is known for its rapid growth and tendency to spread to other parts of the body easily. Luckily, SCLC readily responds to chemotherapy and/or radiation as well as plant-based therapies, often times reducing or eliminating initial tumors rather quickly. The reason it has such a poor prognosis is because this cancer can regularly return a few months to a year later to form new tumors which are drug resistant and grow even more quickly. NET tumors have several different and highly effective defense mechanisms that allow them to hide from detection and recur.

The estimated five-year overall survival rate is 42.9% with chemo/radiation followed by immunotherapy. The five-year survival rate for limited-stage small cell lung cancer (LS-SCLC) without it is typically around 25–30%. Unfortunately, approximately 70% of new SCLC diagnoses are extensive-stage (the cancer has already spread outside the lungs), which has a survival rate without treatment of 2–4 months and 7–11 months with standard chemo/radiation treatment. Immunotherapy has increased the five-year survival rate from 1–2% to around 12% in extensive late-stage SCLC.

Natural Remedies for Small Cell Lung Cancer

The natural remedy plan is to use the plants in the N-Tense formula to fight the tumor(s) (including previously treated and drug-resistant tumors) and to add plants that will target the specific mechanisms that this cancer uses to return and to become drug resistant. The graviola in the N-Tense formula can address one defense mechanism and one type of drug resistance, and adding more espinheira santa (already in N-Tense) can better address a third defense mechanism. Importantly, adding picão preto and pau d'arco can help the N-Tense ingredients target and/or kill cancer stem cells and another defensive molecule in two different ways (the fourth and strongest mechanism that enables the cancer to return). See the plant information in Part 3 (pages 284 and 294) for more on these defense mechanisms. Only purchase an alcohol tincture of pau d'arco as the active plant chemicals needed are not water soluble and must be extracted in alcohol.

The Small Cell Lung Cancer Plan

Recipe

10 parts graviola	1 part bitter melon fruit extract
3 parts espinheira santa	1 part vassourinha
2 parts picão preto	1 part mullaca
1 part guacatonga	1 part cat's claw

Dosages

Capsules: 2–3 g, three times daily, based on stage/grade (see page 82); *or*

Tincture or glycerin extract: 1 teaspoon, three times daily; *or*

Infusion/tea: 1 cup, three times daily.

Pau d'arco tincture: 2 ml, three times daily.

Instructions

- These natural remedies can be taken either with or between meals.
- When/if you achieve remission, take the remedies for two months longer.
- Discontinue use for three months; then follow the instructions for the maintenance dosage and schedule provided on page 82.

LUNG CANCER (NON-SMALL CELL)

Non–small cell lung cancer (NSCLC) is a type of lung cancer that includes several subtypes, the most common being adenocarcinoma, squamous cell carcinoma, and large cell carcinoma. It is the most prevalent form of lung cancer, accounting for roughly 85% of cases. NSCLC is characterized by uncontrolled growth of epithelial cells in the lungs. NSCLC is categorized into three main subtypes: adenocarcinoma, squamous cell carcinoma, and large cell carcinoma. Smoking is the leading risk factor, but NSCLC can also occur in nonsmokers. Treatment options vary based on the stage and subtype of NSCLC, and it may include surgery, chemotherapy, radiation therapy, and targeted therapy. Advances in treatment, including targeted therapies and immunotherapies, have improved survival rates, especially for certain subtypes and stages of NSCLC. Adenocarcinomas have a better prognosis than squamous cell carcinomas.

Around 65% of patients with localized NSCLC (cancer confined to the lung) survive five years or longer. The survival rate decreases to about 37% for stage 2 and 3 and drops to 6% at stage 4. Early-stage NSCLC (stage 1) can have recurrence rates between 5% and 19% and between 11% and 27% for stage 2. Advanced stages may experience recurrence in 24–40% of cases in stage 3 and around 66% for stage 4.

Natural Remedies for Non–Small Cell Lung Cancer

N-Tense had a very good response to NSCLC and has been used for more than 20 years as a natural remedy for this cancer. Newer research indicates that adding anamu and chanca piedra to the plan might help reduce recurrences and address specific defense mechanisms that this cancer uses to become drug resistant, proliferate, and metastasize.

THE NON–SMALL CELL LUNG CANCER PLAN

Recipe

10 parts graviola

2 parts chanca piedra

2 parts anamu

2 parts espinheira santa

1 part bitter melon fruit extract

1 part guacatonga

1 part mullaca

1 part vassourinha

1 part cat's claw

Dosages

Capsules: 2–3 g, three times daily, based on stage/grade (see page 82); *or*

Tincture or glycerin extract: 1 teaspoon, three times daily; *or*

Infusion/tea: 1 cup, three times daily.

Instructions

- This natural remedy can be taken either with or between meals.
- When/if you achieve remission, take the remedy for two months longer.

- Discontinue use for three months; then follow the instructions for the maintenance dosage and schedule provided on page 82.

LYMPHOMA

Lymphoma is a cancer that originates in the lymphatic system, a part of the body's immune system, and specifically affects lymphocytes, a type of white blood cell. It's characterized by the abnormal growth and multiplication of lymphocytes, which can lead to the formation of tumors in lymph nodes and other parts of the body. There are more than 20 different types of lymphoma with the two main types being Hodgkin lymphoma (HL) and non-Hodgkin lymphoma (NHL). In the United States, NHL is one of the most common cancers, accounting for about 4% of all cancers.

Aggressive lymphomas are fast-growing types of NHL that require prompt treatment. Common aggressive NHL subtypes include diffuse large B-cell lymphoma, Burkitt lymphoma, mantle cell lymphoma, peripheral T-cell lymphoma, and lymphoblastic lymphoma. B-cell lymphomas account for the vast majority (85%) of all NHL cases and are formed in a type of white blood cell called a B-cell.

The lymphatic system includes lymph nodes, lymphatic vessels, and other tissues that help fight infections. Lymphoma disrupts the normal function of this system. It is classified as a "hematological" or blood cancer. NHL is more common in men, individuals over 65, and those with autoimmune diseases or family history of blood cancers. HL often affects young adults (20–34 age group) and older adults (55+). HL is more common in males and individuals with a history of certain infections (like Epstein-Barr virus) or autoimmune diseases.

Lymphoma treatment varies based on the specific type and stage of the cancer, but common approaches include chemotherapy, radiation therapy, immunotherapy, targeted therapy, and stem cell transplantation (bone marrow transplant). For certain lymphomas, particularly early-stage or slow-growing types, watchful waiting or active surveillance may be appropriate. Treatment for lymphoma, particularly with chemotherapy and radiation, can increase the risk of developing a second cancer later in life (especially leukemia).

The five-year survival rate for HL is generally very high, often around 90%, while the five-year survival rate for NHL is around 74%. These are general statistics, however, and the actual survival rate can vary significantly based on several factors, including the specific type of lymphoma, the stage at diagnosis, the patient's age and overall health, and how well the lymphoma responds to treatment. HL has a recurrence rate of around 5% (early stage) to 30% (late stage). The recurrence rate of lymphoma also varies significantly based on several factors, including the specific type of lymphoma, the stage at diagnosis, and the type of initial treatment received.

Natural Remedies for Lymphoma

NTense-2 was designed specifically for blood cancers such as lymphomas and leukemias. It has long been used as a natural remedy for most of the common lymphomas for many years with good results. The plan then and now is to add graviola to this formula. Graviola has specific ways it can find the lymphoma cells and kill them; it also shuts down defense mechanisms that allow the cells to become drug resistant and metastasize.

THE LYMPHOMA CANCER PLAN

Recipe

1 part mullaca	1 part picão preto
1 part anamu	1 part graviola
1 part vassourinha	1 part cat's claw
1 part simarouba	1 part espinheira santa

Dosages

Capsules: 2–3 g, three times daily, based on stage/grade (see page 82); *or*

Tincture or glycerin extract: 1 teaspoon, three times daily; *or*

Infusion/tea: 1 cup, three times daily.

Instructions

- This natural remedy can be taken either with or between meals.
- When/if you achieve remission, take the remedy for two months longer.
- Discontinue use for three months; then follow the instructions for the maintenance dosage and schedule provided on page 82.

MELANOMA

Melanoma is a type of skin cancer that develops in melanocytes, the cells that produce melanin (the pigment that gives skin its color). Melanoma is the most serious type of skin cancer, but it is highly curable if detected and treated early. Regular skin self-exams and sun protection measures are essential for early detection and prevention. While melanoma is less frequent than other types of skin cancers, it is responsible for the majority of skin cancer–related deaths. Rates of melanoma are rising rapidly, especially in younger people. In fact, cases of melanoma have tripled in the last 30 years, at a time when cancer rates for other common cancers have declined. Melanoma can be broadly categorized into cutaneous (on the skin), mucosal (in mucus membranes), and ocular melanoma (in the eye). Cutaneous melanoma, the most common type, is further classified into subtypes like superficial spreading, nodular, lentigo maligna, and acral lentiginous melanoma.

The five-year survival rate for melanoma varies significantly based on stage at diagnosis. When detected and treated early (stages 0, 1, 2), the survival rate is very high, often exceeding 99%. When melanoma has spread to nearby lymph nodes (stage 3), the five-year survival rate is around 66% and when it has spread to distant sites, the survival rate drops to 15–50%. Overall, 2–5% of melanomas are estimated to recur, but this can be higher for advanced stages. Higher-stage melanomas (thicker, with ulceration, or involving lymph nodes) have a higher risk of recurrence and tend to recur faster. While many recurrences happen within two to three years, some can occur much later—even more than 10 years after the initial diagnosis. Recurrences can happen in the same skin area or in distant sites (lungs, liver, brain, or other organs).

Natural Remedies for Melanoma

N-Tense capsules have been used as a natural remedy for melanoma for more than 20 years. Results have varied with about 50% seeing benefits. Based on all the new research on chanca piedra, I would try adding it to the cancer plan to see if better results are achieved. Newer research reports that chanca piedra has six different ways to kill melanoma cancer cells, and it prevents several defense mechanisms.

The Melanoma Cancer Plan

Recipe

10 parts graviola

2 parts mullaca

2 parts chanca piedra

2 parts espinheira santa

1 part bitter melon fruit extract

1 part vassourinha

1 part guacatonga

1 part cat's claw

Dosages

Capsules: 2–3 g, three times daily, based on stage/grade (see page 82); *or*

Tincture or glycerin extract: 1 teaspoon, three times daily; *or*

Infusion/tea: 1 cup, three times daily.

Instructions

- This natural remedy can be taken either with or between meals.
- When/if you achieve remission, take the remedy for one month longer.
- Discontinue use for three months; then follow the instructions for the maintenance dosage and schedule provided on page 82.

MULTIPLE MYELOMA

Multiple myeloma (MM) is a cancer that develops from plasma cells, a type of white blood cell in the bone marrow. MM is classified as a blood cancer. These cancerous plasma cells, called myeloma cells, multiply uncontrollably and produce abnormal antibodies. The abnormal antibodies can lead to various complications like bone damage, kidney problems, and immune system issues. Multiple myeloma is considered treatable but is generally not curable. Treatments can induce remission and manage symptoms. Many people with multiple myeloma live for many years with treatment and support. Survival rates vary depending on factors like the stage of the disease, age, and overall health. Early-stage multiple myeloma has a higher five-year survival rate (around 82% for stage 1 and 69% for stage 2) than later stages (around 60% for stage 3 and 40% for stage 4).

Multiple myeloma is known to relapse, and the rate can vary based on factors like the initial stage and individual patient characteristics. Most people with multiple myeloma will experience periods of remission and relapse throughout the course of their disease. While some patients may experience remission for several years, others may relapse sooner, even within the first year. Unlike many other cancers, MM doesn't have as many defense mechanisms to become drug resistant. If a patient relapses, doctors will often consider reusing the same therapy that induced the initial remission, as it may still be effective, especially if the remission lasted for a year or longer.

Natural Remedies for Multiple Myeloma

NTense-2 capsules were specially designed for blood cancers like multiple myeloma and have been used as a natural remedy for blood cancers for more than 20 years with good results. Adding a pau d'arco alcohol tincture to the plan should help avoid relapse because it disables most of the defense mechanisms this cancer uses as well as targets cancer stem cells. The beneficial plant chemicals in pau d'arco must be extracted from the bark in alcohol, so avoid buying capsules and instead buy an alcohol tincture.

THE MULTIPLE MYELOMA CANCER PLAN

Recipe

1 part mullaca	1 part picão preto
1 part anamu	1 part suma
1 part vassourinha	1 part cat's claw
1 part simarouba	1 part espinheira santa

Dosages

Capsules: 2–3 g, three times daily, based on stage/grade (see page 82); *or*

Tincture or glycerin extract: 1 teaspoon, three times daily; *or*

Infusion/tea: 1 cup, three times daily.

Pau d'arco tincture: 2 ml, three times daily.

Instructions

- Take both remedies together at the same time (for synergistic/additive effects), three times daily.
- They can be taken either with or between meals.
- When/if you achieve remission, take the remedies for one month longer.
- Discontinue use for three months; then follow the instructions for the maintenance dosage and schedule provided on page 82.

NASOPHARYNGEAL CANCER—see LARYNGEAL CANCER

ORAL CANCER

Oral cancer is a malignant tumor that can develop on the lips, tongue, gums, floor of the mouth, and other areas of the mouth and throat. Early detection is crucial for successful treatment, so regular dental checkups are recommended. The most common type is squamous cell carcinoma (representing about 90% of oral cancers), which originates in the thin, flat squamous cells lining the mouth and throat. Risk factors include tobacco use, excessive alcohol consumption, and HPV infection. Other types of oral cancers include verrucous carcinoma, salivary gland cancers, lymphomas (which can occur in the tonsils or base of the tongue), and melanomas (which occur in the gums or roof of the mouth).

If the cancer is found and treated before it spreads (stage 1), the five-year survival rate can be as high as 80–90%. The survival rate drops to around 60–70% for cancers that have spread to nearby areas or nearby lymph nodes in the neck (stage 2 and 3). If the cancer has spread to distant parts of the body, survival rates drop to around 30–40%. Approximately 20–47% of patients experience recurrence after initial treatment, depending on the stage at diagnosis and initial treatment. Recurrence can manifest as local recurrence in the same area, second primary tumors, or metastases to lymph nodes or distant sites like the lungs or bones.

Natural Remedies for Oral Cancer

N-Tense has been used for many years as a natural remedy for oral cancers. It is best to prepare this remedy as a tea/infusion. This increases efficacy and speed by getting the anti-cancerous plant chemicals in direct contact with the cancer. It really is worth it, despite the bad taste of the tea. See page 140 for instructions on making a tea/infusion. Once the tea has cooled to lukewarm, drink slowly, swishing around in the mouth before swallowing. Avoid drinking or eating for at least one hour afterward.

Adding chanca piedra to the tea will be very beneficial as it addresses several of the defense mechanisms this cancer uses to become drug resistant and recur.

For oral lymphomas see the cancer plan and instructions in the "Lymphoma" section.

For oral melanomas, see the cancer plan and instructions in the "Melanoma" section.

THE ORAL CANCER PLAN
Recipe

10 parts graviola	1 part mullaca
3 parts espinheira santa	1 part vassourinha
2 parts chanca piedra	1 part guacatonga
1 part bitter melon fruit extract	1 part cat's claw

Dosages
Infusion/tea: 1 cup, three times daily. Use one rounded teaspoon of the plant powder combination per 6 ounces of boiling water in a teacup.

Instructions
- This natural remedy can be taken either with or between meals.
- When/if you achieve remission, take the remedy for one month longer.
- Discontinue use for three months; then follow the instructions for the maintenance dosage and schedule provided on page 82.

OVARIAN CANCER

Ovarian cancer is a disease where cancerous cells form in the ovaries, the female reproductive organs that produce eggs. It is often called a "silent disease" because symptoms may not appear until later stages. Most ovarian cancers are epithelial ovarian carcinomas, which originate in the cells covering the ovaries. Other types include germ cell tumors and stromal cell tumors. Ovarian cancer ranks as the eighth most common cancer among women globally. While not the most common cancer, it is the deadliest gynecologic cancer.

The five-year survival rate for ovarian cancer varies significantly based on the stage at diagnosis. If the cancer is found early (localized to the ovary), the five-year survival rate can be as high as 90–92%. For advanced stages, the five-year survival rate is much lower, around 30%. Ovarian cancer grows quickly and can progress from early stages to an advanced stage within a year. Most patients are diagnosed after the cancer has spread (metastasized) from the ovaries to other areas of the body (stages 3 and 4). This is because early-stage ovarian cancer often has vague or no symptoms. The large majority of ovarian cancer cases are diagnosed in postmenopausal women, with 63 being the average age at diagnosis.

About 10–20% of women with early-stage ovarian cancer will experience a recurrence (stages 1 and 2). Recurrence rates for advanced-stage ovarian cancer (stages 3 and 4) are 70% and 95%, respectively.

Natural Remedies for Ovarian Cancer

N-Tense has long been used as a natural remedy for ovarian cancer with mixed results. This particular cancer is hard to treat conventionally as well as naturally. In my personal experience, it benefited about 45–50% who took it. Those benefits, however, were mostly disease stabilization (the tumor reduced in size and then stopped growing but didn't disappear) in late-stage cancers. Or, in earlier stages, the cancer disappeared but then recurred in a year or two. It seemed as long as they continued to take the N-Tense, their results were sustained, with several patients I knew personally remaining stable for longer than five years. The disease progressed quite rapidly, however, when they stopped taking it.

With all the new information on how cancer behaves on a molecular and genetic level and what signaling pathways they use to thrive and survive, when I started really looking at the new research, I quickly understood why this particular cancer was so hard to treat. Researchers have discovered (to date) at least 32 different mechanisms that ovarian cancer uses to avoid death, recur, and metastasize in 22 different signaling pathways. And it's likely to be much more than that—researchers just haven't found them all. It has 12 different mechanisms to choose from just to become drug resistant (which it does quite well).

Based on all the new research, I would have to add four more plants to the cancer plan to hope to address the majority of the defense mechanisms this cancer uses. These plants include chanca piedra, picão preto, anamu, and pau d'arco. These plants are available in capsules; however, only purchase an alcohol tincture of pau d'arco. The beneficial plant chemicals in the plant aren't water soluble and need alcohol to extract them.

THE OVARIAN CANCER PLAN
Recipe

10 parts graviola

2 parts mullaca

2 parts picão preto

2 parts espinheira santa

1 part bitter melon fruit extract

1 part anamu

1 part guacatonga

1 part vassourinha

1 part cat's claw

Dosages

Capsules: 3 g, three times daily; *or*

Tincture or glycerin extract: 1 teaspoon, three times daily; *or*

Infusion/tea: 1 cup, three times daily.

Chanca piedra in capsules: 1.5 g, three times daily.

Pau d'arco tincture: 2 ml, three times daily.

Instructions

- Take all products together at the same time (for synergistic/additive effects), three times daily.
- They can be taken either with or between meals.
- When/if you achieve remission, take the remedies for two months longer.
- Discontinue use for three months; then follow the instructions for the maintenance dosage and schedule provided on page 82.

PANCREATIC CANCER

Pancreatic cancer is a disease where cancer cells form in the tissues of the pancreas, a gland located behind the stomach. It's often difficult to detect early, and the prognosis is generally poor, though survival rates vary depending on the stage at diagnosis. Pancreatic cancer is primarily categorized into exocrine and neuroendocrine tumors, with exocrine being more common and neuroendocrine harder to treat. The most prevalent type is adenocarcinoma, originating in the cells lining the pancreatic ducts. Neuroendocrine tumors develop from hormone-producing cells in the pancreas and are less frequent.

In the United States, pancreatic cancer rates are rising (probably due to an aging population and rising rates of type 2 diabetes) and has a high mortality rate. This is because it often doesn't cause noticeable symptoms in the early stages. Many patients are diagnosed after the cancer has already spread to the liver, lungs, or other locations (stage 4). It is the third leading cause of cancer-related death and is expected to be the second leading cause by 2030. While it can take a decade or more for the initial cancer cell to develop into a detectable tumor, the transition from an early stage to a more advanced and inoperable state can be rapid (a little over a year).

The life expectancy for pancreatic cancer varies significantly based on stage at diagnosis. Early-stage pancreatic cancer (stage 1 and 2) has a five-year survival rate of around 44%, while stage 3 pancreatic cancer has a survival rate of 13%. In advanced cancers (stage 4), survival rate drops to just 3%. Pancreatic cancer recurrence is unfortunately common, with up to 80% of patients experiencing it after potentially curative surgery (usually stages 1 and 2 before the cancer spreads outside of the pancreas). Many recurrences happen within the first two years following surgery. A small percentage (around 10%) of patients, however, can achieve long-term disease-free survival after surgery. Recurrences can be local (within the pancreas or surrounding tissues), distant (in other organs like the liver or lungs), or a combination of both. Recurrent tumors are usually drug resistant and grow quickly.

Natural Remedies for Pancreatic Cancer

N-Tense has long been used as a natural remedy for pancreatic cancer with mixed results. This particular cancer (like ovarian cancer) is particularly hard to treat conventionally as well as naturally. In my personal experience, it benefited about 40–50% who took it. Those benefits, however, were mostly disease stabilization (the tumor reduced in size and then stopped growing but didn't disappear) in late-stage cancers. Or, in earlier stages, the cancer disappeared but then recurred in a year or two. It seemed as long as they continued to take the N-Tense, their results were sustained, with several I knew personally remaining stable for longer than five years.

Based on all the new research, I would have to add several more plants to the cancer plan to address the majority of the defense mechanisms this cancer uses. This is an aggressive cancer needing an aggressive approach. First, add pau d'arco. A natural pau d'arco chemical is a new small-molecule drug in human trials showing it seeks out and selectively kills pancreatic cancer cells in a novel manner. Other chemicals in pau d'arco directly kill the cancer, as well as stem cells in several different ways. Only purchase an alcohol tincture of pau d'arco since this chemical is not water soluble and needs alcohol to extract it.

Bitter melon juice provides six different mechanisms of action against pancreatic cancer; however, there is not enough of this ingredient in N-Tense to replicate the compelling newer research on it targeting and killing cancer stem cells to avoid relapse. Therefore, I'm adding a concentrated spray-dried or freeze-dried extract of bitter melon juice. Quite a few of these products are available in capsules and are the easiest to take (many find the concentrated juice has an unpleasant bitter taste and avoid liquid extracts).

Finally, I added anamu to the formula recipe. Based on earlier test-tube and animal studies, a new anamu herbal drug was created and is now in human Phase II clinical trials for pancreatic and gastric cancers in Colombia. Other research shows anamu can kill pancreatic cancer in at least five different ways, including stem cells.

The Pancreatic Cancer Plan

Recipe

10 parts graviola

3 parts espinheira santa

2 parts mullaca

2 parts anamu

1 part vassourinha

1 part guacatonga

1 part cat's claw

Dosages

Capsules: 3 g, three times daily; *or*

Tincture or glycerin extract: 1 teaspoon, three times daily; *or*

Infusion/tea: 1 cup, three times daily.

Pau d'arco tincture: 2 ml, three times daily.

Bitter melon fruit juice extract capsules: 1 g, three times daily.

Instructions

- Take all remedies together at the same time (for synergistic/additive effects), three times daily.
- They can be taken either with or between meals.
- When/if you achieve remission, take the remedies for two months longer.
- Discontinue use for three months; then follow the instructions for the maintenance dosage and schedule provided on page 82.

PROSTATE CANCER

Prostate cancer is a type of cancer that develops in the prostate gland, a small gland in males that produces seminal fluid. It's one of the most common cancers in men, and while it often grows slowly and can be successfully treated, some types can be more aggressive and spread to other parts of the body. Prostate cancer is a significant health concern, being the second leading cause of cancer death in American men. Prostate cancer is primarily classified into types based on cell origin. The most common type is adenocarcinoma, which develops from the gland cells of the prostate. Other, less common types include small cell carcinoma, neuroendocrine tumors, transitional cell carcinoma, and sarcomas.

The Gleason score, along with Grade Groups, helps doctors assess the aggressiveness of prostate cancer. The Gleason score is a system used to grade prostate cancer based on how abnormal the cancer cells look under a microscope. It ranges from 2 to 10, with lower scores indicating less aggressive cancer. Nonaggressive prostate cancer, also known as low-grade (grade 1), is a type of prostate cancer that is characterized by its slow progression and low risk of spreading (Gleason score of 6 or less). Many men with this type of cancer may not require immediate treatment and can be managed with active surveillance (monitoring the cancer's progression). A Gleason score of 7 in prostate cancer indicates intermediate-grade cancer, with a higher likelihood of tumor growth. A score of 8, 9, or 10 represents high-grade tumors that are likely to grow and spread quickly and are treated more aggressively.

The five-year survival rate for prostate cancer in the United States is generally very high but varies significantly based on the stage of the cancer at diagnosis. For localized and regional prostate cancer (cancer contained within the prostate or surrounding areas), the five-year survival rate is nearly 100%. When the cancer has spread to distant parts of the body (distant stage), the five-year survival rate drops to around 37%. Approximately 20–30% of men treated for prostate cancer will experience a recurrence, even after initial successful treatment like surgery or radiation. The risk of recurrence varies based on factors like the initial cancer's stage, grade, and individual patient characteristics.

Natural Remedies for Prostate Cancer

Raintree probably helped more men with prostate cancer than any other type of cancer because it is so common. Word-of-mouth referrals reporting how well it worked is what fueled the sale of N-Tense capsules as an effective natural remedy for prostate cancer. It was routinely combined with another Raintree formula called Amazon Prostate Support. This formula helped direct the anti-cancer plants to the prostate more efficiently, reduced inflammation, and relieved some of the symptoms of prostate cancer. Some of the ingredients of Prostate Support are also the subject of research for prostate cancer as well. This combination of products always worked faster and more efficiently than N-Tense alone. (More information on this product can be found on page 330.)

THE PROSTATE CANCER PLAN

Recipe

10 parts graviola

2 parts mullaca

2 parts guacatonga

2 parts espinheira santa

1 part bitter melon fruit extract

1 part vassourinha

1 part mutamba

1 part cat's claw

Dosages

Capsules: 2–3 g, three times daily; *or*

Tincture or glycerin extract: 1 teaspoon, three times daily; *or*

Tea/infusion: 1 cup, three times daily.

Amazon Prostate Support capsules: 1.5 g in capsules, three times daily. (See page 330 for more information about this product.)

Instructions

- Take both remedies together at the same time (for synergistic/additive effects), three times daily.
- They can be taken either with or between meals.
- When/if you achieve remission, take the remedies for two months longer.
- Discontinue use for three months; then follow the instructions for the maintenance dosage and schedule provided on page 82.

SARCOMAS—*see* BONE CANCERS

SKIN CANCERS

Skin cancer is an abnormal growth of skin cells, often caused by sun exposure. The main types are basal cell carcinoma, squamous cell carcinoma, and melanoma. See the separate "Melanoma" section. The type of skin cancer a person gets is determined by where the cancer begins. If the cancer begins in skin cells called basal cells, the person has basal cell skin cancer (BCC). BCCs often look like a flesh-colored round growth, pearl-like bump, or a pinkish patch of skin. They usually develop after years of frequent sun exposure or indoor tanning and are common on the head, neck, and arms; however, they can form anywhere.

Squamous cell carcinoma (SCC) of the skin is the second most common type of skin cancer. Squamous cells are located in the upper layers of the skin, near the surface. People who have light skin are most likely to develop SCC. It often looks like a red firm bump, scaly patch, or a sore that heals and then reopens. While generally treatable, it can be more likely to grow deeper and spread than BCC.

The five-year relative survival rate for skin cancer is generally excellent, with 100% for BCC and 95% for SCC, when detected early. Approximately 20% of patients with skin cancer will experience a recurrence at some point, especially if the BCC or SCC was large, deeply invasive, or not completely removed.

Natural Remedies for Skin Cancer

After many practitioner requests, I developed an N-Tense formula that could be used topically on standard skin cancers such as basal cell and squamous cell carcinomas. It had a huge following and worked well. If it doesn't react at all to the extract, it's probably a non-cancerous spot on the skin. Depending on the size of the cancer, it can take as little as a week and up to a month or a little longer to disappear. If the spot reacted to the topical extract but still isn't healed completely after a month, schedule an appointment with your dermatologist. The spot may be a melanoma and needs to be biopsied (see the information in the "Melanoma" section).

Please note, this product will temporarily stain the skin and may permanently stain other surfaces and clothing reddish-brown. Also note this product is unlike other skin cancer products on the market called "black salves" or "drawing salves" that are corrosive to the skin, leave scars, and/or can remove flesh. This product leaves no scars and the "reaction" seen looks like a minor irritation with a tad of inflammation, not the corrosive damage the black salves create.

THE SKIN CANCER PLAN

N-Tense Topical Recipe

See the full recipe and instructions on page 138.

Instructions

- Soak the affected area with a wet, warm wash rag or paper towel to gently remove any scab.

- Place 3–4 drops of the extract on the affected area to cover completely and let dry completely.

- See full instructions on page 138.

TESTICULAR CANCER

Testicular cancer is a disease where cancerous cells form in one or both testicles. It's the most common cancer in young and middle-aged men, typically diagnosed between the ages of 20 and 34. While rare overall, it's highly treatable and often curable, especially when detected early. The majority of testicular cancers are called germ cell tumors, which originate from cells that produce sperm. There are two main types of germ cell tumors: seminomas and non-seminomas. Seminomas tend to grow slower and respond well to radiation and chemotherapy. Non-seminomas are more common in younger men and tend to grow faster.

Testicular cancer generally has a very high survival rate, with most patients experiencing a normal life expectancy after treatment. More than 95% of men diagnosed with testicular cancer survive at least five years, and the cure rate can be as high as 90%. Localized testicular cancer (confined to the testicle) has a 99% five-year survival rate, while even regional cancer (spread to nearby lymph nodes) has a 96% five-year survival rate. Treatment typically involves surgery (removing the cancerous testicle), and sometimes chemotherapy or radiation therapy, and is often successful in curing the cancer. The overall crude relapse rate is 8–19.3%, with most relapses occurring in the first two years.

Natural Remedies for Testicular Cancer

N-Tense has been used as a natural remedy for testicular cancer with good results for numerous years. It worked well on its own and with a low relapse rate, there wasn't a need to add anything else. Most of the N-Tense ingredients addressed the defense mechanisms this cancer uses. If you are dealing with a recurrence of testicular cancer, or worry about a relapse based on the type of testicular cancer you have, you can add a concentrated spray-dried or freeze-dried extract of bitter melon juice. Research reports that, in dosages higher than what N-Tense provides, this juice can selectively target testicular cancer stem cells and kill them in various ways. These concentrated fruit extracts of bitter melon are available from several larger manufacturers and are sold as dry extract powders in capsules or bulk. Capsules are typically preferred, and as the name indicates, the juice tastes bitter. See the plant information in Part 3 (page 207) for more on the new research.

The Testicular Cancer Plan

Recipe

10 parts graviola	1 part bitter melon fruit extract
2 parts mullaca	1 part vassourinha
2 parts guacatonga	1 part mutamba
2 parts espinheira santa	1 part cat's claw

Dosages

Capsules: 2–3 g, three times daily, based on stage/grade (see page 82); *or*

Tincture or glycerin extract: 1 teaspoon, three times daily; *or*

Infusion/tea: 1 cup, three times daily.

If needed/desired:

Bitter melon fruit extract in capsules: 1 g, three times daily.

Instructions

- Take both remedies together at the same time (for synergistic/additive effects), three times daily.
- They can be taken either with or between meals.
- When/if you achieve remission, take the remedies for two months longer.
- Discontinue use for three months; then follow the instructions for the maintenance dosage and schedule provided on page 82.

THYROID CANCER

Thyroid cancer is a disease where malignant (cancerous) cells form in the tissues of the thyroid gland. The thyroid, a butterfly-shaped gland at the base of the neck, produces hormones that regulate the body's energy use. There are multiple types of thyroid cancer, including papillary, follicular, medullary, anaplastic, and Hurthle cell thyroid cancers. Papillary thyroid cancer is the most common type, which is often slow growing and typically affects one lobe of the thyroid. Anaplastic thyroid cancer is the deadliest; average median survival is generally four to five months after diagnosis. All anaplastic thyroid cancers are considered stage 4 at diagnosis because they are aggressive and can spread quickly.

Women are three times more likely to get thyroid cancer than men. In the United States, thyroid cancer is relatively common. While it's not one of the most prevalent cancers overall, it's the 13th most commonly diagnosed cancer and the sixth most common in women. Although it can occur at any age, it generally affects people ages 30 to 50. The incidence of thyroid cancer has been increasing, particularly in women, though mortality rates remain low.

The overall five-year survival rate for thyroid cancer is very high, around 98%. Survival rates vary significantly, however, depending on the stage and type of cancer. For example, localized (early stage) papillary and follicular thyroid cancers have survival rates near 100%. Papillary and follicular thyroid cancer recurrence rates vary depending on several factors, but generally, it's considered to have a high survival rate with a lower recurrence risk (2–20%).

Natural Remedies for Thyroid Cancer

N-Tense has long been used as a natural remedy for thyroid cancer with good results. It worked well on its own and with a low relapse rate, there wasn't a need to add anything else. Most of the N-Tense ingredients address the defense mechanisms this cancer uses. If you are dealing with a recurrence of thyroid cancer, or worry about a relapse based on the type of cancer you have, you can add chanca piedra to the cancer plan. Research reports that it can selectively target cancer stem cells and kill them in various ways. See the plant information in Part 3 (page 226) for more.

THE THYROID CANCER PLAN

Recipe

10 parts graviola

2 parts mullaca

2 parts guacatonga

2 parts espinheira santa

1 part bitter melon fruit extract

1 part vassourinha

1 part mutamba

1 part cat's claw

The Testicular Cancer Plan

Recipe

10 parts graviola

2 parts mullaca

2 parts guacatonga

2 parts espinheira santa

1 part bitter melon fruit extract

1 part vassourinha

1 part mutamba

1 part cat's claw

Dosages

Capsules: 2–3 g, three times daily, based on stage/grade (see page 82); *or*

Tincture or glycerin extract: 1 teaspoon, three times daily; *or*

Infusion/tea: 1 cup, three times daily.

If needed/desired:

Bitter melon fruit extract in capsules: 1 g, three times daily.

Instructions

- Take both remedies together at the same time (for synergistic/additive effects), three times daily.
- They can be taken either with or between meals.
- When/if you achieve remission, take the remedies for two months longer.
- Discontinue use for three months; then follow the instructions for the maintenance dosage and schedule provided on page 82.

THYROID CANCER

Thyroid cancer is a disease where malignant (cancerous) cells form in the tissues of the thyroid gland. The thyroid, a butterfly-shaped gland at the base of the neck, produces hormones that regulate the body's energy use. There are multiple types of thyroid cancer, including papillary, follicular, medullary, anaplastic, and Hurthle cell thyroid cancers. Papillary thyroid cancer is the most common type, which is often slow growing and typically affects one lobe of the thyroid. Anaplastic thyroid cancer is the deadliest; average median survival is generally four to five months after diagnosis. All anaplastic thyroid cancers are considered stage 4 at diagnosis because they are aggressive and can spread quickly.

Women are three times more likely to get thyroid cancer than men. In the United States, thyroid cancer is relatively common. While it's not one of the most prevalent cancers overall, it's the 13th most commonly diagnosed cancer and the sixth most common in women. Although it can occur at any age, it generally affects people ages 30 to 50. The incidence of thyroid cancer has been increasing, particularly in women, though mortality rates remain low.

The overall five-year survival rate for thyroid cancer is very high, around 98%. Survival rates vary significantly, however, depending on the stage and type of cancer. For example, localized (early stage) papillary and follicular thyroid cancers have survival rates near 100%. Papillary and follicular thyroid cancer recurrence rates vary depending on several factors, but generally, it's considered to have a high survival rate with a lower recurrence risk (2–20%).

Natural Remedies for Thyroid Cancer

N-Tense has long been used as a natural remedy for thyroid cancer with good results. It worked well on its own and with a low relapse rate, there wasn't a need to add anything else. Most of the N-Tense ingredients address the defense mechanisms this cancer uses. If you are dealing with a recurrence of thyroid cancer, or worry about a relapse based on the type of cancer you have, you can add chanca piedra to the cancer plan. Research reports that it can selectively target cancer stem cells and kill them in various ways. See the plant information in Part 3 (page 226) for more.

THE THYROID CANCER PLAN

Recipe

10 parts graviola

2 parts mullaca

2 parts guacatonga

2 parts espinheira santa

1 part bitter melon fruit extract

1 part vassourinha

1 part mutamba

1 part cat's claw

HOW TO PREPARE YOUR OWN NATURAL ANTI-CANCER REMEDIES

Dosages

Capsules: 2–3 g, three times daily, based on stage/grade (see page 82); *or*

Tincture or glycerin extract: 1 teaspoon, three times daily; *or*

Infusion/tea: 1 cup, three times daily.

If needed/desired:

Chanca piedra capsules: 1 g, three times daily.

Instructions

- Take both remedies together at the same time (for synergistic/additive effects), three times daily.
- They can be taken either with or between meals.
- When/if you achieve remission, take the remedies for two months longer.
- Discontinue use for three months; then follow the instructions for the maintenance dosage and schedule provided on page 82.

UTERINE CANCER—*see* ENDOMETRIAL CANCER

Summary

Learning to make your own natural herbal remedies is a rewarding skill to have. It certainly can save a great deal of money over buying manufactured herbal supplements. It's understandable, however, why the majority just opt to purchase available herbal supplements to save time. Finding and ordering the plants, shipping time, buying the necessary supplies, and then, in the case of extracts, waiting two to four more weeks to extract the plants, may not be what most people who are fighting cancer want to do. Some choose to buy already manufactured products first, make sure they're working for them, and then choose to make their own to save money. To each his/her own . . . do what's best for you. Just keep in mind when choosing to make infusions, decoctions, or extracts, these particular combinations of plants don't taste very good at all. You don't want to invest in bulk plants and make an extract that you detest tasting. Try preparing a cup of tea with the blended formula first to see how it tastes to you before deciding how you want to prepare your herbal remedy.

PART 3

The Anti-Cancerous Plants of the Rainforest

The 13 anti-cancer plants featured in this book can be found in the following table. Next to each plant name is a link to a site that will provide the research references used for each plant. The second link goes to the database file for the plant in the Tropical Plant Database referenced in this section.

Plant	Page #	Reference File
Anamu	198	https://rain-tree.com/Anamu-Cancer-Research.pdf https://rain-tree.com/anamu.htm
Bitter melon	207	https://rain-tree.com/Bitter-Melon-Cancer-Research.pdf https://rain-tree.com/bitmelon.htm
Cat's claw	217	https://rain-tree.com/Cats-Claw-Cancer-Research.pdf https://rain-tree.com/catclaw.htm
Chanca piedra	226	https://rain-tree.com/Chanca-Piedra-Cancer-Research.pdf https://rain-tree.com/chanca.htm
Espinheira santa	238	https://rain-tree.com/Espinheira-Santa-Cancer-Research.pdf https://rain-tree.com/espinheira.htm
Graviola	252	https://rain-tree.com/Graviola-Cancer-Research.pdf https://rain-tree.com/graviola.htm
Guacatonga	267	https://rain-tree.com/Guacatonga-Cancer-Research.pdf https://rain-tree.com/guacatonga.htm

THE ANTI-CANCEROUS PLANTS OF THE RAINFOREST

Plant	*Page #*	*Reference File*
Mullaca	274	https://rain-tree.com/Mullaca-Cancer-Research.pdf https://rain-tree.com/mullaca.htm
Pau d'arco	284	https://rain-tree.com/Pau-d-Arco-Cancer-Research.pdf https://rain-tree.com/paudarco.htm
Picão preto	294	https://rain-tree.com/Picao-Preto-Cancer-Research.pdf https://rain-tree.com/picaopreto.htm
Simarouba	304	https://rain-tree.com/Simarouba-Cancer-Research.pdf https://rain-tree.com/simaruba.htm
Suma	311	https://rain-tree.com/Suma-Cancer-Research.pdf https://rain-tree.com/suma.htm
Vassourinha	318	https://rain-tree.com/Vassourinha-Cancer-Research.pdf https://rain-tree.com/vassourinha.htm

In Part 2, we provided the instructions for using the rainforest plants to combat various cancers. In Part 3, we will discuss each of the 13 plants. Each of these entries are divided into the following 10 sections:

- An overview with a plant description detailing family, genus, species, and common names, as well as parts of the plant used.
- Traditional herbal medicine uses.
- Anti-cancerous actions.
- Anti-cancerous plant chemicals.
- Cancer pathways and mechanisms of action.
- Other researched benefits that may be helpful.
- Availability of products.
- Safety.
- Summary of benefits the plant has to fight cancer.
- Online links to more information.

The following is a detailed breakdown of what each of these sections will include.

An Overview with a Plant Description

The first paragraph provides a quick overview on each plant. This information generally includes what the plant looks like; where and how it grows; and sometimes alternate scientific and common names the plant may be referred to or used for product names in the marketplace, if any.

Traditional Herbal Medicine Uses

Plants used in herbal medicine systems around the world have been recorded for thousands of years, and the uses of plants can be very important, especially to researchers. If a plant has been used in a specific way for a specific purpose for many years, and in many different geographical areas, there is probably a reason for it. It works! It is these traditional medicine uses that help scientists target which plants to research first and what to study them for.

In fact, the majority of our plant-based drugs or pharmaceuticals were discovered through this research and documentation process of traditional uses. Readers should keep in mind, however, that although a plant may have a long history of being used for a particular purpose, scientific evidence proving its efficacy for that purpose may be lacking. The information provided in this section gives a quick overview or summary of how the plant has been used as a specific natural remedy around the world. Much more detailed information on traditional uses can be found in the plant's database file in the Tropical Plant Database online (link provided in the "Online Links to More Information" section for each plant).

Anti-Cancerous Actions

An overview of scientific research and clinical data about each plant is provided in the text as it pertains to cancer research. Complete citations of any studies referenced in the text will be found in separate reference files that can be accessed online (shown in each plant's "Online Links to More Information" section). These downloadable files contain programmed links to the available published research articles and clinical studies cataloged at the National Library of Medicine's PubMed Database, which has been provided for convenience and to keep the information timely and updated as new research is published. Nonprofessionals should use care in evaluating these research studies and get help from a qualified professional in their interpretation and meaning if necessary. Nonprofessionals may find them difficult to understand.

Anti-Cancerous Plant Chemicals

Often, the plant's documented uses or researched actions will be closely tied to specific chemicals found in the plant that have been tested and verified to have specific pharmacological and biological activities. In other words, it helps explain why the plant works for, or is used for, certain things like cancer. Rainforest plants have a remarkable number of active plant chemicals (usually around 300–400 chemicals total; half of which or more are considered as "active"). While some chemicals may have a well-researched anti-cancer action, the total amount of that chemical may not be found in large enough amounts to provide a therapeutic anti-cancer benefit. Therefore, this section may not provide the names of, or research on, every single anti-cancer plant chemical found in the plant.

Instead, it will provide an overview of the research on those chemicals in the plant that are most likely providing the anti-cancer benefits and actions of the plant. You'll quickly note, however, that each plant detailed herein generally contains numerous anti-cancer chemicals that work in different ways that do provide real benefits. Some of these rainforest plant chemicals are so powerful that they can provide a benefit in very low dosages—as little as 1 part per million! Some plant chemicals discovered in the plants in this book have already been turned into new drugs, and others are somewhere in the long process of becoming a new cancer drug. This information, if applicable, will appear in this section.

Cancer Pathways and Mechanisms of Action

This section details how the plant and/or its active plant chemicals are working on a molecular level to treat cancer, which particular genes or chemicals in signaling pathways might be affected in treating particular types of cancer, and/or the results of newer biological testing methods, as well as computer models that are predicting how the plant/chemical is making changes on molecular levels, which may help describe in greater detail why it is treating cancer. None of the information in this section should be considered as "settled science" as it is constantly evolving; scientists are still learning of all the complicated interactions that happen when cancer can change the function of 400 different genes and all the many signaling pathways connected to the function of all those genes.

Also keep in mind that studying this in a medicinal plant with 200 or more different individual active chemicals is much more complicated. There are typically just a handful of chemicals that have been studied in this manner in a plant so far, and the hundreds of ways all these chemicals might affect many cancer types just haven't been tested completely yet. Based on reading this type of research on these plants so far, it helps explain why these rainforest plants can treat so many different types of cancer. Oftentimes different chemicals are providing a specific benefit for one type of cancer, while different chemicals are being activated to treat a different type of cancer in a different way. This section will provide an overview of what is known today based on the research performed to date on how the plant might treat cancer but will probably never be considered fully complete or settled science.

Other Researched Benefits That May Be Helpful

As I've described often in this book, many different active chemicals equate to diverse and different benefits for many different conditions when using these powerful rainforest plants. The text in this section will detail other confirmed properties and actions that a plant might possess, which would be helpful or beneficial to someone fighting cancer (or preventing or relieving some side effects of traditional cancer therapies). For example, this might be sharing information on the plant being confirmed with pain-relieving actions. This book focuses on the cancer research performed on these plants. More complete information on all the research performed on the plant can be found in the plant database file, including the actions and benefits that are detailed in this section.

Availability of Products

Information is provided concerning what products are available in the marketplace: how to find them; the type of available products (capsules, tinctures, bulk tea-cut, etc.); and possible quality control issues to watch out for, if any.

Safety

This section will provide an overview of the safety or toxicity studies performed on the plant, which usually are always conducted in animals in a standardized way initially. It will also provide the dosages used in traditional herbal medicine systems that are considered safe and effective based on those studies and/or traditional uses. Also included is information on possible contraindications and drug interactions. This particular information is usually extrapolated from animal studies and may not have specifically been tested in humans. For example, a plant may have traditionally been used for high blood pressure, an animal study confirmed it lowered blood pressure in mice, and several chemicals in the plant were shown to lower blood pressure in animals. This section might say that the plant might be contraindicated for people with low blood pressure (and to use with caution or seek professional advice prior to use) and that the plant may increase the effect of drugs to lower blood pressure. It has not, however, been studied specifically in people.

Summary of Benefits the Plant Has to Fight Cancer

This final section will provide a brief overview of why the plant can fight cancers, my personal experiences with it, and/or other formulas I developed using the plants.

Online Links to More Information

Here readers will find the links to the Tropical Plant Database file on the plant, the reference file for the book text on the plants in the Tropical Plant Database, and any other helpful links to more information on the plants or formulas that incorporate the plants.

The amount of new research and interest in these rainforest plants over the last 10 years has been extensive. It was especially rewarding to see that all the new research methods figuring out new cancer pathways were also, without exception, performed on these important rainforest plants. It is also quite a testament to the power of these plants to see how many new small-molecule drugs have been developed from these plants in the long process of creating new approved chemotherapy drugs. I am excited to share all this new knowledge on the plants I've used for so many years!

ANAMU

Family: Phytolaccaceae

Genus: *Petiveria*

Species: *alliacea*

Common Names: Anamu, apacin, apacina, apazote de zorro, aposin, ave, aveterinaryte, calauchin, chasser vermine, congo root, douvant-douvant, esperanza, emeruaiuma, garlic weed, guine, guinea, guinea hen leaf, guinea henweed, gully root, herbe aux poules, hierba de las gallinitas, huevo de gato, kojo root, kuan, kudjuruk, lemtewei, lemuru, mal pouri, mapurit, mapurite, mucura, mucuracaa, mucura-caa, ocano, payche, pipi, tipi, verbena hedionda, verveine puante, zorillo

Parts Used: Whole herb

Anamu is an herbaceous perennial that grows up to 3 feet in height. It is indigenous to the Amazon rainforest and tropical areas of Central and South America, the Caribbean, and Africa. It produces dark green leathery leaves that lie close to the ground and tall spikes lined with small white flowers that float airily above the leaves. It is sometimes called "garlic weed," as the plant, and especially the roots, have a strong garlic odor. It is called *mucura* in the Peruvian Amazon, *anamu* or *tipi* in Brazil, *esperanza* in Colombia, and in English-speaking areas in the West Indies, Jamaica, and the Caribbean it's called guinea hen weed or garlic weed.

TRADITIONAL HERBAL MEDICINE USES

Anamu has a long history in herbal medicine in all of the tropical countries where it grows. In Brazilian herbal medicine, it is considered an antispasmodic, diuretic, menstrual promoter, stimulant, and sweat promoter. Herbalists and natural health practitioners there use anamu for edema, arthritis, malaria, rheumatism, and poor memory, as well as a topical analgesic and anti-inflammatory for skin afflictions. Anamu is commonly used in big cities and towns in South and Central America as a natural remedy to treat colds, coughs, influenza, respiratory and pulmonary infections, and cancer, and to support the immune system. In Cuba, herbalists decoct the whole plant and use it to treat cancer and diabetes; it is also used as an anti-inflammatory and abortive. Various research published over the years has validated some of these traditional remedy uses. More complete information on anamu's traditional uses and this research can be found in the Tropical Plant Database (see the link provided in anamu's "Online Links to More Information" section).

Anti-Cancerous Actions

The anti-cancerous actions of anamu were first reported in Cuba in 1976. They reported that a leaf decoction demonstrated very good anti-tumorous actions in laboratory animals with several types of tumors. In a plant-screening program at the University of Illinois at Chicago that evaluated more than 1,400 plant extracts as novel therapies for the prevention and treatment of cancer, anamu was one of 34 plants identified with active properties against cancer.

Other research published on anamu reveals that it has a broad range of therapeutic properties, including anti-leukemic, anti-tumorous, and anti-cancerous activities against various types of cancer cells, including ovarian, breast, prostate, lung, liver, gastric, uterine, cervical, melanoma, pancreatic, and brain tumor cells. In a test-tube study by Italian researchers in 1990, water extracts and ethanol extracts of anamu retarded the growth of leukemia cells and several other strains of cancerous tumor cells. Three years later, the researchers followed up with another study, which showed that the same extracts had a cytotoxic effect, actually killing some of these cancer cells, rather than just retarding their growth. This study indicated that whole herb water extracts of anamu were toxic to leukemia and lymphoma cancer cells but only inhibited the growth of breast cancer cells.

In another test-tube study published in 2002, researchers reported a toxic effect against a liver cancer cell line; another test-tube study in 2001 reported that anamu retarded the growth of brain cancer cells. A German study documenting anamu's activity against brain cancer cells related its actions to the sulfur compounds found in the plant including one named dibenzyl trisulfide. Most of the research reports that anamu's toxic actions to cancer cells are highly selective, without any harm to healthy cells.

Colombia researchers first reported that anamu has anti-cancer action against lymphoma, leukemia, and melanoma in a test-tube study in 2008. In 2009, they published another study using new laboratory methods to track which genes were involved or changed when anamu was introduced to cancer cells in test tubes. They reported when anamu was introduced to chronic myeloid leukemia cells, the gene expression of 21 different genes were affected and/or modified. The authors suggested that the identification of modulated genes treated with anamu could provide new targets in cancer therapy.

The Colombian researchers publishing the animal and test-tube studies on anamu's anti-leukemic actions filed a U.S. patent on their extract of anamu in 2011, which was awarded in 2014. Their patent was on treating cancer with their extract, and data provided as supporting documentation in the patent were their studies with leukemia, breast cancer, and melanoma. They then registered a Phase 1 clinical trial in 2014, and registered a Phase 1b/2 human clinical trial in 2023 in Colombia.

Anamu's common name in Colombia is *esperanza*. The Phase 2 study was designed to "evaluate the safety profile of an Esperanza extract in patients with metastatic gastrointestinal tumors and acute leukemias, while exploring its potential efficacy in conjunction with standard treatment for these pathologies." The extract used is termed a *phytomedicine* in Colombia, and it is a water extract of anamu leaves that has been spray dried and encapsulated into 500 mg capsules. Online information says they are still recruiting patients, so no results of the trial have been published yet.

Their research published in 2023 and 2024 is still confirming anamu can kill leukemia cells, but we now have a better understanding how. Their new data reports cancer cells are well known to change metabolic processes inside their cells, usually controlled and orchestrated by cell components called mitochondria. Anamu seems to be addressing many metabolic changes specifically made by leukemia cells that promote their growth, proliferation, and survival. The researchers began referring to anamu as a *mitocan* since much of its actions on leukemia happen within the mitochondria. A mitocan is a type of anti-cancer substance that specifically targets the mitochondria of cancer cells, disrupting their energy production and triggering cell death pathways; the term is a combination of the words *mitochondria* and *cancer*. Anamu has long been known to have immune modulation actions and these actions have also been reported to address some of the signaling pathways leukemia cells change in immune cell function to promote lymphocyte blastogenesis, a hallmark of leukemia.

These Colombian researchers published several prior studies in animals and test tubes and one human *ex vivo* study (extracting bone marrow from acute leukemia patients and introducing it to anamu) demonstrating anamu's anti-leukemic action. They also published various animal toxicity studies showing anamu is nontoxic in animals as part of their Phase 1 clinical trial. One study they published in 2023 describes how leukemia cells were sensitized to a standard cancer drug named doxorubicin in test tubes, suggesting that anamu might increase the effectiveness of the drug if combined together. They also reported that anamu was selectively toxic to just leukemia cells while doxorubicin was toxic to all cells tested.

Anti-Cancerous Plant Chemicals

Anamu contains an enzyme called *alliinase*, which is also found in garlic. This is the main chemical in both plants responsible for their garlic odor. While garlic uses this enzyme to make a large amount of an organosulfur compound called *allicin*, anamu uses the enzyme to make a large amount of a different organosulfur compound called *petivericin*. As the plant metabolizes petivericin utilizing other compounds in the plant, new organosulfur compounds are created. Chemical analysis of anamu indicates it contains up to 18 different organosulfur compounds. Some of these compounds are attributed to anamu's antimicrobial actions against various bacteria, viruses, and fungi. One in particular (*dibenzyl trisulfide*), however, is only found in anamu. This novel plant chemical (which anamu produces a lot of) has been widely touted as the main reason anamu has anti-tumorous and anti-leukemic actions. About 80% of all organosulfur compounds anamu produces is dibenzyl trisulfide.

Dibenzyl trisulfide has been documented with broad-spectrum anti-cancer and immune modulation benefits in studies published over the years. It has shown to kill various types of tumorous cancers and several types of leukemia and lymphoma. Researchers from the West Indies reported in 2007 that dibenzyl trisulfide exhibited potent anti-proliferation and cytotoxic activity on a wide range of cancer cell lines (some cell lines with up to 100% mortality!) with little to no toxicity to healthy cells. Then, just two years later, a Chinese company created a derivative (changed this natural plant chemical in anamu slightly) and patented it in 2009 as a new chemotherapy drug for cancer.

Their initial test-tube research indicated it was effective for several types of leukemias and breast cancers as well as ovarian, liver, and lung cancers and fibrosarcomas. They've called this new derivative of dibenzyl trisulfide *fluorapacin* and applied for Phase I human clinical trials in 2010 in China. It was approved in China; however, the Chinese company has not applied for human clinical trials for the approval of a new cancer drug in the United States. Instead, they registered it as an investigational small-molecule drug in the United States that U.S. cancer researchers can purchase from the American bioscience division of the Chinese pharmaceutical company.

In 2021, researchers also reported that dibenzyl trisulfide could inhibit an enzyme (CYP1A1) in test tubes and animals. CYP1A1 metabolizes xenobiotics, drugs, procarcinogens, and other substances. Inhibiting CYP1A1 may be beneficial for cancer prevention and overcoming drug toxicity and resistance.

Daucosterol is an active natural sterol compound that has anti-inflammatory, anti-cancer, and immunomodulatory activities. Anamu's anti-inflammatory and immune modulation actions might relate to this natural chemical.

Polyphenols: Anamu contains a wide variety of polyphenols (including flavonoid and flavonoid glycosides). Polyphenols in anamu include astilbin, catechin, cinnamic acid, coumarin and its metabolites, epicatechin, engeletin, kaempferol and its metabolites, myricetin, protocatechuic acid, quercetin and its metabolites, and a novel polyphenol called petiveral and its metabolite 4-ethylpetiveral.

Astilbin: Astilbin is found in many plants and is the subject of research reporting it has anti-cancer, immune modulation, antioxidant, and anti-inflammatory actions. Several researchers attributed anamu's immune modulation and anti-inflammatory actions to the astilbin content (as well as the daucosterol) in the plant. Many of anamu's other common polyphenols have also been the subject of anti-cancer and/or antitumor research.

Cancer Pathways and Mechanisms of Action

More complete information on these genes, signaling pathways, cancer pathways, and new chemical targets for cancer therapy can be found in chapter 5.

- Anamu has the ability to modify certain molecular targets that allow it to seek out and kill cancer stem cells, which are attributed as a main cause of tumor recurrences in many cancers.

- Anamu was found to change the structure of the cell's internal framework (called the actin cytoskeleton), stop cells from dividing at a specific stage (called the G2 phase), and cause the cells to die in a way that doesn't involve the mitochondria.

- Anamu was found to lower the activity or number of certain proteins. These proteins help maintain the cell's structure, assist in folding proteins correctly, carry signals inside the cell, and support metabolism. At the same time, there was an increase in proteins that help create new proteins and break down unwanted materials inside the cell.

- Anamu reduces energy to cancer cells in two ways. It affects genes linked to energy production through glycolysis (hexokinase, phosphofructokinase, and lactate dehydrogenase), which stops cancer cells from taking in glucose and lowers their energy levels. It also targets mitochondrial proteins (like β-F1-ATPase), which block the production of ATP, another important energy source for cells.

- Anamu has also been reported to modify the apoptotic genes and proteins (Bax and caspase-3), which flips the suicide switch back on, causing cancer cells to die through the apoptosis pathway.

- Dibenzyl trisulfide's main action in actually killing cancer cells has been reported as inhibiting microtubules. This can suppress or block cell cycle progression and results in apoptosis.

- Daucosterol inhibits cancer cell proliferation by inducing autophagy through a ROS-dependent manner. Daucosterol was also reported to inhibit colon cancer growth by inducing apoptosis, inhibiting cell migration and invasion, and targeting the caspase signaling pathway.

- Anamu can block the epidermal growth factor receptor (EGFR) protein, which can be overexpressed or mutated in some cancer cells, leading to uncontrolled growth.
- Other research reports anamu inhibits the following: Hsp90, PI3K/AKT/mTOR, Notch, P2X7, p53, Bcl-2, ATP, and GLUT1, while activating Bax, and caspase-3. These molecular targets are detailed more fully in chapter 5.

OTHER RESEARCHED BENEFITS THAT MAY BE HELPFUL

Several animal studies suggest that anamu has pain-relieving effects that might be beneficial for some cancer patients. Quite a few test-tube and animal studies report anamu's immunostimulant and antimicrobial actions, including against common cold and flu strains. This might be helpful for immunocompromised cancer patients to protect against infections.

It is also possible that anamu is making changes in the inflammation and immune pathway that cancer uses to survive and thrive. In several early studies, anamu was reported to have immune stimulant actions, which may relate to its active chemical, dibenzyl trisulfide. In a critical review published in 2007 on dibenzyl trisulfide, West Indian researchers (who call the plant *guineahen weed* and the chemical *dibenzyl trisulphide*) describe this action to be more of an immune modulation action rather than a stimulatory action. They explained: "Dibenzyl trisulphide seems to have a cytokine switching mechanism in which it down regulates immune cells from the Type I helper cells (Th-1 cell) pathway which contain several pro-inflammatory immune cells and up-regulates those of the Type 2 helper cells (Th-2) pathway." Basically, this means it increases the actions of the immune cells that are responsible for tracking down and removing foreign cells like bacteria and cancer, and its previously documented anti-inflammatory action might be from suppressing other pro-inflammatory immune cells that cause inflammation.

AVAILABILITY OF PRODUCTS

Anamu has become quite popular in the United States as an herbal remedy. It is available under quite a few labels and offered in capsules, tablets, tinctures, and extracts under the "anamu" common name. Several cut and sifted whole herb or root products are available to make tea with, usually referred to by its Jamaican name *Guinea Hen Tea* or *Guineahen weed*. Usually the whole plant (i.e., leaves, stems, and vine parts) is harvested in South America and imported into the United States as "anamu," but some available products just say "anamu leaves." The beneficial plant chemicals discussed herein can be found in all parts of the anamu plant, including its root. Research has shown that the active sulfur compounds are water soluble and easily digested and absorbed, so taking it in capsules is fine.

SAFETY

Anamu has long been used in South America's traditional herbal medicine system and has been considered a safe herbal remedy, with no toxicity or negative side effects. The research studying anamu's toxic action to cancer cells reports little to no toxicity to healthy cells. In two independent toxicity studies, oral doses of anamu leaf and root extracts did not cause any toxicity in rats and mice at up to 5 g/kg of body weight. Methanol extracts of the plant did, however, cause uterine contractions in an early study; such contractions can lead to abortion, one of anamu's well-documented uses in traditional herbal medicine.

Dosages

In South America, a standard decoction is generally prepared with the aerial parts (leaves, stems, vines) and sometimes the root and taken two or three times daily in ½-cup doses. (It tastes quite horrible, however!) The natural remedy in North American herbal medicine systems is generally 1 or 2 grams of the powdered plant in tablets or capsules two or three times daily, or 2–3 mgs of a standard tincture or water/glycerin extract twice daily, or as needed.

Contraindications

Anamu has been documented to lower blood pressure in two animal studies; therefore, anamu is probably contraindicated for people with low blood pressure. Those with a heart condition or taking heart medications should consult with their doctor before using this plant.

Anamu has demonstrated to be a uterine relaxant and traditionally employed as a childbirth aid. A pregnant woman should use it only under the supervision of a qualified health care practitioner.

Drug Interactions

Animal studies suggest anamu might potentiate prescription heart medications for high blood pressure.

SUMMARY OF BENEFITS THE PLANT HAS TO FIGHT CANCER

With the many documented properties and actions of this tropical plant, it is no wonder that anamu has enjoyed such a long history of use in herbal medicine. Continuing research on this plant's attributes is quantifying and qualifying the richness of indigenous herbal traditions. As of this writing, anamu is being used in South America, for its immune stimulant and anti-cancerous properties as a support aid for cancer and leukemia patients. This use is catching on here in the United States, and it is now considered a natural cancer remedy.

The easiest way to summarize the compelling data compiled in research thus far is that anamu can significantly influence the expression of various genes in tumor cells, primarily by downregulating genes involved in cell proliferation and survival, by inhibiting tumor cell growth and inducing apoptosis. It is also being employed in various formulas for its antimicrobial actions against bacteria, viruses, yeast, and fungi, as well as in other formulas supporting immune function.

Anamu is an ingredient in the NTense-2 herbal formula I developed more than 20 years ago for leukemias, lymphomas, and other blood cancers. See chapter 8 to learn how to make this formula. It was also a main ingredient in a formula I developed to support and enhance immune system function, which I called Amazon Immune Support. I often recommended this formula to those fighting cancer in my naturopathic protocols, especially if they were also using immune-suppressing chemotherapy drugs to fight their cancer.

ONLINE LINKS TO MORE INFORMATION

- Tropical Plant Database file for anamu: https://rain-tree.com/anamu.htm.
- Research references for this text: https://rain-tree.com/Anamu-Cancer-Research.pdf.
- Anamu was an ingredient in a Raintree Nutrition formula called Amazon Immune Support, which was often used in fighting cancer. Instructions on making this formula can be found at https://rain-tree.com/amazon-immune-support.htm.

BITTER MELON

Family: Cucurbitaceae

Genus: *Momordica*

Species: *charantia*

Synonyms: *Momordica chinensis, M. elegans, M. indica, M. operculata, M. sinensis, Sicyos fauriei*

Common Names: Bitter melon, karela, balsam apple, balsam pear, bitter-gourd, kor-kuey, ku gua, k'u kua kurela, melao de sao caetano, papailla, pare, pava-aki, peria, peria laut, salsamino, sorci, sorossi, sorossie, sorossies

Parts Used: Whole plant, fruit, seed

Bitter melon grows in tropical areas, including parts of the Amazon, east Africa, Asia, and the Caribbean, and it is cultivated throughout South America as a food and medicine. It's a slender, climbing annual vine with long-stalked leaves and yellow, solitary male and female flowers borne in the leaf axils. The fruit looks like a warty gourd, usually oblong and resembling a small cucumber. The young fruit is emerald green, turning to orange-yellow when ripe. At maturity, the fruit splits into three irregular valves that curl backwards and release numerous reddish-brown or white seeds encased in scarlet arils. The Latin name *Momordica* means "to bite," referring to the jagged edges of the leaves, which appear as if they have been bitten. All parts of the plant, including the fruit, taste bitter.

TRADITIONAL HERBAL MEDICINE USES

In Brazilian herbal medicine, bitter melon is used for tumors, wounds, rheumatism, malaria, vaginal discharge, inflammation, menstrual problems, diabetes, colic, fevers, and worms. It is also used to induce abortions and as an aphrodisiac. It is prepared into a topical remedy for the skin to treat vaginitis, hemorrhoids, scabies, itchy rashes, eczema, leprosy, and other skin problems. In Mexico, the entire plant is used for diabetes and dysentery; the root is a reputed aphrodisiac. In Peruvian herbal medicine, the leaf or aerial parts of the plant are used to treat measles, malaria, and all types of inflammation.

In Nicaragua, the leaf is commonly used for stomach pain, diabetes, fevers, colds, coughs, headaches, malaria, skin complaints, menstrual disorders, aches and pains, hypertension, infections, and as an aid in childbirth. Dried extracts of bitter melon fruits have become quite popular as a natural remedy for diabetes, diabetic complications, and high cholesterol in North, South, and Latin American herbal medicine systems.

Anti-Cancerous Actions

Bitter melon and its active ingredients were tested in laboratory cancer cell models and in animals. Studies focused on preventing various types of cancer, including blood, breast, colon, head and neck, liver, prostate, skin, and stomach cancers, using bitter melon extracts. These extracts were made from the leaves, fruit, seeds, and seed oil of bitter melon, using water, methanol, or ethanol. Additionally, therapeutic studies using these crude extracts or specific compounds were conducted in lab and animal models of cancers such as blood, brain, breast, colon, stomach, head and neck, kidney, liver, lung, nasopharyngeal, ovary, pancreas, prostate, skin, and cervical/uterine cancers.

Several animal studies have demonstrated the anti-tumorous activity of the entire plant of bitter melon. In one study, a water extract blocked the growth of rat prostate carcinoma; another study reported that a hot water extract of the entire plant inhibited the development of mammary tumors in mice. Numerous *in vitro* studies have also demonstrated the anti-cancerous and anti-leukemic activity of bitter melon leaves, fruits, and fruit seeds against numerous cell lines, including liver cancer, human leukemia, melanoma, and solid sarcomas. A 2019 test-tube study reported that a whole fruit extract inhibited 90% of the growth of chronic myeloid leukemia in 72 hours with a very small dosage (0.082 mg/ml).

Researchers in Japan published a study in 2024 reporting a water extract of bitter melon leaves prevented melanoma proliferation and infiltration into the lungs of mice and determined through new research methods that it suppressed tumor survival genes by regulating PAX3. Other research on bitter melon dried fruit extracts reports that it is active against chronic myelogenous leukemia, T-cell leukemia, breast cancer (estrogen positive and negative), cervical cancer, colorectal cancer, lung cancer, liver cancer, and nasopharyngeal carcinoma in test tubes and/or animals.

In addition to treating cancer, several research groups report that fruit extracts can prevent many types of cancers by enhancing reactive oxygen species (ROS) generation; inhibiting cancer cell cycle, cell signaling, cancer stem cells, glucose and lipid metabolism, invasion, metastasis, hypoxia, and angiogenesis; inducing apoptosis and autophagy cell death; and enhancing immune function defenses. One research group summarized their study by saying, "Thus, bitter melon may serve as a promising cancer preventive and as a therapeutic agent." Another research group in China reported in 2015 that a crude fruit juice extract could overcome drug resistance in test tubes and mice with ovarian cancer when they combined the juice with a chemo drug named cisplatin. In 2020, they repeated this ovarian/mouse test with MAP30 extracted from the fruit seeds and reported similar results.

In addition to cancer prevention actions, bitter melon extracts are also reported to inhibit or prevent metastases of various types of cancer by affecting matrix metalloproteinases (MMPs). MMPs are special proteins that help break down the extracellular matrix—the support structure that surrounds and holds cells together. While this process is normal and necessary for the body, too much activity from MMPs can cause problems. In diseases like cancer, MMPs can help tumors grow, spread to other parts of the body, and form new blood vessels. Because of this, scientists are now focusing on ways to stop MMPs from working too much, as a new approach to treating cancer.

Studies found that ethanol extracts of bitter melon leaves can significantly reduce the transfer and invasion of prostate and lung cancer cells by depressing the secretion of MMP-2 and MMP-9. Its methanolic extracts inhibited the motility of human lung adenocarcinoma CL1 series of cell lines in a dose-dependent manner and depressed the activity of enzymes related to metastases.

Some exciting news about bitter melon juice was published in 2018 by American researchers concerning their studies on pancreatic cancer. Pancreatic cancer is one of the deadliest malignancies worldwide and frontline treatment (with gemcitabine) eventually becomes ineffective due to increasing drug resistance. This cancer research group at a U.S. university cancer research clinic first reported the efficacy of bitter melon juice against pancreatic cancer cells, including those already resistant to gemcitabine in animals and test tubes in two 2018 studies.

Since cancer stem cells are actively involved in cancer initiation, progression, relapse, and drug resistance, these researchers next assessed the juice's ability in targeting pancreatic cancer–associated cancer stem cells. They found good efficacy in killing the stem cells in animals and test tubes as well as increasing the sensitivity of gemcitabine-resistant stem cells. Their mechanism of action studies reported bitter melon juice decreases protein expression by reducing stem cell–associated transcription factors (including SOX2, OCT4, NANOG, and cancer stem cell marker CD44) in associated regulatory pathways.

Their earlier research (in 2013) reported the bitter melon juice evidenced strong anti-cancer efficacy against four human pancreatic carcinoma cell lines in test tubes and in mice. They reported the juice employed a different mechanism of action (triggering apoptosis) and reduced tumor sizes by 60% without noticeable toxicity in nude mice (immunodeficient mice grafted with human pancreatic tumors). They suggested several other actions (inhibiting cellular energy in pancreatic cancer cells and stem cells) two years later.

In 2020, they combined bitter melon juice treatment with gemcitabine and gave it to mice with three different types of grafted pancreatic tumors (extracted from humans) and reported the combination-regimen displayed enhanced and sustained efficacy over gemcitabine alone. They suggested: "Study outcomes, highlighting significantly higher and sustained efficacy of GEM in combination with BMJ, make a compelling case for a clinical trial in PanC patients, wherein BMJ could be combined with GEM to target and overcome GEM resistance."

Anti-Cancerous Plant Chemicals

Bitter melon contains an array of biologically active plant chemicals, including triterpenes, proteins, steroids, polyphenols, and saponins. At latest count, approximately 420 different compounds with possible medicinal properties, acting alone or in combination, have been isolated from bitter melon fruit, seeds, leaves, stems, pericaps, endosperm, callus tissues, and cotyledons. More than 260 cucurbitane-type triterpenoids have been reported in bitter melon, and these are considered the plant's main active medicinal compounds. Some of the isolated compounds—including charantagenins A–E, cucurbitacin B, charantin, goyaglycosides B and D, kuguaoside A, kuguacin J, karaviloside XI, kuguaglycoside C, momordin, momordicoside Q–U, momordicoside F1, F2, I, K, α-momorcharin, β-momorcharin, α-eleostearic acid, α-momorcharin, RNase MC2, and MAP30—possess potent biological activity against cancer in very low dosages.

A chemical analog of a bitter melon protein discovered in the fruit seeds has been developed, patented, and named "MAP-30." Its developers reported that MAP-30 was able to inhibit tumor growth among many types of cancer and provides good antiviral actions. It is sold as a small-molecule drug and reported to kill various tumor cells through N-glycosidase activity (inhibiting glucose uptake in cancer cells which lowers available energy stores inside the cancer cell and irreversibly inhibits protein synthesis, which kills the cancer cell).

Another chemical (α-eleostearic acid), which is known as the major component in bitter melon fruit seeds, as well as its dihydroxy derivative, has proven to be the most effective antitumor agent extracted by ethanol; it strongly inhibited the growth of some cancer and fibroblast cell lines, including leukemia and colon cancer. Eleostearic acid inhibited the proliferation of both breast cancer cell lines of estrogen receptor (ER) α-negative and ER α-positive and induced G2-M block in the cell cycle and apoptosis in other research.

Indian researchers reported in 2024 that bitter melon contains five plant sterol derivatives that were effective CHK-1 inhibitors. Checkpoint kinase 1 (Chk-1) is a protein that is an emerging target in cancer research owing to its crucial role in cell cycle arrest. Another chemical has clinically demonstrated the ability to inhibit the enzyme guanylate cyclase that is necessary for the growth of leukemia and cancer cells. In addition, a protein found in bitter melon has clinically demonstrated anti-cancerous activity against Hodgkin lymphoma in animals.

Polyphenols: Like most rainforest plants, bitter melon is rich in polyphenols. Catechin and epicatechin are the highest phenolic acids contained in bitter melon (46.16 mg/g of dry weight, 72–86% of the total phenolic contents in water extracts). Studies have demonstrated that catechins can inhibit cancer cell proliferation, induce cell cycle arrest, and promote apoptosis across multiple cancer types, including skin, breast, lung, liver, prostate, and colon cancers. Furthermore, catechins have shown the ability to inhibit angiogenesis, a critical process for tumor growth and metastasis, by restricting new blood vessel formation. Catechin's impact on cancer extends beyond its direct effects on cancer cells. It also modulates various signaling pathways involved in cancer progression, such as those associated with cell survival, inflammation, and metastasis. Bitter melon fruit and leaves also contain a polyphenol named verbascoside, which has been demonstrated to exert cytotoxic and apoptotic effects in human cancers, including colorectal cancer, oral squamous cell carcinoma, breast cancer, and glioblastoma.

Cancer Pathways and Mechanisms of Action

More complete information on these signaling pathways, cancer pathways, and new chemical targets for cancer therapy shown here can be found in chapter 5.

- Bitter melon was shown to inhibit matrix metalloproteinases (MMPs) enzymes, which are linked to occurrence and promotion of tumor invasion, metastasis, and angiogenesis.
- Bitter melon interferes in a survival mechanism many cancers use to become drug resistant. It shuts down P-glycoprotein (P-gp), a protein that acts like a "drug pump" on the surface of cancer cells. P-gp pushes chemotherapy drugs out of the cells, making the drugs ineffectual and leading to multidrug resistance.
- Chemicals in bitter melon (momordins) have shown to stop AP-1 from working. When AP-1 is overactive, it can contribute to the development and spread of cancer cells.
- Prostate cancer cells treated with bitter melon fruit extracts experienced S-phase cell cycle arrest by modulating cyclin D1, cyclin E, and p21 expression. It also enhanced Bax expression, induced PARP cleavage, and delayed the progression to high-grade prostatic intraepithelial neoplasia in TRAMP (transgenic adenocarcinoma of mouse prostate) in mice.
- In breast and liver cancer cells, bitter melon juice was reported to cause cell cycle arrest in the G0/G1 phase.
- Bitter melon was shown to block signaling in the MAPK pathway, a key target for cancer therapies to prevent cancer cell growth.
- Ribosome-inactivating proteins (RIPs) have been reported to exert antitumor and antiviral activities. A Chinese patent has developed a new

method to prepare Momordica anti-HIV protein called MAP30. MAP30 is a type I RIP, which kills various tumor cells through N-glycosidase activity and irreversibly inhibits protein synthesis.

• Momordicine-1 was found to be nontoxic and stable in the blood of mice, even after being injected. Treatment with Momordicine-1 slowed the growth of head and neck cancer tumors in mice and stopped the activity of a protein called c-Met and its related signaling pathways.

• In estrogen positive and negative breast cancers, bitter melon induced a significant decrease in the cell viability (greater than 80%) at concentrations of only 2% and 5% while toxicity to healthy cells was negligible. It caused the breakdown of PARP and activated caspases in the cancer cells. It also blocked certain proteins (survivin, XIAP, and claspin) that normally help the cells survive.

• Bitter melon inhibits glycolysis and lipid metabolism and induces ER and oxidative stress-mediated cell death in oral cancer.

• Bitter melon juice restricts the ability of pancreatic cancer cells to metabolize glucose, thus cutting the cells' energy source and eventually killing them.

• In lung and breast cancer cells, bitter melon caused cancer cell death by disrupting energy metabolism and increasing reactive oxygen species (ROS) generation.

• Cucurbitacin chemicals in bitter melon have been reported to suppress JAK-STAT 3, mTOR, VEGFR, Wnt/β-catenin, and MAPK signaling pathways, all of which are crucial for the survival and destruction of cancer cells.

• A methanol extract of bitter melon fruit can activate AMPK by reducing intracellular ATP levels, leading to tumor cell autophagy (and resulting death) of colon cancer stem cells and ancestral cells.

• Overall, bioactive chemicals in bitter melon act as antitumor agents mainly through inhibiting tumor cell proliferation, inducing tumor cell apoptosis, influencing energy metabolism, depressing tumor cell metastasis, and enhancing relevant tumor suppressor gene activity. Bitter melon can inhibit PAK1, NOTCH, Wnt/β-catenin signaling, TGF-β-associated EMT progression, MAPK pathway signaling, and ABCB, while killing various types of cancer by triggering autophagy.

Other Researched Benefits That May Be Helpful

Quite a few test-tube and animal studies report bitter melon's immunostimulant and antimicrobial actions, including against common cold and flu strains. This might be helpful for immune-compromised cancer patients to protect against infections during conventional immunosuppressive chemotherapy. The plant and the fruit juice are also reported to possess antioxidant and anti-inflammatory actions, which many may find helpful. Several studies report that bitter melon provides anti-ulcerous actions as well as ulcer-preventative actions (and even protects animals from toxic chemicals meant to induce ulcerative colitis). This might prove helpful to avoid these side effects of some chemotherapeutic drugs.

Availability of Products

Over the years, scientists have verified many of the traditional uses of this bitter plant that continues to be an important natural remedy in herbal medicine systems. Bitter melon capsules and tinctures are becoming more widely available in the United States and are employed by natural health practitioners for diabetes, viruses, colds and flu, cancer and tumors, high cholesterol, and psoriasis. The majority of available products are concentrated fruit and fruit and seed extracts in capsules and tablets, which are commonly marketed and used to enhance blood sugar regulation in diabetics and in people with pre-diabetes. Many of the active beneficial chemicals occur in both the fruit as well as leaves; however, there are very few bitter melon leaf products sold in the United States.

If you have a vegetable or flower garden, bitter melon vine is easy to grow as an annual. It loves the heat and full sun but is also shade tolerant, looks much like its cousin, the cucumber vine, and is fast growing—producing an abundance of both leaves and fruit to use for a natural remedy. Like a cucumber, harvest the entire plant before the first frost.

Safety

Many animal studies and a handful of human clinical studies have demonstrated the relatively low toxicity of all parts of the bitter melon plant when ingested orally. Toxicity and even death in laboratory animals, however, have been reported when extracts are injected intravenously. Other studies have shown extracts of the fruit and leaf (ingested orally) to be safe during pregnancy. The seeds, however, have demonstrated the ability to induce abortions in rats and mice, and the root has been documented as a uterine stimulant in animals. The fruit and leaf of bitter melon have demonstrated an antifertility effect in female animals; and in male animals; it has been shown to affect the production of sperm negatively. Read product labels carefully. Some fruit juice extract product manufacturers juice the entire fruit, including the seeds (which can have a higher toxicity), while others remove the seeds from the fruit before juicing them.

Dosages

One cup of a standard leaf or whole herb decoction is taken one or two times daily, or 1–3 mgs of a 4:1 tincture is taken twice daily. Powdered leaf in tablets or capsules, 1–2 grams can be substituted, if desired. The traditional South American remedy for diabetes is to juice one to two fresh bitter melon fruits and drink twice daily. For concentrated fruit extracts in capsules, follow the instructions in the cancer plans in chapters 7 and 8.

Contraindications

- Bitter melon traditionally has been used as an abortive and has been documented with weak uterine stimulant activity; therefore, it is contraindicated during pregnancy.
- This plant has been documented to reduce fertility in both males and females and should therefore not be used by those undergoing fertility treatment or seeking pregnancy.
- The active chemicals in bitter melon can be transferred through breast milk; therefore, it is contraindicated in women who are breastfeeding.
- All parts of bitter melon (especially the fruit and seed) have demonstrated in numerous *in vivo* studies that they lower blood sugar levels. As such, it is contraindicated in persons with hypoglycemia. Diabetics should check with their physicians before using this plant and use with caution while monitoring their blood sugar levels regularly, as the dosage of insulin medications may need adjusting.
- Although all parts of the plant have demonstrated active antibacterial activity, none have shown activity against fungi or yeast. Long-term use of

this plant may result in the die-off of friendly bacteria with resulting opportunistic overgrowth of yeast (*Candida*). Cycling off the use of the plant (every 21–30 days for one week) may be warranted, and adding probiotics to the diet may be beneficial if this plant is used for longer than 30 days.

Drug Interactions

Bitter melon fruit may potentiate insulin and antidiabetic drugs and cholesterol-lowering drugs.

SUMMARY OF BENEFITS THE PLANT HAS TO FIGHT CANCER

Almost 200 studies detail how bitter melon's most widespread herbal medicine use, to lower blood sugar for diabetics, is explained, categorized, and validated. It's no real surprise that researchers eventually discovered how bitter melon affects diabetes, glucose, and insulin metabolism, which might provide effective strategies to treat pancreatic cancers as well as other fast-growing tumors that need extra glucose to fuel their rapid growth. Interfering with the uptake of glucose in cancer cells slows down their growth, shuts down intercellular pumps created to pump chemotherapy drugs out of cancer cells before the drugs can kill them, and disables some cancer cells' ability to metastasize.

This research on pancreatic cancer has prompted me to add a bitter melon juice product to the pancreatic cancer protocols. See chapter 6 for more information on dosages and types of products to purchase. The multi-plant formula I developed more than 20 years ago (N-Tense) contains bitter melon, and rather than reduce the ratios and amounts of other important anti-cancer plant formulas, I just added bitter melon fruit supplements to the protocols on the types of cancer it will help the most. See chapter 6 for more information on dosage and types of products to purchase.

ONLINE LINKS TO MORE INFORMATION

- Tropical Plant Database file for bitter melon: https://rain-tree.com/bitmelon.htm.

- Research references for this text: https://rain-tree.com/Bitter-Melon-Cancer-Research.pdf.

CAT'S CLAW

Family: Rubiaceae

Genus: *Uncaria*

Species: *tomentosa*

Synonyms: *Uncaria surinamensis, Nauclea aculeata, N. tomentosa, Ourouparia tomentosa*

Common Names: Cat's claw, uña de gato, garabato, garbato casha, hawk's claw, paraguayo, samento, tambor huasca, toroñ, uña de gavilan, uña huasca

Parts Used: Vine bark, root

Cat's claw (*U. tomentosa*) is a large, woody vine that derives its name from hook-like thorns that grow along the vine and resemble the claws of a cat. Two closely related species of *Uncaria* are used almost interchangeably in the rainforests: *U. tomentosa* and *U. guianensis*. Both species can reach more than 100 feet high into the canopy. *U. tomentosa* has small, yellowish-white flowers, whereas *U. guianensis* has reddish-orange flowers and thorns that are more curved. Cat's claw is indigenous to the Amazon rainforest and other tropical areas of South and Central America, including Peru, Colombia, Ecuador, Guyana, Trinidad, Venezuela, Suriname, Costa Rica, Guatemala, and Panama.

TRADITIONAL HERBAL MEDICINE USES

The Ashaninka Indian tribe in central Peru has the longest recorded history of use of the plant. They are also the largest commercial source of cat's claw from Peru today. The Ashaninka use cat's claw to treat asthma, inflammations of the urinary tract, arthritis, rheumatism, and bone pain; to recover from childbirth; as a kidney cleanser; to cure deep wounds; to control inflammation and gastric ulcers; and for cancer. Cat's claw has been used in Peru and Europe since the early 1990s as an adjunctive treatment for cancer and AIDS as well as for other diseases that target the immune system. In herbal medicine today, cat's claw is employed around the world for many different conditions, including immune disorders, gastritis, ulcers, cancer, arthritis, rheumatism, rheumatic disorders, neuralgias, chronic inflammation of all kinds, and such viral diseases as herpes zoster (shingles).

Test-tube and animal research over the years has validated many of the plant's traditional uses. This research reports that cat's claw has anti-inflammatory, anti-ulcerous, anti-cancerous, antidepressant, anti-leukemic, antimutagenic (cellular protector), antioxidant, anti-tumorous, antiviral, contraceptive, and immune stimulant actions. More complete information on cat's claw's traditional uses and this research can be found in the Tropical Plant Database (see the link provided in the "Online Links to More Information" section for this plant).

Anti-Cancerous Actions

Research on cat's claw began in the early 1970s when Klaus Keplinger, a journalist and self-taught ethnologist from Innsbruck, Austria, organized the first definitive work on cat's claw. Keplinger's work in the 1970s and 1980s led to several extracts of cat's claw being sold in Austria and Germany as herbal drugs, as well as the filing of four U.S. patents describing extraction procedures for the immune-stimulating oxindole alkaloids. These herbal drugs were prescribed as an adjunctive cancer therapy in combination with many types of chemotherapy drugs to prevent or reduce the immunosuppressive actions of the cancer drugs.

Several small-scale human studies were published indicating that cat's claw potentiated the toxic effects of the cancer drugs in cancer cells, but protected immune cells from toxicity, as well as increased the number of and actions of NK immune cells (natural killer cells whose role are targeting and removing harmful cells like cancer and microbes). These novel oxindole alkaloids fueled worldwide interest in the medicinal properties of this valuable vine of the rainforest.

Other independent researchers in Spain, France, Japan, Germany, and Peru followed Keplinger, many of them confirming his research on the immunostimulating alkaloids in the vine and root. Many of these studies published from the late 1970s to early 1990s indicated that the whole oxindole alkaloid fraction, whole vine bark and/or root bark extracts, or six individually tested oxindole alkaloids, when used in relatively small amounts, increased immune function by up to 50%. Early reports on Keplinger's observatory trials with cancer patients taking cat's claw in conjunction with such traditional cancer therapies as chemotherapy and radiation reported fewer side effects to the traditional therapies (such as hair loss, weight loss, nausea, secondary infections, and skin problems).

Brazilian research in the early 2000s performed in humans and animals, including a human clinical trial, confirmed the early European Union research and reported cat's claw can avoid two common side effects of chemotherapy: neutropenia and leukopenia. In 2012, however, they used a patented water extraction process for the cat's claw product they gave breast cancer patients in the study that was alkaloid free and in a low dosage of 300 mg daily. They did not record any real differences in tumor status (all 40 patients had stage 2 invasive ductal carcinoma). They attributed the immunostimulant actions they achieved to other chemicals in cat's claw called carboxyl alkyl esters.

A Brazilian university published another human clinical trial with 51 cancer patients with advanced solid tumors who had no further therapeutic options and a life expectancy of at least two months in 2015. This study also used the same 300 mg daily dosage of an alkaloid-free water extract. They reported the treatment improved the patients' overall quality of life and social functioning and reduced fatigue. Again, no changes in tumor status were noted at this low dosage, but the disease stabilized for more than eight months in four participants. Since the actual antitumor actions of cat's claw are attributed to its alkaloids (which were missing in the product given), one does have to wonder how the results would have been different with a higher and more therapeutic dosage of cat's claw containing all of its beneficial plant chemicals.

Italian researchers reported in a 2001 study that cat's claw directly inhibited the growth of a human breast cancer cell line by 90% in test tubes, while another research group reported that it inhibited the binding of estrogens in human breast cancer cells in test tubes. Other researchers confirmed that cat's claw could also inhibit the binding of progesterone in breast cancer cells. In newer research, it was reported that P2X7 receptors stimulate breast cancer cell invasion and migration via the AKT pathway, and as such, it has become a new molecular chemical target in breast cancer drug research. More recent studies have shown that cat's claw is a new P2X7 receptor inhibitor, which can inhibit P2X7 receptor-mediated breast cancer invasion, and is expected to be used clinically as such.

In addition to its immunostimulating activity, anti-cancerous properties have been documented for these alkaloids and other constituents in cat's claw in test-tube research. Five of the oxindole alkaloids have been clinically documented with anti-leukemic properties in test tubes, and various root and bark extracts have demonstrated anti-tumorous and anti-cancerous properties in test tubes against various cancer cells, including bladder, lung, colon, liver, gastric, cervical, breast, and prostate cancers; medullary thyroid carcinoma; and squamous cell skin cancer. Swedish researchers documented cat's claw inhibited the growth of lymphoma and leukemia cells *in vitro* in 1998. In 2006, researchers reported that in 48 hours, an alkaloid extract of cat's claw induced cell cycle arrest (at G0/G10) in 57% of the acute lymphoblastic leukemia cells tested.

Anti-Cancerous Plant Chemicals

Cat's claw has several groups of plant chemicals that account for much of the plant's actions and uses. First and most studied is a group of oxidole alkaloids that has been documented with immune-stimulant, anti-cancer, and anti-leukemic properties. Another group of chemicals called quinovic acid glycosides has documented anti-inflammatory and antiviral actions. Antioxidant chemicals (tannins, catechins, and procyanidins), as well as plant sterols (beta-sitosterol, stigmasterol, and campesterol), account for the plant's anti-inflammatory properties. A class of compounds known as carboxyl alkyl esters found in cat's claw has been documented with immunostimulant, anti-inflammatory, anti-cancerous, and cell-repairing properties.

Cat's claw contains more than 40 different polyphenols, including 15 proanthocyanidins, seven procyanidin type-B dimers, two procyanidin type-B trimers, four propelargonidin dimers, seven hydroxybenzoic acids, three hydroxycinnamic acids, chlorogenic acid, epicatechin, (+)-catechin, and

(−)-epicatechin flavan-3-ol monomers. Many of these polyphenols have been the object of different studies due to their potential health benefits, mainly considering their antioxidant activity and the important role they may play by acting as cancer chemo-preventive agents. Cat's claw provides a significant amount of proanthocyanidin B2, which has reported strong toxicity to breast cancer and liver cancer cells in animal and test-tube research.

Cancer Pathways and Mechanisms of Action

More complete information on these signaling pathways, cancer pathways, and new chemical targets for cancer therapy shown here can be found in chapter 5.

- More than two dozen animal studies and two human studies confirm cat's claw anti-inflammatory actions. See the plant database file (in this plant's "Online Links to More Information" section) for more information on this research. Cat's claw achieves these actions through inhibiting the production of Interleukin 6 and NF-κB. Many types of cancer cells specifically increase these two chemicals inside their cells to help them replicate and proliferate. NF-κB activity not only promotes tumor cells' proliferation but also suppresses apoptosis, attracts angiogenesis, and facilitates distant metastasis.

- Cat's claw's anti-cancer activities are also related to its ability to inhibit JAK/STAT3, which plays a crucial role in cancer by regulating cell proliferation, survival, and immune responses.

- Cat's claw increases reactive oxygen species (ROS) and oxidative stress in cancer cells but acts as an antioxidant in healthy, normal cells. This can reduce the toxicity to healthy cells that chemotherapy drugs cause.

- Cat's claw can inhibit P2X7 receptor-mediated breast cancer invasion and migration.

- In breast cancer and colorectal cancers, cat's claw inhibits the Wnt-signaling pathway, which plays a role in the maintenance and self-renewal of cancer stem cells.

- Cat's claw acts as an LDH-A inhibitor. Less glucose is absorbed in cancer cells when this enzyme is inhibited, which lowers energy—energy the cancer needs to keep replicating and proliferating at a much faster pace than normal cells.

- Cat's claw can also inhibit glycolysis and Glut1, which prevents the mitochondria's use of glucose to manufacture the ATP energy all cancer cells need to survive.
- In acute lymphoblastic leukemia cells, cat's claw alkaloids arrested the cell cycle at the G0/G1 stage, triggering apoptosis.
- In some cancer cells, cat's claw was reported to have a pro-apoptosis effect by activating caspase-3 and caspase-8.

OTHER RESEARCHED BENEFITS THAT MAY BE HELPFUL

Many studies confirm that cat's claw has cellular- and organ-protective actions. This research is detailed in the main plant database file (see the link provided in this plant's "Online Links to More Information" section). This extends to protecting the gastric tract, nerves, heart, and liver from chemical agents well known to damage them, including chemo drugs. Cancer patients taking cat's claw in combination with chemotherapy may notice fewer side effects, through this protective action.

Cat's claw antioxidant benefits are also very well studied. Since cat's claw can protect healthy cells from the oxidative stress and resulting death caused by chemo drugs without protecting or interfering in the death of cancer cells, chemotherapy patients may also notice less toxicity and resulting side effects in this area as well.

AVAILABILITY OF PRODUCTS

The most common forms used today are cat's claw capsules and tablets, both of which have become widely available in most health food stores at reasonable prices. There are also newer (and more expensive) proprietary extracts of cat's claw in tablets and capsules, some backed by research—albeit paid-for research.

A good-quality, natural cat's claw vine bark with naturally occurring chemicals is the best value, money wise. It contains all the natural chemicals that nature provides in the proper ratio (including immune-stimulating alkaloids, anti-inflammatory glycosides, and antioxidant polyphenol chemicals), without chemical intervention. Some invasive extraction and manufacturing techniques may only extract one particular type of chemical, or change the complex ratio of naturally occurring chemicals in the plant, which ignores the efficiency and synergy of the plant. Scientists do not fully know how all these complex chemicals work together in harmony. In fact, scientists are still discovering new and novel active chemicals in this plant, even after 30-some-odd years of research on cat's claw.

As the market demand has increased for this rainforest plant, more companies have gone into the business of harvesting it, and the quality of the bulk materials coming in from South America can be sometimes questionable. Oftentimes, a combination of *U. tomentosa* and *U. guianensis* is harvested and sold as "cat's claw" (as, presently, the *guianensis* species is found more easily). Pick a good-quality and trusted label and manufacturer for the best results and the best value.

Safety

Several human clinical trials conducted using varying dosages of cat's claw have reported it was well tolerated and without toxic effects. Many animal studies have reported the same over many years, even in chronic dosages as well as large dosages (4 g/kg of body weight).

Dosages

For general immune and prevention benefits, practitioners usually recommend 1 gram daily of vine powder in tablets or capsules. Therapeutic dosages of cat's claw are reported to be as high as 20 grams daily and average 2–3 grams two or three times daily. Generally, as a natural aid for arthritis and bowel and digestive problems, 3–5 grams daily is recommended, if a good product is obtained.

Alternatively, a standard vine bark decoction can be used much the same way Indigenous peoples of the Amazon use it. The dosage for a standard decoction for general health and maintenance is ½ to 1 cup of a decoction once daily and up to 1 cup three times daily in times of special need. Adding lemon juice or vinegar to the decoction when boiling will help extract more alkaloids and fewer tannins from the bark. Use about ½ teaspoon of lemon juice or vinegar per cup of water. For standardized and/or proprietary extract products, follow the label instructions.

Contraindications

- Cat's claw has been clinically documented with immunostimulant effects and is contraindicated before or following any organ or bone marrow transplant or skin graft.

- Cat's claw has been documented with antifertility properties and is contraindicated in persons seeking to get pregnant. This effect has not been proven to be sufficient for the product to be used as a contraceptive, however, and it should not be relied on as such.
- Cat's claw has chemicals that can reduce platelet aggregation and thin the blood. Check with your doctor first if you are taking blood-thinning drugs and discontinue use one week to 10 days prior to any major surgical procedure.
- Cat's claw vine bark requires sufficient stomach acid to help break down the tannins and alkaloids during digestion and to aid in absorption. Avoid taking bark capsules or tablets at the same time as antacids. Avoid taking high tannin (dark-colored) liquid extracts and tinctures directly by mouth and dilute first in water or acidic juice (such as orange juice).
- Large doses of cat's claw (3-gram or 4-gram dosages at a time) have been reported to cause some abdominal pain or gastrointestinal problems, including diarrhea (due to the tannin content of the vine bark) in some people. The diarrhea or loose stools tend to be mild and go away with continued use. Discontinue use or reduce dosage if diarrhea persists longer than three or four days.

Drug Interactions

- Due to its immunostimulant effects, cat's claw should not be used with medications intended to suppress the immune system, such as cyclosporin or other medications prescribed following an organ transplant. (This theory has not been proven scientifically.)
- Based upon rat studies, cat's claw may protect against gastrointestinal damage associated with nonsteroidal anti-inflammatory drugs (NSAIDs) such as ibuprofen.
- Cat's claw may potentiate blood-thinning drugs.

SUMMARY OF BENEFITS THE PLANT HAS TO FIGHT CANCER

Cat's claw holds a special place in my heart, since it was responsible for taking me to the Amazon rainforest for the first time. The whole idea of making cat's claw available in the United States and sharing the European cancer research on it here to help cancer and AIDS patients was the main reason I created my company, Raintree Nutrition, in 1995. I am gratified to still see it helping cancer patients in the same manner, so many years later, with research still continuing.

Cat's claw has long been in my cancer protocols and natural remedies for cancer. It is an ingredient in the NTense-2 formula due to its anti-leukemic and anti-lymphoma actions. It is also in the main N-Tense formula for its immune benefits and other antitumor actions. I've also long recommended taking extra cat's claw while undergoing chemotherapy (2 grams twice daily) or when fighting hormone-positive breast cancers (2 grams twice daily).

In Brazil, cat's claw is prepared into an herbal medicine that is available free of charge from the Brazilian Public Health System for the treatment of arthritis. This important rainforest vine can also effectively contribute to improving the quality of life and the recovery of people undergoing chemotherapy treatments, and it is often given out free of charge to cancer patients in Brazil for that purpose as well.

Online Links to More Information

• Tropical Plant Database file for cat's claw: https://rain-tree.com/catclaw.htm.

• Research references for this text: https://rain-tree.com/Cats-Claw-Cancer-Research.pdf.

CHANCA PIEDRA

Family: Euphorbiaceae

Genus: *Phyllanthus*

Species: *niruri, amarus, lathyroides*

Synonyms: *Phyllanthus carolinianus, P. sellowianus, P. fraternus, P. kirganella, P. lathyroides, P. lonphali, Nymphanthus niruri*

Common Names: Chanca piedra, quebra pedra, stone-breaker, arranca-pedras, punarnava, amli, bhonya, bhoomi amalaki, bhui-amla, bhui amla, bhuianvalah, bhuimy-amali, bhuin-amla, bhumyamalaki, cane peas senna, cane senna, carry-me-seed, creole senna, daun marisan, derriere-dos, deye do, elrageig, elrigeg, erva-pombinha, evatbimi, gale-wind grass, graine en bas fievre, hurricane weed, jar amla, jar-amla, kizha nelli, malva-pedra, mapatan, para-parai mi, paraparai mi, pei, phyllanto, pombinha, quinine weed, sacha foster, shka-nin-du, viernes santo, yaa tai bai, yah-tai-bai, ya-taibai, yerba de san pablo

Parts Used: Entire plant

Chanca piedra is a small, erect, annual herb that grows 12–18 inches in height. It is indigenous to the rainforests of the Amazon and other tropical areas throughout the world, including the Bahamas, southern India, and China. The *P. niruri* plant is quite prevalent in the Amazon and other wet rainforests, growing and spreading freely (much like a weed). *P. amarus* and *P. sellowianus* are closely related to *P. niruri* in appearance, phytochemical structure, and history of use, but they typically are found in the drier tropical climates of India, Brazil, and even Florida and Texas. *P. amarus* and

P. sellowianus are often considered a variety of *P. niruri*, or no distinction is made among these three species in published clinical research. Oftentimes one name is indicated to be synonymous with another, and sometimes, both names are used interchangeably as if referring to one plant. It became so confusing that, in the 1990s, a major reorganization of the *Phyllanthus* genus was conducted (which classified *P. amarus* as a type of *P. niruri*). The plant's name in Peru is chanca piedra, and in Brazil, it's named quebra piedra; both names translate to "stone-breaker," which refers to its very long history of treating kidney stones.

Traditional Herbal Medicine Uses

Chanca piedra has a long history in herbal medicine systems in every tropical country where it grows. For the most part, it is employed for similar conditions worldwide. Its main uses are for many types of biliary and urinary conditions, including kidney and gallbladder stones; for hepatitis, colds, flu, tuberculosis, and other viral infections; liver diseases and disorders including anemia, jaundice, and liver cancer; and for bacterial infections such as cystitis, prostatitis, venereal diseases, and urinary tract infections. It is also widely employed for diabetes and hypertension, as well as for its diuretic, pain-relieving, digestive-stimulant, antispasmodic, fever-reducing, and cellular-protective properties in many other conditions. Various research published over the years has validated many of these traditional remedy uses. More complete information on chanca piedra's traditional uses, and this research can be found in the Tropical Plant Database (see the link provided in this plant's "Online Links to More Information" section).

Anti-Cancerous Actions

Chanca piedra's cancer-preventative and anti-cancer actions have been documented in many test-tube studies, and there has been an increase in animal studies over the last five years that validate many of the test-tube studies. This data reveals that the types of cancer cells most susceptible to the actions of the chanca piedra in these studies include leukemia, breast, colorectal, lung, melanoma, liver, cervical, prostate, and ovarian cancer cells. Some of this research reported that chanca piedra could kill these cancer cells in dosages as small as 8 mcg (0.08 mg).

This research also reports that chanca piedra selectively kills the cancer cells in a dose-dependent manner without damage or cell death to healthy cells. The research suggests that, when the plant or its chemicals can directly kill cancer cells, it's usually by causing cell cycle arrest when the cancer cells are trying to make another copy of itself. In several test-tube and animal studies, chanca piedra has also been shown to have anti-metastatic and anti-proliferative actions against breast, lung, prostate, melanoma, and osteosarcoma cancers. It didn't kill these types of cancer outright; rather, it inhibited the growth and/or spread.

A 2000 study documented that chanca piedra increased the lifespan of mice with liver cancer from 33 weeks (control group without treatment) to 52 weeks. Another research group tried to induce liver cancer in mice that had been pretreated with a water extract of chanca piedra. Their results indicated the chanca piedra extract dose-dependently lowered tumor incidence, levels of carcinogen-metabolizing enzymes, levels of liver cancer markers, and levels of liver injury markers. Other *in vitro* and animal studies suggest that chanca piedra can reduce the risk of developing liver cancer.

Researchers in India reported in 2009 and again in 2011 that chanca piedra protected mice from skin cancer when they gave animals oral dosages of chanca piedra before, during, or after inducing skin cancer in the animals. Tumor incidence was greatly reduced in all three administration periods. Their 2011 study reported that chanca piedra's strong antioxidant actions were measured and verified, and the cancer-prevention abilities with regard to skin cancers were probably due to chanca piedra's strong antioxidant abilities to prevent the cellular damage that would result in the mutation of skin cells into cancerous cells.

Several *in vitro* studies, as well as the animal studies, report that chanca piedra might provide cancer-preventative actions due to its antimutagenic actions. When healthy cells are exposed to various cancer-causing toxic chemicals and/or exposed to free radical damage, it can cause DNA damage to the cell, which promotes the cell to mutate into a cancer cell.

Several test-tube studies report that chanca piedra prevented healthy cells from mutating into cancerous cells when given a substance known to create mutations. The animal studies reported cancer-prevention abilities along the same lines for skin cancer and liver cancer as well. Many of the strong cellular-protective antioxidant polyphenols in chanca piedra have been shown to have good antimutagenic actions in other studies, so it is not surprising that chanca piedra evidenced this cancer-preventative action. Tens of thousands of studies over the last 20 years confirm the general cancer-prevention abilities of polyphenols, including several found in chanca piedra.

It may well be that chanca piedra's documented ability to stop cells from mutating plays an important factor in this reported anti-cancerous activity. In several animal studies (as well as within test tubes), extracts of chanca piedra have stopped or inhibited cells (including liver cells) from mutating in the presence of chemical substances known to create cellular mutations and DNA strand breaks (which can lead to the creation of cancerous cells). Again, one of these studies indicated that chanca piedra inhibited several enzyme processes peculiar to cancer cells' replication and growth—rather than a direct toxic effect of killing the cancer cell (sarcoma, carcinoma, and lymphoma cells were studied). This cellular-protective quality was evidenced in other research, which indicated that chanca piedra protected against chemically induced bone marrow damage in mice, as well as against radiation-induced damage in mice.

This cellular-protective ability did not go unnoticed by cancer researchers. Quite a few studies report that chanca piedra can protect the kidneys, liver, gastric and digestive tract, heart, and nerves from known substances that cause cellular damage. They started studying the possible benefits of combining chanca piedra with various frontline chemotherapy drugs and reported that it reduced the toxic effect of the drugs on healthy cells without affecting the cancer-killing ability of the drugs. In fact, some researchers reported that chanca piedra enhanced or increased the efficacy of the chemo drugs while protecting healthy cells.

Anti-Cancerous Plant Chemicals

Chanca piedra's anti-cancer actions are largely attributed to its diverse and novel polyphenols. While chanca piedra contains a handful of regular polyphenols found in many fruits and vegetables (such as gallic acid, chlorogenic acid, rutin, and quercetin), the majority of the polyphenols in chanca piedra are not found in fruits and vegetables, and you won't be getting these beneficial compounds from regular dietary sources.

Certain polyphenols are found *only* in chanca piedra, and others are found only in related medicinal *Phyllanthus* plants. These novel chemicals fall into a category of polyphenols called lignans and tannins. Chanca piedra contains quite a few lignans, and when we digest them, these lignans regularly form bonds with other polyphenols and with other natural compounds in our bodies to form many more polyphenol chemicals (called metabolites and derivatives). In fact, more than 80 new polyphenols and their derivatives and metabolites were discovered in *Phyllanthus* plants between 2016 and 2018—in just two years.

While the polyphenol content in plants can vary based on growing and harvesting conditions, overall, chanca piedra delivers an average of 220–250 mgs of polyphenols in just 1 gram of dried whole-herb chanca piedra. All told, chanca piedra delivers more than 70 polyphenols, including some of the derivatives and metabolites that were created in the herb before it was harvested for use. There is simply no way to determine how many other beneficial polyphenol metabolite compounds are formed inside our bodies when we ingest and digest chanca piedra.

Some of chanca piedra's novel polyphenol compounds have been the subject of research to determine their pharmacological effects. A few of these chemicals have been synthesized by scientists (copied in the laboratory without using the plant) and are the subject of ongoing pharmaceutical drug company research in an effort to create new drugs. The table on page 231 highlights a few of chanca piedra's unique polyphenols and their effects that have been documented in research.

Crude extracts of chanca piedra have been the subject of a great deal of research on the plant's immune modulation action, which reports the modulation of both innate and adaptive immune systems through various mechanisms and their possible therapeutic benefits for treatment of immune-related diseases, including cancer. This research is further detailed in the Tropical Plant Database file on chanca piedra (see the link in this plant's "Online Links to More Information" section). Research reports that, again, chanca piedra's polyphenols are the main players delivering this benefit. These include corilagin, geraniin, gallic acid, phyllanthin, hypophyllanthin, ellagic acid, phyltetralin, niranthin, catechin, quercetin, astragalin, and chebulagic acid.

THE ANTI-CANCEROUS PLANTS OF THE RAINFOREST

Compound	*Documented Pharmacological Effect*
Amariin	Antioxidant, hepatoprotective, **radioprotective**
Chebulagic acid	Antioxidant, anti-inflammatory, antidiabetic, **anti-cancer**, antiviral
Corilagin	Analgesic, antidiabetic, antifungal, anti-HIV, anti-inflammatory, antioxidant, antiplatelet, **antitumor**, antiviral, hypotensive **immunomodulating**, **radioprotective**, thrombolytic, vasorelaxant
Dioscin	**Antimetastatic, anti-cancerous**
Furosin	Analgesic, antioxidant, wound healing
Geraniin	Analgesic, antioxidant, anti-HIV, antimalarial, **antitumor**, antiviral, hepatoprotective, hypotensive, **immunomodulating**, **radioprotective**, wound healing
Hinokinin	Antioxidant, antiviral
Hypophyllanthin	**Anti-cancer**, anti-genotoxic, **antitumor**, antiviral, hepatoprotective, hypotensive
Isocorilagin	Antioxidant, **antitumor**, cholinesterase inhibitor
Lintetralin	Anti-inflammatory, antiviral
Methyl brevifolin carboxylate	Antiplatelet, anti-inflammatory, antioxidant, hypotensive
Niranthin	Analgesic, anti-inflammatory, antioxidant, antiparasitic, **antitumor**, antiviral, **immunomodulating**
Nirtetralin	Anti-inflammatory, antioxidant, **antitumor**, antiviral, hypotensive; **reverses multidrug resistance**
Phyllanthin	Antiaging, anti-amnestic, antibacterial, **anti-cancer**, anti-genotoxic, antioxidant, antiviral, hypouricemic, anti-inflammatory, **anti-leukemic**, antioxidant, **antitumor**, cellular protective, liver protective, hypotensive, kidney and renal protective, **immunomodulating**, reverse transcriptase inhibitor (anti-HIV)
Phyltetralin	Anti-inflammatory, antioxidant, antiviral, **immunomodulating**

Note: Terms in bold denote an application or benefit for cancer.

New research on cancer has reported a connection between inflammation and certain types of cancer, and it has become a subject of much research interest. Researchers are looking for compounds able to modulate inflammation-related signaling pathways in anti-cancer drug development programs as a new way to treat cancer. Chanca piedra has surfaced in this new search as a possible candidate. A group of researchers from the United States, Malaysia, and India published a study in 2020 that reported that the flavonoids (astragalin, kaempferol, quercetin, rutin), lignans (phyllanthin, hypophyllanthin, and niranthin), tannins (corilagin, geraniin, ellagic acid, gallic acid), and triterpenes (lupeol, oleanolic acid, ursolic acid) found in chanca piedra exert various anti-cancer and anti-inflammatory activities via perturbation of the NF-κB, MAPKs, PI3K/Akt, and Wnt signaling pathways.

Research on chanca piedra reveals that it can significantly increase the production and activation of specific immune cells responsible for killing foreign invaders (like cancer, viruses, and bacteria), while lowering the production of immune cells and chemicals called cytokines that cause inflammation. This has been confirmed by human studies. The human research reports adults and children with pneumonia, tuberculosis, hepatitis, chicken pox, and Hanson's disease (leprosy) mounted a much stronger immune response to fight these infections, which sped healing and viral/bacterial clearance when using chanca piedra.

It was also noted in these clinical studies that immune cells responsible for immunity were also increased, and those taking chanca piedra for their infections had no relapses or secondary infections and had higher levels of antigens (cells responsible for immunity). See "The Inflammation/Immune Pathway" section in chapter 5 for more information on how cancer uses the inflammatory/immune pathway to promote its growth and spread.

Several of chanca piedra's anti-cancer lignan chemicals have been copied and synthesized into small-molecule drugs for cancer by a major pharmaceutical company in the United States. Collectively, they called this group of now synthetic and patented chemicals *phyllanthusmins*. One in particular, called PHY34, will probably yield the first new approved cancer drug based on natural compounds found in chanca piedra. Their research shows it has real promise for ovarian cancer.

Cancer Pathways and Mechanisms of Action

More complete information on these signaling pathways, cancer pathways, and new chemical targets for cancer therapy shown here can be found in chapter 5.

- Chanca piedra can turn back on the "kill switch" by restoring p53 function, which cancer cells turned off to ignore apoptosis signals.

- Chanca piedra was shown to inhibit P-glycoprotein, which prevents the formation of intercellular pumps to expel chemo drugs out of cancer cells before the drugs can kill them, allowing them to become multidrug-resistant.

- A variety of polyphenol chemicals in chanca piedra exert both anti-cancer and anti-inflammatory activities via perturbation and/or modulation of the NF-κB, MAPKs, PI3K/Akt, and Wnt signaling networks. Activation of these cell-signaling pathways can lead to various aspects of cancer-related inflammation. See the "Inflammation/Immune Pathway" section in chapter 5 for more information.

- Chanca piedra induced S-phase cell cycle arrest and apoptosis in leukemia cells. One of the plant's polyphenols (phyllanthin) was shown to inhibit leukemic cancer cell growth and induced apoptosis through the inhibition of AKT and JNK signaling pathways. It also decreased the expression of anti-apoptotic genes and increased pro-apoptotic gene expression.

- Chanca piedra induced cell cycle arrest in ovarian cancer cells in the S phase.

- In leukemic cells, chanca piedra demonstrated G1 cell arrest, and an increase in p53 expression.

- In liver cancer cells, chanca piedra induced G2/M cell cycle arrest.

- Corilagin inhibited the growth of ovarian cancer cells via the TGF-β/AKT/ERK signaling pathways. It also induced apoptosis and autophagy by reducing NRF2 expression in glioma brain tumors.

- Geraniin suppresses ovarian cancer growth through inhibition of NF-κB activation and downregulation of Mcl-1 expression.

- Chanca piedra inhibited angiogenesis by decreasing the levels of vascular endothelial growth factor (VEGF) and hypoxia-inducible factor-1α (HIF-1α) in breast cancer tumor cells.

- Chanca piedra suppressed breast carcinoma metastasis and proliferation by suppressing matrix metalloprotein 2 and 9 expression via inhibition of the extracellular signal-related kinase (ERK) pathway.

- Chanca piedra inhibited tumor metastasis and angiogenesis through the suppression of four MMP (matrix metalloproteinase) enzymes in prostate and melanoma cancers.
- In research on melanoma, chanca piedra modified five different signaling pathways (NFκB, Myc/Max, Hypoxia, MAPK/ERK, and MAPK/JNK) to prevent proliferation, metastasis, and angiogenesis.
- Geraniin inhibited osteosarcoma cell migration and invasion by reducing the expression of MMP-9 through the PI3K/Akt and ERK1/2 signaling pathways.
- Chanca piedra has been reported to inhibit a protein called AP-1. Because AP-1 is often overactive in cancer cells, inhibiting it can potentially suppress tumor growth, induce apoptosis, inhibit metastasis, and sensitize cancer cells to chemotherapy.
- Chanca piedra was shown to alter cancer stem cell–specific signaling pathways (including NOTCH signaling) to make stem cells of multiple cancer types easier to find and kill.
- Chanca piedra also exhibited telomerase-inhibitor actions. This protein is generated by cancer cells to allow them to replicate indefinitely and avoid apoptosis.
- Chanca piedra was shown to kill various cancer cells by triggering autophagy.

Other Researched Benefits That May Be Helpful

Chanca piedra is one of the great Amazon plants that provides strong cellular-protective actions. Whether it's the heart, kidneys, liver, or gastric tract, many studies over the years have demonstrated that chanca piedra can protect organs from chemicals (and chemotherapy drugs) well known to damage them. Chanca piedra also reduces pain and inflammation, which can be helpful for some. For more information on this research, consult the Tropical Plant Database file on chanca piedra (see the link in this plant's "Online Links to More Information" section).

Availability of Products

Chanca piedra is available under many manufacturers' labels and includes capsules, liquid extracts, and whole herb powders. It is sold using the chanca piedra name as well as its translated-to-English name: stone-breaker. Since many of chanca piedra's active chemicals are polyphenols, which are water soluble, it's best to choose an alcohol-free extract. The extracts taste grassy and aren't overly objectionable to most; however, most prefer capsules since they are easier to take and are generally cheaper.

SAFETY

Chanca piedra has a long history of use in traditional medicine systems around the world where it is generally considered safe and nontoxic. Many animal studies and some human studies reported no toxicity or side effects even in very high dosages of 5,000 g/kg of body weight in animals.

Dosages

A standard herb infusion or weak decoction is prepared as the traditional remedy. Depending on what it's employed for, 1–3 cups are taken daily. Since most of the active chemicals are water soluble (and broken down during digestion), 2 grams in tablets or capsules twice daily can be substituted if desired. Concentrated fluid extracts or water/glycerine extracts are available in the marketplace. Depending on the concentration of the extracts, 2–4 mgs are taken two to three times daily. Alcohol tinctures (and spray-dried extracts that use alcohol) have not been traditionally used with chanca piedra (as the more fragile, water-soluble plant chemicals and sterols are thought to be damaged in alcohol).

Contraindications

• Chanca piedra has demonstrated hypotensive effects in animals and humans. People with a heart condition and/or taking prescription heart medications should consult their doctor before taking this plant. It may be contraindicated for some individuals with low bood pressure, and/or heart medications may need monitoring and adjusting.

• Chanca piedra has been considered in herbal medicine to be abortive (at high dosages) as well as a menstrual promoter. While not studied specifically in humans or animals, animal studies do indicate it has uterine relaxant effects. It should therefore be considered contraindicated during pregnancy.

- Chanca piedra has been documented with female antifertility effects in one mouse study (the effect was reversed 45 days after cessation of dosing). While this effect has not been documented in humans, the use of the plant is probably contraindicated in women seeking pregnancy or taking fertility drugs. This effect has not been substantiated sufficiently to be used as a contraceptive, however, and should not be relied on as such.
- Chanca piedra has demonstrated hypoglycemic effects in animals and humans. It is contraindicated for people with hypoglycemia. Diabetics should consult their doctor before taking this plant as insulin medications may need monitoring and adjusting.
- Chanca piedra has been documented in human and animal studies with diuretic effects. Chronic and acute use of this plant may be contraindicated in various other medical conditions where diuretics are not advised. Chronic long-term use of any diuretic can cause electrolyte and mineral imbalances; however, human studies with chanca piedra (for up to three months of chronic use) have not reported any side effects. Consult your doctor if you choose to use this plant chronically for longer than three months concerning possible side effects of long-term diuretic use.

Drug Interactions
- Chanca piedra may potentiate insulin and antidiabetic drugs.
- This plant contains a naturally occurring plant chemical called geraniin. This chemical has been documented with negative chronotropic, negative inotropic, hypotensive, and angiotensin-converting enzyme inhibitor effects in animal studies with frogs, mice, and rats. As such, this plant may potentiate antihypertensive drugs, beta-blocker drugs, and other heart medications (including chronotropic and inotropic drugs). This has not been confirmed in humans.

Summary of Benefits the Plant Has to Fight Cancer

After poring through all the new cancer research on chanca piedra, my original opinions formed before this new research was conducted haven't changed very much. I never used or recommended chanca piedra as a stand-alone remedy to treat cancer. Based on the research I'm reading today, it might slow cancer growth (anti-proliferative) and reduce or prevent some cancers from metastasizing or spreading. I did, however, often use chanca piedra or one of the chanca piedra multi-herb formulas as an adjunctive supplement for liver cancer and urinary tract cancers in combination with the N-Tense formula.

I knew chanca piedra was having a beneficial effect on the liver and kidneys and had an anti-proliferative effect. But I was mainly relying on the anti-cancer actions of the N-Tense formula to find and kill the cancer cells, and not chanca piedra directly. I must note, however, liver cancer was one of the most remarkable results I have seen in all my years of helping cancer patients. The combination of the chanca piedra–rich liver support formula (called Amazon Liver Support) in combination with the N-Tense formula created more remissions and cures than I've seen in any other type of cancer.

Since chanca piedra is one of the rainforest's best cellular-protective plants, I often recommended that people who were taking standard chemotherapy drugs add chanca piedra to help reduce chemo drugs' well-known toxic effects to the heart, liver, gastric/digestion, nerves, and/or kidneys. Newer research now validates that use as well (in both animal and test-tube research) by combining chanca piedra with chemo drugs like cisplatin and doxorubicin, in addition to helping avoid damage to healthy cells from radiation. See chapter 5 for dosages and more naturopathic protocols on how to incorporate this valuable little herb to help fight cancer and reduce normal side effects of conventional treatments and even enhance the efficacy of some conventional cancer drugs.

Online Links to More Information

• Tropical Plant Database file for chanca piedra: https://rain-tree.com/chanca.htm.

• Research references for this text: https://rain-tree.com/Chanca-Piedra-Cancer-Research.pdf.

ESPINHEIRA SANTA

Family: Celastraceae

Genus: *Maytenus*

Species: *ilicifolia*

Synonyms: *Celastrus ilicinus, Gymnosporia ilicina, Maytenus ilicina, Monteverdia ilicifolia*

Common Names: Espinheira santa, cancerosa, cangorosa, maiteno, limaosinho

Parts Used: Leaves

Espinheira santa is a small, shrubby evergreen tree growing to 16 feet in height with leaves and berries that resemble holly. It is native to many parts of South America, and in southern Brazil, it's even found in city landscapes for its attractive, holly-like appearance. With more than 200 species of *Maytenus* distributed in temperate and tropical regions throughout South America and the West Indies, there are many *Maytenus* species that are indigenous to the Amazon region that have been used medicinally by Indigenous tribes. Espinheira santa has been classified as *Maytenus ilicifolia* for many years. However, some Brazilian researchers began using a different name: *Monteverdia ilicifolia*. This name occasionally appears in research studies conducted in that country and some of their herbal products and drugs. Both names refer to the exact same species.

TRADITIONAL HERBAL MEDICINE USES

Espinheira santa has a long-documented history of use in South American herbal medicine practices. In Brazil, the leaves of the plant are brewed into a tea for the treatment of cancer, stomach ulcers, indigestion, chronic gastritis, and dyspepsia (with a recorded history of use for these purposes dating back to the 1930s). The leaf tea is also applied topically to wounds, rashes, and skin cancer. Espinheira santa is listed in the Brazilian Pharmacopoeia and in the National List of Essential Medicines (the list of approved pharmaceutical and herbal drugs in use in the country's public sector).

In other herbal medicine systems in South America, espinheira santa is used for anemia, asthma, stomach and gastric ulcers, cancer, constipation, gastritis, dyspepsia, heartburn, acid reflux, liver disorders, respiratory and urinary tract infections, and diarrhea, as well as a contraceptive, pain reliever, and antiseptic wound healer. More information on traditional uses and herbal remedies of espinheira santa can be found in the Tropical Plant Database (see link in this plant's "Online Links to More Information" section).

Anti-Cancerous Actions

Early research performed in Brazil in the early 1970s revealed that espinheira santa, as well as a few other species in the *Maytenus* plant family, contains chemical compounds that showed potent antitumor and anti-leukemic activities in animal and test-tube studies at very low dosages. They named this group of chemicals "maytansinoids." Then, in a 1976 plant screening program by the National Cancer Institute (NCI), an alcohol and water extract of espinheira santa leaves was documented with toxicity to cancer cells at very low dosages, and U.S. and European pharmaceutical companies began to show an interest in it.

Brazilian companies were using topical preparations of espinheira santa for skin cancers soon after the NCI research. Today, an espinheira santa herbal drug (an ointment) is manufactured in Brazil and is prescribed for basal and squamous cell skin cancers.

Quite a few scientists have reported that espinheira santa has anti-cancerous action in test tubes across various human and animal cell lines. More recently, Brazilian researchers published a study on espinheira santa reporting that it killed colorectal and liver cancer cells in test tubes and in animals in 2013. More important, using new laboratory testing methods, they determined espinheira santa had the ability to kill these cancer cells by manipulating an important gene (BCL2) in the intrinsic apoptosis pathway (programmed cell death). More information is found in this plant's "Cancer Pathways and Mechanisms of Action" section.

Pretty quickly after the first test-tube studies reported anti-cancer actions, researchers started evaluating the plant's chemicals to determine which ones were responsible. As usual, there have been many more studies published on espinheira santa's active chemicals instead of the plant itself. While we may not know specifically which chemical or chemicals are responsible for the anti-cancerous action demonstrated in the first test-tube and animal studies on the plant, we certainly have numerous chemicals to choose from! And as is usual, it's probably a combination of more than just one. It's also very possible that one group of chemicals may be affecting one type of cancer, while other chemical(s) play different roles with other types of cancer. This might explain espinheira santa's broad spectrum action against many types of cancer.

Anti-Cancerous Plant Chemicals

Espinheira santa contains quite a few natural chemicals with remarkable anti-cancerous actions and most fall into categories of plant chemicals called alkaloids and triterpenes. Triterpenes are produced in plants as specialized plant defense compounds, which usually have more specialized actions than polyphenols (discussed in chapter 2). They are often produced in plants growing in tropical climates because polyphenols can't address all extreme growing conditions. Some plants produce triterpenes by using polyphenols as starting materials to make them.

In the 1990s, Japanese researchers discovered a group of triterpene chemicals in espinheira santa, which they named cangorins (cangorin A through J). These new chemicals showed selective toxicity and/or inhibitory activity against various leukemia and cancer tumor cells in test tubes, and the researchers have published more than eight studies on their discovery and results. These researchers then reported in 2004 that they discovered four new triterpenes (named maytefolins A–C and uvaol-3-caffeate), which demonstrated significant anti-cancer actions against epithelial carcinoma, squamous cell carcinoma, and renal cell carcinoma.

Other important triterpene chemicals occurring in the plant include pristimerin, celastrol, and friedelin, which have been documented with remarkable anti-cancer actions and will be described later in this section. But let's look at the two most famous alkaloid chemicals targeted first for cancer drug development many years ago.

Following the NCI research, maytansine and mayteine (alkaloids) were extracted from espinheira santa and tested in cancer patients in the United States and South America in the 1970s. Mostly they were studied in patients with advanced cancer with limited available standard chemotherapy options. Although there were some significant regressions in ovarian carcinomas and some lymphomas with maytansine, further research was not continued due to the toxicity at the dosages used.

Maytansine: Renewed interest in this toxic anti-cancer chemical started again after cancer researchers learned how to chemically target cancer cells in all the road maps discovered in gene research (discussed in chapter 4). They found they could chemically bond this plant chemical to another substance found in a particular cancer cell or chemical in an aberrant signaling pathway that would help direct the toxicity to the cancer cells. This new knowledge resulted in new cancer drugs called "targeted chemotherapy drugs." Scientists started creating derivatives of maytansine for this purpose. Mertansine (DM1) and ravtansine (DM4) emerged as new maytansine derivative small-molecule approved drugs for further research. These were called maytansinoid derivatives. Their main mechanism of action is to bind to a protein called tubulin (present in all cells), causing cells to arrest in the G2/M phase of the cell cycle, which leads to cell death.

A Swiss pharmaceutical company changed mertansine slightly (enough to be patented), and named it emtansine. They got it approved as a new chemical (named DM1) for research, and the changes made to the original plant chemical made it even more toxic to both cancer and healthy cells. Eventually, a combination of emtansine and another antibody drug used to target HER2 + breast cancer (trastuzumab) resulted in a new drug called T-DM1 to use for human clinical trials. Years later, it was approved as a new cancer drug for breast cancer in 2019 and is now named Kadcyla. Other FDA-approved clinical trials are under way studying other types of tumors with T-DM1. A different antibody was combined with DM1 to target acute myelogenous leukemia (AML).

While these new drugs are generally less toxic than other cancer drugs because they are directed to cancer cells, it still has some of the same side effects due to damage to healthy cells along the way. The original maytansine derivatives, ravtansine and mertansine, are presently in various human studies in the same fashion for other types of tumors.

Maytenin/Tingenone/Maitenin (all three names are used for the same natural plant chemical): The early NCI research indicated, unlike maytansine, maytenin was killing cancer cells without toxicity to healthy cells. Researchers in the United States reported in 1998 that tingenone was toxic to liver cancer cells in the test tube. Researchers in Brazil published two 2021 test-tube studies reporting the mechanism by which tingenone killed acute myeloid leukemia cells and melanoma cells.

In 2020, researchers reported that they extracted two chemicals from espinheira santa (maytenin and a maytenin metabolite, 22-β-hydroxymaytenin) and treated mice with head and neck squamous cell carcinomas (including a metastasis-derived cell line). They compared the effects of these two natural plant chemicals with a common chemotherapy drug called cisplatin. Their results indicated that the natural chemicals were able to kill almost as many cancer cells as the drug did but without any toxicity to the kidneys.

Cisplatin and other platinum chemotherapy drugs can regularly cause renal failure due to kidney injury. In fact, half of the animals given just cisplatin died of renal failure in this study. Another study reported in 2011 that two chemicals in espinheira santa (tingenone and pristimerin) were more effective at killing breast cancer cells than the standard chemotherapy drug used to treat breast cancer (paclitaxel) in test tubes and animals.

Pristimerin: Pristimerin is another important anti-cancerous triterpene found in espinheira santa. It was first discovered in a tropical plant in 1951, and over the years, research has reported anti-cancer, antioxidant, anti-inflammatory, antibacterial, antimalarial, and insecticidal activities. The anti-tumorous activities of pristimerin have been demonstrated in various cancer cell lines and animal models in research over many years. New research on this natural chemical has been extensive and, lately, largely conducted in China. Unlike the United States, China regularly approves plant-based drugs for use by prescription as well as over-the-counter products in their well-established Chinese Traditional Medicine system. Some of these products are produced by Chinese pharmaceutical companies. Reviewing all the new research reveals that pristimerin may soon become a new cancer drug in China.

This extensive research (more than 175 studies so far) has shown that pristimerin has very strong anti-tumorous actions against a wide variety of different types of cancerous tumors as well as strong anti-cancerous actions against blood cancers such as leukemia and multiple myeloma. In test tubes, these studies report potent antitumor activity against various cancers such as breast cancer, bile duct cancer, gastric cancer, pancreatic cancer, prostate cancer, esophageal cancer, glioblastoma, ovarian cancer, colorectal cancer, oral squamous cell carcinoma, cervical cancer, osteosarcomas, and lung cancer.

Animal studies report very good efficacy in treating breast, cervical, prostate, lung, skin, and colorectal cancers, as well as osteosarcoma, leukemia, and multiple myeloma. One study in 2015 with mice also reported that it prevented prostate cancer bone metastasis. No toxicity to healthy cells, animal deaths, or side effects were reported in any of these animal studies.

Researchers have been conducting studies on adding the natural pristimerin plant chemical to their standard chemotherapy drugs. They report better efficacy in killing the cancer while reducing toxicity to healthy cells in the heart, kidneys, and liver (which usually results in halting the cancer drug treatment). One of these animal studies reported that adding pristimerin to a cancer drug named Adriamycin prevented the usual toxicity to the heart that the drug is known to cause.

Multiple studies report that pristimerin can prevent the process that cancer cells use to become resistant to chemotherapy drugs. This mechanism is the same as graviola's—it inhibits the formation of the small intercellular pumps that cancer cells create to expel chemotherapy drugs before it can kill them. Once these pumps are formed, the tumor cells can be totally resistant to any type of chemotherapy drug used. More information on these P-glycogen pumps can be found in chapter 5. Newer research also suggests that pristimerin has the ability to shut down these pumps previously created due to drug exposure as well as target the cancer cell and kill it.

This is especially good news for people fighting multidrug-resistant tumors. Research is being published now that shows if you add pristimerin to a cancer drug that cancer became resistant to, it overcomes the drug resistance, and the same cancer drug can begin treating the tumor again.

Espinheira santa contains another natural triterpene chemical, which is also found in some other medicinal plants, called *friedelin*. The plant makes several natural isomers and metabolites of friedelin, including friedelinol, friedoolean, friedooleanan, and friedelan. In fact, the plant uses friedelin to actually make pristimerin. Friedelin is well studied and reported with anti-inflammatory, antioxidant, anti-cancer, and antimicrobial activities. In recent cancer research, this compound was found to interfere with a protein (CYP17A1) involved in prostate cancer. In animal studies, friedelin reduced prostate tumor weight, prostate indexes, serum PSA levels, and testosterone levels in tumor-bearing mice. Other research indicates that friedelin can inhibit the growth and spread of breast and brain tumors and leukemia in animals and test tubes.

Espinheira santa has yet another triterpenoid plant chemical called *celastrol*, which is also found in a handful of Chinese medicinal plants in the same plant family. This chemical has been on the radar of cancer drug researchers for almost 10 years now. Their preliminary animal and test-tube research shows it exhibits significant broad-spectrum anti-cancer activities in the treatment of a variety of cancers, including lung cancer, liver cancer, colorectal cancer, hematological (blood) malignancies, gastric cancer, prostate cancer, renal carcinoma, breast cancer, bone tumors, brain tumors, cervical cancer, and ovarian cancer.

The data from published literature suggests that celastrol modulates multiple molecular targets such as TNF-α, NF-κB COX-2, VEGF, Akt, CXCR4, and pro-inflammatory cytokines and chemokines. These molecules play a major role in all three steps (initiation, proliferation, and progression) of cancer as described in chapter 5. Some researchers are presently creating analogs and derivatives of celastrol to study further in cancer research. Scientists report, however, that the action of celastrol is not specific to only cancer cells, and some toxicity to healthy cells was reported in animal studies.

Polyphenols: The polyphenols in espinheira santa that occur in the highest amounts include kaempferol, quercetin, catechins (including epicatechin and epigallocatechin), and myricetin. Metabolites of these polyphenols are also well documented in chemical analyses of espinheira santa. These compounds and their benefits for cancer are discussed in chapter 2.

While espinheira santa does contain maytansine and celastrol, which demonstrate toxic effects to both cancer cells and healthy cells, the use of the plant, full of many different plant chemicals, has shown repeatedly in animals and humans to be nontoxic. This might indicate that there is not enough of these chemicals in the plant to cause toxicity or that the chemicals are poorly absorbed during digestion of the plant. Therefore, theoretically, the anti-cancerous action of the plant may not be attributed to these chemicals at all.

There is also the possibility that the polyphenols (and pristimerin) in espinheira santa (which demonstrate protective effects in normal cells but not cancer cells) could possibly prevent the damage these two chemicals cause to healthy cells. For example, pristimerin protected healthy cells from the toxicity caused by toxic cancer drugs such as cisplatin and Adriamycin without affecting the toxicity of the drugs in cancer cells.

Many polyphenols, including those found in espinheira santa, have been combined with various toxic cancer drugs in newer research reporting that they also protected healthy cells from damaging cancer drugs. With a lack of motivation/profits on natural plants that can't be patented, we'll probably never determine which theory is more plausible by any significant human research.

Cancer Pathways and Mechanisms of Action

• When a plant extract of espinheira santa was tested *in vitro* and then new biological scientific methods were used, Brazilian researchers reported in 2013 that the plant mediated the induction of apoptosis by downregulating Bcl-2, which affected caspase-3 in human liver and colorectal cancer cells. They also reported this mechanism of action occurred only in the cancer cells tested. When healthy cells were combined with espinheira santa, it had a beneficial protective effect. See chapter 5 for more information on how Bcl-2 and caspase-3 are new chemical targets for cancer therapies in the "Apoptosis Pathway" section.

• Espinheira santa has shown anti-cancerous actions through the following genes and substances involved in gene function (and new chemical targets): NF-κB, PARP-1, JNK, Bax, p27, Bcl-2, Bcl-xL, Bcr-Abl, caspase-3, and ROS/JNK. See chapter 5 for more information.

• Pristimerin has demonstrated a stunning number of mechanisms of action in how it specifically treats cancer. Interestingly, it often uses different mechanisms of action and pathways for different types of cancer. Some of these include apoptosis, autophagy, cell migration and invasion, angiogenesis, and targeting several crucial signaling pathways (see chapter 5 for definitions and more information). Pristimerin has been reported to affect cancer in animals and test tubes through the following pathways.

• Pristimerin was reported to arrest the cell cycle (at G1) during cancer cell division, which results in cell death by triggering apoptosis.

• Pristimerin was also shown to reduce cancer stem cell activity, which may prevent metastases of many tumor types and address drug resistance.

• Research reports that espinheira santa is affecting the PI3K/AKT pathway. This pathway is a signaling network that controls cell growth, survival, and metabolism. It's often overactive in cancer, which can lead to tumor growth and resistance to cancer treatments.

• It is also affecting the nuclear factor-kappaB (NF-κB) pathway. This pathway typically enhances inflammation in the tumor microenvironment by increasing the secretion of pro-inflammatory chemicals, which eventually leads to rapid proliferation of tumor cells.

• Pristimerin affects the reactive oxygen species (ROS)/mitogen-activated protein kinase (MAPK) pathway. Research indicates that pristimerin actually increases ROS inside of cancer cells, damaging them enough to trigger apoptosis, much like chemotherapy drugs do. Unlike many chemotherapy drugs, however, it only increases ROS damage in cancer cells, while protecting normal healthy cells from ROS damage.

• Pristimerin was shown to alter the Shh/Gli1 pathway. This signaling cascade regulates the expression of genes involved in cell proliferation, differentiation, and survival. Dysregulation of this pathway is often associated with various cancers.

• Pristimerin was reported to affect several proteins in HIF-1α/SPHK1 pathways. Both pathways are involved in tumor growth and spread.

• Pristimerin was reported to inhibit Akt/NF-kappaB/mTOR signaling proteins. This is one of the pathways that cancer cells use to turn off the programmed cell death code (apoptosis), which allows them to keep multiplying indefinitely.

• It was reported that pristimerin significantly impacts the complex interaction between proteasome functioning and telomerase activity. The data suggests that one of its mechanisms of action in the inflammation pathway is eliciting cellular responses closely resembling those elicited by proteasome inhibitors (the usual chemotherapy drugs for multiple myeloma and lymphomas) but without any toxicity to healthy cells. Again, these mechanisms and pathways are explained in chapter 5.

- Pristimerin induces autophagy-mediated cell death in some types of cancer through the ROS/JNK signaling pathway. In other cancer types, pristimerin affected the miR 23a/Akt/GSK3β signaling pathway to inhibit autophagy, which triggered apoptosis.
- Pristimerin was reported to modulate the epithelial-mesenchymal transition (EMT) process, leading to decreased expression of key EMT-related proteins like vimentin, N-cadherin, and matrix metalloproteinases (MMPs), thereby reducing the cancer cells' ability to detach, move, and invade surrounding tissues.
- It has also been reported to inhibit tumor cells from forming new blood vessels (angiogenesis) to bring more nutrients to fuel the tumor's rapid growth.
- Pristimerin causes a loss of mitochondrial membrane potential. Some cancer cells have an abnormally high mitochondrial membrane potential than normal cells do. This can contribute to cancer cell invasion and metastasis.
- Pristimerin was also able to limit colorectal cancer invasion and metastasis. It caused downregulation of PI3K/AKT/mTOR pathway and its subsequent downstream p70S6K and E4-BP1 proteins.
- Pristimerin suppressed the invasion of human prostate cancer cells through inhibition of epithelial-to-mesenchymal transition (EMT), which was confirmed by the EMT-related markers including N-cadherin, fibronectin, vimentin, and ZEB1.
- MMP2 and MMP9, which are important proteins regulating invasion and metastasis, were decreased by pristimerin in esophageal cancer cells in a dose-dependent manner, resulting in inhibition of migration and invasion.

Other Researched Benefits That May Be Helpful

Many of espinheira santa's uses in traditional herbal medicine have been verified by research. Its most popular use has been for the treatment of stomach ulcers and digestive complaints. Quite a few animal studies indicated that espinheira santa not only treated gastric ulcers but also protected the animals from known ulcer-causing chemicals and drugs. These actions were shown to be related to other natural chemicals in the plant called polysaccharides and alkaloids. See espinheira santa's database file in the Tropical Plant Database (link provided later in this plant's "Online Links to More Information" section) to learn more about the uses and research on the plant's anti-ulcer and gastroprotective actions.

Based on these uses and researched actions, it's possible that cancer patients taking cancer drugs might notice additional beneficial effects when they take espinheira santa if the drug is known to cause stomach damage, pain, and ulcers or mouth ulcers (called mucositis, which some chemo drugs cause). If used for this purpose, the research indicates it is advisable to prepare a simple espinheira tea (infusion) and drink 30 minutes to an hour prior to taking known chemicals and drugs that cause stomach or mouth ulceration. The natural plant chemicals known to be beneficial for stomach pain and ulcers are different than the anti-tumorous chemicals. They are more delicate and don't like high prolonged heat. Preparing an infusion is just like making tea. Bring the water to boil and turn off the heat. Add the plant to the pot/cup, cover it, and allow it to steep for at least 10 minutes. Use the same quantities of plant and water as described in the decoction instructions.

Research indicates that espinheira santa has anti-inflammatory actions, which also include modulating pro-inflammatory immune cells to reduce inflammation. The plant database file will provide more information and the research on espinheira santa's anti-inflammatory and immune modulation actions. As described in chapter 5, many types of cancers create an inflammatory state inside their cells or within the tumor microenvironment, which facilitates cancer growth and progression. These actions reported by other research may prove beneficial to espinheira santa's anti-cancer benefits.

Availability of Products

While the cancer benefits of espinheira santa have not been widely disseminated in the United States, it has been used as a digestive herbal remedy here for quite a while. It is available from several U.S. companies, which provide products in capsules, liquid extracts, tinctures, and tea-cut leaves used to prepare natural teas and herbal decoctions. It is probably best to rely on a U.S. supplier to purchase products. U.S. manufacturers are required to follow good manufacturing practices established by the Food and Drug Administration (FDA), which confirms the identity of the actual plant species in their products with standardized tests. It has been noted by research in Brazil that several *Maytenus* species are sold as "espinheira santa." In addition, it was reported that one adulterant has been identified in some products sold in Brazil that is an entirely different plant with much different properties and actions than espinheira santa and even other *Maytenus* species.

SAFETY

The very long history of traditional uses in herbal medicine reports the plant decoction or a simple infusion (herbal tea) was well tolerated by people taking it without any reported side effects noted. The many animal studies performed on the plant and its active chemicals did not report any toxicity or side effects. Acute toxicity studies in 1978, 1991, and 2002 showed no toxicity in rats and mice in dosages up to 1 g/kg of body weight.

A research group in Brazil conducted Phase I and II human clinical studies in 2017 to study toxicity in people taking espinheira santa (presumably in the approval of a new anti-ulcer/antacid herbal drug). Twenty-four healthy volunteers were given espinheira santa tablets in increasing weekly dosages, from an initial dose of 100 mg to a final dose of 2,000 mg. They reported "the administration of up to 2,000 mg of the extract was well tolerated, with few changes in biochemical, hematological or psychomotor function parameters, and no significant adverse reactions." A few subjects reported dry mouth and/or increased urination, but these resolved during the study without any intervention. The same researchers published acute and chronic toxicity studies in rats, mice, and dogs in the same year that reported no toxic effects in animals, even if given in high doses or over a long period (180 days).

A group of university researchers in Brazil, however, published a paper on a test-tube toxicity study in 2024 that reported when they soaked slices of rat liver in an espinheira santa extract and the polyphenol, quercetin, for six hours in test tubes "[t]he intracellular enzymes leakages, CYP2D6, LDH and AST, were increased." They suggested these results might suggest liver toxicity. They recommended that "patients with liver disorders must have care using *M. ilicifolia* tea and products."

This effect wasn't reported in live animals fed espinheira santa by mouth or in other toxicity studies in humans. Animals given quercetin by mouth by other researchers reported a liver protective effect at normal dosages and a rise in all liver enzymes (not just three) in only very high dosages. The amount of quercetin in espinheira santa would be considered a low to normal dose based on the research on orally ingested quercetin (studied in humans and animals). Some might suggest that the effects of soaking slices of rat liver for six hours in a test tube may not completely correlate with the same effects of espinheira santa being ingested as a natural remedy by humans, undergoing normal digestive processes and then filtered through the liver.

Dosages

The traditional herbal remedy usually recommends 1 cup of a standard leaf decoction twice daily. To prepare a standard decoction, boil 2 teaspoons of the herb in 1 cup of water (or 2 tablespoons per liter of water) for 10 minutes. If desired, 2–3 grams of leaf powder in tablets, capsules, or stirred into juice or water twice daily can be substituted. A standard leaf decoction or a tincture can also be applied directly to the skin for topical use for skin cancers, wounds, and rashes. The tincture can be taken orally at a dosage of 30–60 drops (1–2 milliliters), depending on body weight, twice daily.

Contraindications

None reported.

Drug Interactions

None reported.

SUMMARY OF BENEFITS THE PLANT HAS TO FIGHT CANCER

Espinheira santa is rather unique since it has so many different chemicals that are active against cancer; these chemicals work in many different ways and in so many pathways. Research indicates it affects so many different types of cancer by using different pathways and mechanisms of action. For example, oftentimes a medicinal plant works well for tumorous types of cancers but not for blood-type cancers (such as leukemias and lymphomas). The research indicates that espinheira santa has a beneficial effect for both types of cancer by impacting different pathways with different natural plant chemicals. For more than 20 years, espinheira santa was an ingredient in all three cancer formulas I developed for Raintree.

The research data concerning protecting healthy cells and preventing intercellular pumps (which create drug resistance) might indicate that using an espinheira santa natural remedy during standard chemotherapy treatment may be helpful. Hopefully, people will learn much more about this important rainforest medicinal plant from this book—when looking for natural remedies for cancer, this is an important one to consider. See more information in chapters 7 and 8 on how it has been used with other rainforest plants for herbal remedies for different types of cancer.

Online Links to More Information

• Tropical Plant Database file for espinheira santa: https://rain-tree.com/espinheira.htm.

• Research references for this text: https://rain-tree.com/Espinheira-Santa-Cancer-Research.pdf.

GRAVIOLA

Family: Annonaceae

Genus: *Annona*

Species: *muricata*

Synonyms: *Annona macrocarpa, A. bonplandiana, A. cearensis, Guanabanus muricatus*

Common Names: Graviola, soursop, Brazilian paw paw, guanábana, guanábano, guanavana, guanaba, corossol épineux, huanaba, toge-banreisi, durian benggala, nangka blanda, cachiman épineux

Parts Used: Leaves, fruit, seeds

Graviola is a small, upright evergreen tree, 16–20 feet high, with large, glossy, dark green leaves. It produces a large, heart-shaped, edible fruit that is 6–8 inches in diameter, is yellow-green in color, and has white flesh inside. Graviola is indigenous to most of the warmest tropical areas in South and North America, including the Amazon rainforest. The fruit is sold in local markets in the tropics, where it is called guanábana in Spanish-speaking countries, soursop in the United States and English-speaking tropics, and graviola in Brazil.

TRADITIONAL HERBAL MEDICINE USES

Traditional medicinal uses of graviola have been identified in tropical regions to treat diverse ailments such as fever, pain, respiratory, heart, and skin illness, internal and external parasites, bacterial infections, hypertension, inflammation, diabetes, and cancer. Test-tube research has confirmed some of these traditional uses; graviola has demonstrated antimicrobial, anti-inflammatory, anti-protozoan, antioxidant, insecticide, larvicide, and anti-cancerous actions. Animal studies of the crude extracts and isolated compounds of graviola were shown to possess anti-cancerous, anti-anxiety, anti-stress, anti-inflammatory, contraceptive, anti-tumoral, anti-ulcerous, wound-healing, liver-protective, neuro-protective, pain-relieving, hypotensive, and hypoglycemic activities.

For the past 25 years graviola has been used as a natural herbal remedy for cancer in many countries around the world. More complete information on all of graviola's traditional uses and this research can be found in the Tropical Plant Database (see the link provided later in this plant's "Online Links to More Information" section).

Anti-Cancerous Actions

In a 1976 plant screening program by the National Cancer Institute (NCI), graviola leaves and stem showed active toxicity against cancer cells, and researchers have been following up on these findings since. Thus far, graviola and/or its active chemicals have been reported to be selectively toxic to these types of tumor cells: lung carcinoma cell lines, human breast solid tumor lines, prostate adenocarcinoma, pancreatic carcinoma cell lines, cervical cell lines, colorectal cell lines, liver cancer cell lines, human lymphoma cell lines, and multidrug-resistant human breast adenocarcinoma.

As graviola became more popular as a natural cancer remedy, many doctors noted their patients were taking it. Several doctors published papers called "case reports," which detailed their patients' use of graviola with some amazing results. In 2020, a doctor in Portugal detailed the case of a 68-year-old patient with liver cancer; the patient refused chemotherapy but had his tumors disappear while taking graviola. He was still cancer free after five years of follow-up when the report was published.

A doctor at a cancer center in NSW Australia also wrote a case report in 2019 on a woman who was 68 years old when she was diagnosed with metastatic ovarian cancer in 2011. She was initially treated with conventional chemotherapy, surgery, and radiation and, a year later, began taking graviola. She experienced a rapid and dramatic decline in her Ca-125 (a tumor marker) from 404 kU/L down to 47 kU/L over 32 months despite no other concurrent anti-cancer therapy.

Over the years, she relapsed several times when stopping the graviola, did more chemotherapy, and restarted the graviola as well. Each time, her cancer marker returned to normal. The doctor summarized the case report saying: "Our case highlights that despite an advanced disease with a poorly differentiated carcinoma at diagnosis, the relatively long periods of disease stability whilst being on graviola our patient experienced remains a remarkable phenomenon. In between her multiple relapses, she continued to show response to graviola. Such a pattern of stability and response achieved with graviola alone during these periods warrants further investigation."

Doctors at a cancer center in Miami, Florida, wrote a case report on a patient with metastatic breast cancer who took graviola. They reported in 2014 the clinical benefit, without side effects, of using graviola in a patient with breast cancer whose disease was resistant to multiple lines of chemotherapy including anthracyclines and taxanes. Multiple rounds of chemotherapy over several years resulted in metastasis to the lungs and liver. The patient began boiling 5–7 graviola leaves in a cup of water and drinking it daily. She was reported to have stable disease several months later and discontinued the graviola. A year later her lung metastases worsened, and she resumed the graviola. Afterward her disease stabilized again, and at the time of the case report's publication, the patient had achieved stable disease and experienced no side effects from just graviola therapy for more than five years.

Researchers in Indonesia conducted a randomized controlled human clinical trial with 30 colorectal cancer patients and published three clinical studies in 2017 reporting their results. The first clinical study was on the safety and tolerability of the graviola product that was used, which reported it was safe and highly tolerable. The second clinical study reported that these patients were given a low dosage of only 300 mg of a graviola leaf water extract daily for eight weeks. They performed an *ex vivo* test that is designed to represent the effect of the extract after it is absorbed and reaches the plasma of the patient.

They tested the patients' blood in test tubes against a type C colorectal adenocarcinoma cell line and a highly tumorigenic Dukes type D colon cancer line. The results indicated that the blood inhibited the cancer cell lines 97% as much as the plant extract did, which represents very high absorption and bioavailability. They also reported the blood had selective inhibitory activity against colorectal cancer cells without inhibiting normal/healthy cell growth.

Their third study, published in 2017, involved 20 of the same colorectal cancer patients and tested whether graviola extract had anti-inflammatory effects. The study was a randomized, double-blind trial, meaning neither the participants nor the researchers knew who was receiving the actual extract or a placebo. After eight weeks of taking graviola, they found a strong link between certain immune system markers of inflammation (TNF-α and IL-18).

They also found a significant relationship between two other markers (IFN-γ and IL-10). This means that IL-10 levels increased in response to inflammation. This was the first human study to confirm that graviola has anti-inflammatory effects.

A compelling animal study was performed in 2012 in the United States that used the graviola leaf powder that researchers obtained from my company, Raintree Nutrition. Pancreatic cancer is one of the hardest cancers to treat. By the time of diagnosis, pancreatic cancer is usually already in advanced stages and is resistant to conventional chemotherapy and radiotherapy.

Their study focused on testing how graviola affects pancreatic cancer by looking at its ability to kill cancer cells, impact cell metabolism, change cancer-related protein and gene expression, and influence tumor growth and spread. First, they employed various assays, in silico methods, and other newer testing methods to determine ATP levels, necrosis, apoptosis, cell cycle arrest, metabolism, and other actions. Then the researchers implanted pancreatic tumors into immunodeficient mice to determine the effect of graviola on pancreatic tumor growth.

The results showed that graviola caused pancreatic cancer cells to die by stopping their metabolism. It also reduced the levels of molecules involved in oxygen and glucose regulation (like HIF-1α, NF-κB, GLUT1, GLUT4, HKII, and LDHA). Additional tests confirmed that graviola blocked the cancer cells' ability to grow and form tumors. In the *in vivo* part of the study, after 35 days of treatment (with 50 mg or 100 mg of graviola water extract), the animals were euthanized, and the pancreatic tumors were removed and weighed.

The results indicated that tumor growth decreased significantly in graviola-treated mice in comparison to the control group. Specifically, the tumor growth inhibition in mice treated with a dose of 100 mg/kg (of body weight) graviola extract was 59.8% whereas in mice treated with a dose of 50 mg/kg (of body weight) graviola extract the inhibition was 50.3%, indicating the efficacy of graviola in cancer regression. They summarized their research reporting: "Overall, the compounds that are naturally present in a Graviola extract inhibited multiple signaling pathways that regulate metabolism, cell cycle, survival, and metastatic properties in PC cells. Collectively, alterations in these parameters led to a decrease in tumorigenicity and metastasis of implanted pancreatic tumors, indicating promising characteristics of the natural product against this lethal disease."

Seven animal studies in rats and mice have reported the inhibitory potential of graviola on breast cancer induced in female rats and mice. The breast cancer studies reveal that graviola significantly reduced the incidence of death, tumor incidence, volume and weight of tumors, total protein levels in tumors, reduced levels of CA 15–3, and a decrease of pro-inflammatory TNF-α, IL-6, and INF-γ levels. These studies suggest that graviola triggered cell cycle arrest, induced apoptosis, and interacted with the estrogen receptor-alpha (ERα) signaling pathway, which is a key regulator of cell growth in breast tumors.

Other animal research reported a 72.5% reduction of colorectal cancer in rats and reduced tumor size and reduced infiltration by tumor cells to liver tissue in mice by significantly improving the abnormalities in the expression of pro-apoptotic (Bax and caspase-3) and anti-apoptotic (Bcl-2) genes. Another group studying liver tumors in rats reported graviola triggered apoptosis in liver tumor cells by significantly decreasing anti-p53 expression in liver cells.

Several studies report that combining graviola with standard chemotherapy drugs may prove beneficial for some patients. In 2023, researchers in South Korea reported the polysaccharides chemicals in graviola protected immune system macrophages from the well-known toxicity and death by cisplatin without interfering with the effectiveness of the drug against lung cancer cells in animals and test tubes. Other researchers reported in 2021 that combining graviola with doxorubicin enhanced the effectiveness of killing breast cancer cells (including triple-negative breast cancer) of both anti-cancer substances.

Anti-Cancerous Plant Chemicals

Thus far, scientists have confirmed a total of 410 plant chemicals in the leaves, stems, fruit, tree bark, and roots of the graviola tree. The main active components with anti-cancer benefits are acetogenins, alkaloids, and polyphenols. Graviola leaves have demonstrated potent anti-cancer effects primarily due to their bioactive chemicals called acetogenins. The acetogenin with the strongest anti-cancer action is called annonacin and it has been the subject of the most research.

Acetogenins: More than 120 Annonaceous acetogenins (now called ACGs) have been isolated from leaves, barks, seeds, roots, and fruits of graviola. Most all of these natural ACG chemicals have been shown in test tubes, animals, and several small-scale human studies to selectively target and kill cancer cells without harming healthy cells across various cancer types, including brain, breast, colorectal, gastric, lung, liver, oral, ovarian, pancreatic, prostate, renal, and skin cancers, as well as melanoma and leukemia. Due to these powerful anti-cancer chemicals, graviola has become a promising natural anti-cancer remedy to use while drug companies are still working on turning some of these acetogenin chemicals into new cancer drugs. Some have already been copied by scientists, and cancer researchers are now creating mimics, derivatives, and metabolites in their quest for new effective cancer drugs. At least two of these derivatives have been turned into small-molecule drugs for further cancer research.

Many of the acetogenins have demonstrated selective toxicity to tumor cells at very low dosages—as little as 1 part per million. Four studies were published in 1998, which further specify the chemicals and acetogenins in graviola that are demonstrating the strongest anti-cancerous and anti-tumorous actions. Mode-of-action studies in three separate laboratories have determined that these acetogenins are superb inhibitors of an enzyme process that is only found in the membranes of cancerous tumor cells (called "tumor-associated NADH oxidase" or tNOX). This is why they are toxic to cancer cells but have no toxicity to healthy cells. ACGs in graviola are drawn to this enzyme.

When they find a cancer cell with it, the ACGs attach to them and stop the enzyme from working. This causes the cell's membrane to break down; the cell's contents then spill out, and the cancer cells die. This process leads to necrosis (instead of apoptosis), which sends a signal for immune cells to come and clean up the damage. Unlike apoptosis, necrosis also causes pro-inflammatory immune cells to respond, and some inflammation may be present.

Other natural chemicals in graviola, however, may mitigate this effect since they are effective anti-inflammatories as previously described. In fact, researchers conducting the animal study on pancreatic cancer previously discussed noted that pancreatic cancer cells in the animals were killed by both necrosis and apoptosis and wondered if the results would have been better if they hadn't used immune-deficient animals.

In addition to this remarkable action, the ACGs in graviola have shown they are effective inhibitors of a substance called Mitochondrial Complex I (also known as ubiquinone-linked NADH oxidase). All cells in the body need energy to do their jobs. This energy is made in a part of the cell called the mitochondria. They make a substance called Complex 1 and then turn it into a chemical called ATP (adenosine triphosphate), which is like fuel for the cell. It's similar to how crude oil is turned into gasoline to power a car.

Since cancer cells are growing and dividing at a much faster rate than normal cells, they need a lot more ATP energy. The ACGs in graviola are especially attracted to high energy/high ATP cells, which help them hunt down cancer cells; when found, they begin inhibiting the chemical process of turning Complex 1 into ATP. The ACGs act on Complex 1 and block the corresponding electron transport chain, which terminates ATP production. This reduced energy stops the cancer cells from dividing/replicating, which initially slows down tumor growth. Over time, with ATP production blocked, the cancer cells lack enough energy to run their life-sustaining processes, and it triggers cell death through apoptosis.

In 1997, Purdue University published information with promising news that graviola was killing tumor cells that were resistant to chemotherapy drugs. They reported that several of the ACGs "not only are effective in killing tumors that have proven resistant to anti-cancer agents, but also seem to have a special affinity for such resistant cells." In several interviews after this information was publicized, the head pharmacologist in Purdue's research explained how this worked. As he explains it, cancer cells that survive chemotherapy can develop resistance to the agent originally used as well as to other, even unrelated drugs. This phenomenon is called multidrug resistance (MDR).

One of the main ways that cancer cells develop resistance to chemotherapy drugs is by creating an intercellular pump, which is capable of pushing anti-cancer agents out of the cell before the drugs can kill it (called a

P-glycoprotein efflux pump). On average, only about 2% of the cancer cells in any given person might develop this pump—but they are the 2% that can eventually grow and expand to create multidrug-resistant tumors.

Some of the research on acetogenins reported that they were capable of shutting down these intercellular pumps, thereby killing multidrug-resistant tumors. Purdue researchers reported that the acetogenins preferentially killed multidrug-resistant cancer cells by blocking the transfer of ATP into them. A tumor cell needs energy to grow and reproduce, and a great deal more to run its pump and expel attacking agents. By inhibiting energy to the cell, it can no longer run its pump. Normal cells seldom develop such a pump; therefore, they don't require large amounts of energy to run a pump and, generally, are not adversely affected by ATP inhibitors.

An interesting animal study was published in 2002 by researchers in Japan, who were studying various acetogenins found in several species of plants. They inoculated mice with lung cancer cells to grow into tumors. One-third received nothing (the control group), one-third received the chemotherapy drug Adriamycin, and one-third received the main graviola acetogenin, annonacin (at a dosage of 10 mg/kg).

At the end of two weeks, five of the six in the untreated control group were still alive, and lung tumor sizes were then measured. The Adriamycin group showed a 54.6% reduction of tumor mass over the control group—but 50% of the animals had died from toxicity (this particular chemo drug causes toxicity to the heart). The mice receiving annonacin were all still alive, and the tumors were inhibited by 57.9%—slightly better than Adriamycin—and without toxicity.

Researchers in Taiwan reported in 2003 that the main graviola acetogenin, annonacin, was highly toxic to ovarian, cervical, breast, lung, bladder, and skin cancer cell lines at very low dosages in test-tube research. Newer research in 2024 reported that combining annonacin with a chemotherapy drug used to treat advanced liver tumors (Sorafenib) demonstrated synergistic actions in test tubes and animals by increasing the drug's ability to induce apoptosis.

Polyphenols: In different studies, when different extraction methods have been used with graviola leaves, the quantity of extractable total polyphenols is considerably different. This is important to mention because the most common medicinal use is an aqueous infusion/tea and the majority of phenols are soluble in water. Phenolic compounds are considered as the major phytochemicals responsible for graviola's antioxidant and anti-inflammatory activity. Many of the 38 different polyphenols in graviola have also been well documented in treating and/or preventing various types of cancers. See the reference file for review articles that provide more information on graviola's polyphenols and their anti-cancerous actions.

The main polyphenols in graviola leaves include argentinine, caffeoylquinic acid, catechin, chlorogenic acid, cinnamic acid, coumaric acid, daidzein, dicaffeoylquinic acid, emodin, epicatechin, feruloylquinic acid, fisetin, gallocatechin, genistein, glycitein, homoorientin, isoferulic acid, Isovitexin, kaempferol, kaempferol 3-O-rutinoside, luteolin 3́7-di-O-glucoside, quercetin, quercetin 3-O-glucoside, quercetin 3-O-neohesperidoside, quercetin 3-O-robinoside, quercetin–O-rutinoside, quercetin 3-O-α-rhamnosyl, robinetin, tangeretin, taxifolin (+), and vitexin.

Curzerenone (also called SF-1603 as an experimental drug): This is a monoterpenoid compound found in graviola leaves with many potential health benefits including anti-cancer (via programmed cell death, loss of mitochondrial membrane potential, reactive oxygen species [ROS], and blocking the ERK/MAPK and NF-κB signaling pathways), anti-inflammatory, antioxidant, liver protective, and antiviral actions. It has been studied in test tubes for liver cancer, which reported it had a strong ability to induce apoptosis in liver cancer cells.

Cancer Pathways and Mechanisms of Action

Graviola has been reported to kill cancer cells through the apoptosis, proliferation, and metastasis pathways. Graviola and its anti-cancerous acetogenins have shown to affect the apoptosis pathway in several highly effective ways, as well as other key pathways. More complete information on these signaling pathways, cancer pathways, and new chemical targets for cancer therapy shown here can be found in chapter 5.

- Graviola inhibits Complex 1, which reduces ATP energy in cancer cells; this slows the cells' growth and, over time, triggers apoptosis. This can also prevent multidrug-resistant tumors (and cancer cells) from forming during chemotherapy. This can also target and kill multidrug-resistant tumors by decreasing the extra ATP required to fuel their pump and continue limiting high energy levels needed to rapidly form new cancer cells, which causes their death.

- Graviola downregulates HIF-1α, GLUT1, GLUT4, and HK2, which decreases cell motility and invasion by downregulating MUC4; this results in tumor regression. It also results with decreased glucose uptake in cancer cells, which lowers ATP energy.

- Graviola inhibits lactate dehydrogenase-A (LDH-A)—an enzyme that is overexpressed in many cancers. LDH-A is a key enzyme in the metabolic pathway in which glucose is broken down to produce energy (ATP), which fuels cancer cell growth and is associated with aggressive tumor outcomes.

- Graviola inhibits a mitochondrial membrane enzyme found in cancer cells, which causes the membrane to fail, and the cell to die, triggering necrosis.

- Graviola inhibits anti-apoptotic proteins Bcl-2, Bcl-w, and Mcl-1.

- Graviola affects the mTOR pathway, which is crucial for cell growth and proliferation. It has been shown to potentially inhibit mTOR activity, similar to the effects of known inhibitors like rapamycin.

- Graviola reactivates apoptosis in cancer cells by activating the programmed-cell-death gene called p53. Research also reports graviola upregulates pro-apoptotic genes, Bax, and Bak, which are involved in the destruction of cancer cells.

- Graviola induces cell cycle arrest at G0/G1 phase in some cancers and in the G2/M phase in other cancer types, which triggers apoptosis. In liver cancer cells, ACGs were shown to regulate the cell cycle in the G1/S transition by inhibiting cyclin D1 expression.

- Graviola significantly and selectively elevates ROS formation in cancer cells (but not healthy cells) followed by attenuation of MMP (mitochondrial membrane potential) via upregulation of Bax and downregulation of Bcl-2 at the gene expression level, accompanied by cytochrome c release to the cytosol. The released cytochrome c triggers the activation of caspase 8 and caspase-9, followed by caspase-3, which triggers apoptosis. When caspase-3 is activated, there is no way to reverse cell death.

- Graviola downregulates EGFR expression, which acts as a tumor suppressor mechanism by limiting cell growth.
- Graviola inhibits hypoxia-induced NADPH oxidase activity in cancer cells, reducing their proliferation and the ability of a cancer cell to replicate itself and form a colony of identical cells (clonogenicity).
- ACGs were shown to downregulate the expression of the MDR1 gene and MRP1 proteins, as well as the expression of topoisomerase IIα and glutathione S-transferase in drug-resistant human liver carcinomas. MRP1 (Multi-drug Resistance Protein 1) is a transporter that forms p-glycoprotein efflux pumps, meaning it transports molecules (and chemo drugs) out of cells.
- Graviola was shown to induce mRNA expression of the anti-cancer gene p21 in breast and colorectal cancer cells.
- Graviola suppresses nuclear factor-κB (NF-κB) signaling. NF-κB is a group of pro-inflammatory proteins that help control many functions in a cell, including cell growth and survival. These proteins also control the body's immune and inflammatory responses. NF-κB may be overactive or found in higher-than-normal amounts in some types of cancer cells. This may lead to faster cancer cell growth.

Other Researched Benefits That May Be Helpful

Several animal and test-tube studies report that graviola leaves have gastroprotective and anti-ulcer actions. This might provide additional benefits to cancer patients taking chemotherapy drugs that cause stomach and/or mouth ulcers or damage to the stomach lining. Graviola has also shown to protect the liver from various chemicals known to damage the liver in animal research. This might be helpful to patients taking chemotherapy drugs that are toxic or that are known to damage the liver.

Availability of Products

Graviola has become quite popular around the world as a natural cancer remedy as well as a remedy for treating diabetes and hypertension, among other things. Graviola leaf and stem products are widely available under many different labels in many countries in capsules, tablets, alcohol extracts, water and glycerin extracts, and in bulk cut and sifted leaves to use to prepare teas and decoctions. Several graviola fruit juice products are also widely sold as well. The fruit contains some of the same anti-cancerous acetogenins that the leaves contain (including annonacin), but leaves contain a larger array of different acetogenins than the fruit provides.

SAFETY

A French research group earlier reported in the early 2000s that a handful of graviola's ACG chemicals and several alkaloids were toxic to dopaminergic brain cells. However, further studies showed that this decreased ATP production and associated neurodegeneration they noted did not change mice behavior or locomotor activity. Besides, most of these early French reports were extracting single chemicals from graviola and injecting them into various laboratory animals (including into their brains), which did not correlate to the traditional medicine uses of ingesting the whole leaf of graviola in capsules or brewing them into a tea.

In addition, they reported that the consumption of graviola by an isolated group of West Indians was associated with the sudden appearance of atypical Parkinson's disease in several early anecdotal observational studies. These observational studies did not scientifically confirm anything, they simply noted graviola fruit was in their diet and leaf teas were ingested as a parasite remedy when needed. This association was immediately questioned by other researchers who claimed vitamin deficiencies were probably to blame instead.

However, a recent study by l'Agence Française de Sécurité des Aliments (France's Food Safety Agency) weighed in to clarify the research that followed, reporting that, based on the amount of various constituents in the graviola, pharmacokinetics studies (which revealed acetogenins did not cross the blood-brain barrier easily) and daily human consumption in many countries indicated that there is no clinical link between graviola and atypical Parkinson's and/or any neurotoxicity.

Overall, a majority of the studies undertaken for dose escalation and to identify the therapeutic efficacy of various extracts and fractions of graviola in many diseases have shown either very mild or no toxicity associated with these extracts suggesting its safety in patients. In 2020, researchers at the Australian Research Centre of Complementary and Integrative Medicine published a guidance paper concerning the safety and toxicity of using graviola and reported: "The overall outcome of the current review suggests that *A. muricata* has a favourable safety and tolerability profile. Future studies investigating its use in people diagnosed with a range of cancers are warranted." They also noted the unsuitable methods of the earlier published reports on the possible neurotoxicity and movement disorders of graviola and dismissed them. The main public health agency in Indonesia came to the same conclusion as the French and Australians.

Researchers in Malaysia published animal toxicity studies that reported the following: "Importantly, the outcomes suggest that *A. muricata* leaf ethanol extract can be safely consumed at a dose of 2,000 mg/kg and the LD50 must be more than 2,000 mg/kg." Researchers in Mexico also reported no toxic effects in an acute toxicity rat study published in 2023.

The United States hasn't kept pace or abreast of newer research, and one can still find warnings of possible neurotoxicity of graviola on various government and conventional health websites, which reference the unsuitable early published reports of atypical Parkinson's symptoms in the West Indies, and neurotoxicity when injecting lab animals with graviola extracts and/or isolated graviola chemicals.

I can attest that my company sold hundreds of thousands of bottles of graviola and N-Tense (which contains graviola), and we never had a single instance of any Parkinson's-like movement disorder reported directly to us or through any of the many practitioners who were using graviola and N-Tense with their patients.

Dosages

The therapeutic dosage in traditional medicine systems is reported to be 2–4 grams of leaves, three times daily, in capsules or tablets. A standard infusion (1 cup, three times daily) or a 4:1 standard tincture (2–4 mgs, three times daily) can be substituted if desired. Follow label recommendations on juice products. More information on dosages for cancer and dosages based on different cancer types can be found in chapters 7 and 8.

Contraindications

• As one of graviola's anti-cancer mechanisms of action is to deplete ATP energy to cancer cells, combining it with other supplements and natural products that increase or enhance cellular ATP may reduce the effect of graviola. The main supplement that increases ATP is a common antioxidant called coenzyme Q10, and for this reason, it should be avoided when taking graviola.

• Graviola has demonstrated uterine stimulant activity in an animal study (rats) and should therefore not be used during pregnancy.

• Graviola has demonstrated hypotensive, vasodilator, and cardiodepressant activities in animal studies and is probably contraindicated for people with low blood pressure. People taking antihypertensive drugs should check with their doctors before taking graviola and monitor their blood pressure accordingly (as medications may need adjusting).

• Graviola has demonstrated significant *in vitro* antimicrobial properties. Chronic, long-term use of this plant may lead to die-off of friendly bacteria in the digestive tract due to its antimicrobial properties. Supplementing the diet with probiotics and digestive enzymes is advisable if this plant is used for longer than 30 days.

• Graviola has demonstrated emetic properties in one animal study with pigs. Large single dosages may cause nausea. Reduce the use accordingly if this occurs or take graviola with a meal.

Drug Interactions

No drug interactions have been reported; however, graviola may potentiate antihypertensive and cardiac depressant drugs. It may potentiate antidepressant drugs and interfere with MAO-inhibitor drugs. See contraindications previously noted.

Summary of Benefits the Plant Has to Fight Cancer

Graviola has scientifically demonstrated that it has the ability to kill many types of cancer cells in quite a few different and important ways. Many of these ways are specific to only cancer cells without harming healthy cells. Just as important, it has been reported to overcome some of the main survival mechanisms that cancer uses that promote cellular proliferation, migration, invasion, metastasis, and survival. I created the first cancer natural remedy with graviola and other anti-cancerous plants found in the Amazon in 1998, which has helped many people over all these years. But it is *not* the be-all and end-all cure for cancer, and it didn't work for everyone. Neither does graviola.

The multi-plant formula always seemed to work better than just taking graviola alone, however. More information on multi-herb formulas for cancers is found in chapter 6.

The main issue is that cancer is complicated and the same type of cancer can behave quite differently from person to person because we are wonderfully complicated living beings. Cancer staging, diet and lifestyle factors, genetics, gut bacteria and absorption differences, and other factors play large roles in who gets cancer and who survives it. I view graviola as an important tool in the toolbox for cancer survival, and we need as many tools as we can get for the best chance for survival.

My personal experience with taking it myself and working with many other practitioners and cancer patients is that it has little to no toxicity, no major side effects (not a single report of any movement disorder in almost 20 years selling it), and it has huge possible benefits. That graviola has become a major herb of commerce offered by many manufacturers over the last 25 years does speak to its possible benefits. If something works, word gets out about it, and sales increase.

Online Links to More Information

• Tropical Plant Database page on graviola: https://rain-tree.com/graviola.htm.

• Research references for this text: https://rain-tree.com/Graviola-Cancer-Research.pdf.

GUACATONGA

Family: Flacourtiaceae

Genus: *Casearia*

Species: *sylvestris*

Synonyms: *Samyda parviflora, Casearia parviflora, Anavinga samyda*

Common Names: Guacatonga, guassatonga, wild coffee, burro-kaa, café-bravo, cafeiillo, café silvestre, congonhas-de-bugre, corta-lengua, crack-open, dondequiera, erva-de-bugre, erva de pontada, guayabillo, mahajo, papelite, pau de lagarto, piraquina, raton, sarnilla, ucho caspi

Parts Used: Bark, leaves

Guacatonga grows as a shrub or small tree usually 6 or 10 feet tall, but sometimes grows up to 30 feet in undisturbed areas of the Amazon. In the clay soils of the Amazon, the plant has adapted for nutrient absorption and support by forming extensive lateral roots that are white, stiff, and covered with a corky bark. The tree produces small white, cream, or greenish flowers (which smell like a mixture of honey and urine) crowded on short stalks on the leaf axils. After flowering it produces small fruits, which split open to reveal three brown seeds covered with a red-to-orange aril. Guacatonga grows wild throughout the tropics, adapting to both forests and plains. It is native to Cuba, Jamaica, Hispaniola, Puerto Rico, the Caribbean, Central America, and South America (including Brazil, Peru, Argentina, Uruguay, and Bolivia).

TRADITIONAL HERBAL MEDICINE USES

Guacatonga has a long history of use in Brazilian herbal medicine, documented in early folk medicine books as an antiseptic and wound healer for skin diseases (in 1939), as a topical pain reliever (in 1941), and as an anti-ulcer drug (in 1958). It is currently used in Brazilian herbal medicine systems as a topical pain reliever, a blood purifier, an anti-inflammatory, and an antiviral. They use guacatonga to treat rheumatism, syphilis, herpes, stomach and skin ulcers, edema, diarrhea, and fevers of all kinds. It has become a natural remedy for cancer over the last 10 years.

The plant is also a popular natural remedy employed in Bolivian herbal medicine, where it is considered useful to relieve pain, reduce inflammation, reduce stomach acid and prevent ulcers, stop bleeding, and heal wounds. There it is used to treat skin diseases, cancer, stomach ulcers, snakebites and bee stings, and herpes, as well as an ingredient in dental antiseptic mouthwash products.

Anti-Cancerous Actions

In 2009, a research group in Brazil screened 50 Brazilian medicinal plants in their search for a new anti-cancer drug. Guacatonga leaves had the strongest anti-cancer action of all of those tested; it was effective at the very smallest of dosages. The IC50 dosage (how much it took to kill 50% of the cancer cells in the test tube) were 0.1 mcg/ml for colon cancer; 0.9 mcg/ml for glioblastoma; 1.2 mcg/ml for melanoma; and 1.3 mcg/ml for human promyelocytic leukemia.

Research published in 2014 reported that a water and alcohol extract of guacatonga had anti-tumorous actions against breast cancer in test tubes and against adenosarcomas in lab animals. In 2017, test-tube research by Brazilian university researchers on a crude extract of guacatonga reported it effectively reduced cell viability of four tumor cell lines (liver, lung, brain, and melanoma). They extracted and tested several casearins in the crude extract and reported that casearin D significantly inhibited cancer cell proliferation and tumorigenesis in liver cancer cells by causing cell cycle arrest.

In 2024, researchers in Brazil prepared an extract of guacatonga leaves that was rich in clerodane diterpenes (see information on these chemicals in the next section) and tested it in mice who had sarcomas and colorectal tumors. They reported that giving mice 10 mg by injection or 25 mg orally once daily reduced tumor size/growth comparable to a standard cancer drug (5-Fluorouracil) that is commonly used for colorectal cancer. Two of the animals in the cancer drug group died, and toxicity to healthy cells was reported in the remainder.

Animals taking guacatonga orally had no toxic effects, and no animals died. They also reported that the extract had a pain-relieving effect without sedation, which they proposed was working by desensitizing several pain molecules and/or their receptor sites. The researchers suggested that more research should be performed on guacatonga and its active chemicals since pain management for cancer patients can be difficult. Several previous studies conducted by other researchers also reported guacatonga's effective pain-relieving actions.

Anti-Cancerous Plant Chemicals

Natural plant compounds, called clerodane diterpenes, are found abundantly in guacatonga, and some have been patented as anti-cancerous agents. Clerodane diterpenes have been documented with a wide range of biological activities ranging from insect antifeedants and HIV replication inhibitors to anti-tumorous, antioxidant, anti-cancerous, anti-inflammatory, anti-ulcer, cancer-preventive, and antibiotic agents.

Some of the clerodane diterpenes documented in guacatonga are novel chemicals, which scientists have named casearins (A thru X); several have shown remarkable anti-cancerous actions in low dosages. Some have been patented as anti-sarcomic agents. Other clerodane diterpenes include casearvestrins, caseazins, and caseargrewiins. Guacatonga also contains a clerodane-type diterpene called hardwickiic acid, which may relate to guacatonga's pain-relieving and anti-inflammatory actions.

The research on guacatonga's anti-cancerous chemicals began in 1988 by Japanese researchers from the Tokyo College of Pharmacy and Pharmacognosy. They published one preliminary study in 1988 on their discovery of these novel clerodane diterpenes and their anti-cancerous and anti-tumorous activities. The study indicated that an ethanol extract of the leaf showed strong anti-tumorous activity in laboratory mice with sarcomas.

As soon as they made this discovery, they rushed to patent it, filing a Japanese patent for the casearin chemicals they'd discovered as new anti-tumorous agents. They published a follow-up study in 1990, again reporting their results from injecting mice with sarcomas with an ethanol extract of guacatonga leaves (100 mg/g of body weight) and confirming their previous findings. They then tested individual casearins against various human cancer cell lines and published two more studies in 1991 and 1992. These studies reported newly isolated casearin chemicals and their anti-tumorous and anti-cancerous actions against various cancer tumor cells.

An extract of guacatonga was developed by a Brazilian university as a possible new herbal drug for cancer, which contains Casearin B, D, and X, as well as Caseargrewiin F. Their research in 2010 reported two of the diterpenes (casearin X and caseargrewiin F) exhibited the strongest anti-tumorous action in test-tube studies against multiple human cancer cell lines, which were comparable to a standard cancer drug called doxorubicin. Other test-tube research reported that casearin D, caseargrewiin F, and casearin X exerted significant toxic activity against promyelocytic leukemia, two types of human breast carcinoma, two types of human prostate adenocarcinoma, and a mouse melanoma cell line.

Polyphenols: Guacatonga contains rutin, quercetin, ferulic acid, ellagic acid, caffeic acid, gallic acid and its metabolites, luteolin, chlorogenic acid, and other glycosylated flavonoids. Research published in 2009 reported that a gallic acid metabolite (gallate-3,5-dimethyl ether) extracted from guacatonga had anti-tumorous actions in mice by completely reversing the effect the cancer had in suppressing natural killer immune cells. This chemical is also named "syringic acid," and more than 100 studies have been published on its anti-cancerous effects and mechanisms of action on a wide range of cancer types in animals and test tubes. See links to research in this plant's "Online Links to More Information" section for the anti-cancerous and cancer-preventative actions of the polyphenols in guacatonga.

Other Chemicals: Guacatonga contains icariside B, which is now a small-molecule drug for research in developing cancer, immunotherapy, and anti-inflammatory drugs. It also contains loliolide: a natural plant chemical found in medicinal plants and some algae. Research suggests this natural plant compound is beneficial for breast cancer, colorectal cancer, and melanoma. Guacatonga contains another triterpene named lupeol. Research on lupeol's anti-cancer and cancer-prevention actions reports it targets many cancer-associated factors, impacting its proliferation, progression, and apoptosis processes. Guacatonga also contains common plant sterols including β-sitosterol, stigmasterol, and campesterol, which have been reported with cancer-preventative actions.

Cancer Pathways and Mechanisms of Action

The signaling pathways, cancer pathways, and molecular targets discussed here are described and discussed in greater detail in chapter 5.

- A water/alcohol extract of guacatonga caused cell cycle arrest (at G2/S), which initiated apoptosis by affecting two molecular targets (p53, p16).
- Guacatonga increases reactive oxygen species (ROS) and oxidative damage in cancer cells, which trigger apoptosis, while acting as an antioxidant in healthy cells.
- Guacatonga and some of its casearins were shown to inhibit AP-1. Because AP-1 is often overactive in cancer cells, inhibiting it can potentially suppress tumor growth, induce apoptosis, inhibit metastasis, and sensitize cancer cells to chemotherapy.
- Guacatonga has shown the ability to modulate specific pathways used by cancer stem cells, which make them easier to target and kill.
- Casearin D significantly inhibited cancer cell proliferation and tumorigenesis by causing G1/S cell cycle arrest by reducing ERK phosphorylation and cyclin D1 expression levels.
- Several chemicals in guacatonga have been reported to disrupt c-Myc activity, leading to reduced tumor cell growth and potentially inducing tumor regression.
- Casearin J demonstrated SERCA inhibition, oxidative stress, and interference with Notch1 signaling (which helps kill cancer stem cells).
- Phospholipase A2 (PLA2) has recently shown to be a possible new molecular target for new cancer drugs. The actions of PLA2 contribute to the development of the tumor microenvironment, promoting immune evasion, angiogenesis, tumor growth, and invasiveness. Guacatonga has shown to be an effective PLA2 inhibitor, which is demonstrated in unrelated research on guacatonga's antivenin actions against snakebites. Eight studies on guacatonga water extracts report that the plant's traditional uses for snakebites were confirmed scientifically since it effectively inhibited PLA2 toxins in snake venom. More information on this research can be found in the Tropical Plant Database file (see the link provided later in this plant's "Online Links to More Information" section).

OTHER RESEARCHED BENEFITS THAT MAY BE HELPFUL

Research published in 2023 reported that a tea made with guacatonga leaves (a water extract) protected lab animals from drugs and toxins known to cause damage in the gastric tract. This confirms prior studies on its anti-ulcer actions as well as traditional uses in herbal medicine. Cancer patients taking cancer drugs may notice this beneficial effect if the drug normally causes damage, ulcers, and pain in the digestive tract, or mouth ulcers (mucositis). Based on animal studies, cancer patients taking guacatonga might also experience less cancer-related pain.

Availability of Products

Guacatonga leaf products are starting to become more popular in the U.S. market. It is now available under several different labels selling capsules, powders, and tea-cut products.

Safety

A rat study published in 2023 showed no toxicity to pregnant rats; however, there were changes in fetal development. Brazilian researchers reported in 2017 that guacatonga did not cause cancer. In 2015, the same researchers studied acute toxicity of guacatonga in rats and reported it as nontoxic in dosages as high as 2,000 mg/kg of body weight.

Dosages

The traditional remedy consists of 20 grams of dried leaves infused in a liter of water, and ¼-cup amounts are taken two to three times daily with meals as a digestive and anti-ulcer aid. Since most of the chemicals are water soluble, powdered leaves in tablets or capsules (1–2 grams twice daily) can be substituted if desired.

Contraindications

Based on animal studies, the use of guacatonga is contraindicated in pregnancy.

Drug Interactions

None known.

Summary of Benefits the Plant Has to Fight Cancer

Guacatonga has been an ingredient in the N-Tense formula since it was first created over 20 years ago. Its ability to directly target and kill various cancer cells, prevent some common side effects of chemotherapy, and relieve pain without side effects should draw the attention of more researchers to study this effective rainforest resource. The fact that recent studies have shown it to be just as effective as a leading drug for colorectal cancer without any of the well-known toxicity and side effects of that chemotherapy drug should stimulate more research as well.

ONLINE LINKS TO MORE INFORMATION

• Tropical Plant Database file for guacatonga: https://rain-tree.com/guacatonga.htm.

• Research references for this text: https://rain-tree.com/Guacatonga-Cancer-Research.pdf.

MULLACA

Family: Solanaceae

Genus: *Physalis*

Species: *angulata, peruviana*

Synonyms: *Physalis capsicifolia, Physalis lanceifolia, Physalis ramosissima*

Common Names: Mullaca, camapu, bolsa mullaca, cape gooseberry, wild tomato, winter cherry, juá-de-capote, capulí cimarrón, battre-autour, k'u chih, 'urmoa batoto bita, cecendet, dumadu harachan, hog weed, nvovo, polopa, saca-buche, thongtheng, tino-tino, topatop, wapotok

Parts Used: Whole plant, leaves, roots

Mullaca is an annual herb indigenous to many parts of the tropics, including the Amazon rainforest. It can be found on most continents in the tropics, including Africa, Asia, and the Americas. It grows up to 3 feet high; bears small, cream-colored flowers; and produces small, light yellowish-orange, edible fruit sometimes referred to as cape gooseberry or ground cherry. The fruit is about the size of a cherry tomato, and like tomatoes, it contains many tiny edible seeds inside. With its papery husk around the fruit, most Americans and Latin Americans might think it is another *Physalis* plant: tomatillo (*Physalis philadelphica*). Mullaca propagates easily from the many seeds the fruit contains; spontaneous clumps of plants can be found along river banks and just about anywhere the soil is disturbed and the canopy is broken (allowing enough sunlight to promote its rapid growth) in the Amazon.

Traditional Herbal Medicine Uses

Mullaca has been employed in traditional medicine in South America for many years. It has been used as an herbal remedy for diabetes, hepatitis, asthma, bronchitis, chronic rheumatism, fever, vomiting, malaria, various types of skin problems, and many types of kidney, liver, and gallbladder problems for many years. Various research published over the years has validated some of these traditional remedy uses. More complete information on mullaca's traditional uses and this research can be found in the Tropical Plant Database (see the link provided later in this plant's "Online Links to More Information" section).

Anti-Cancerous Actions

Mullaca has been the subject of recent research, based on the preliminary studies showing that it is an effective immune modulator, is toxic to numerous types of cancer and leukemia cells, and has anti-inflammatory actions that relate to cancer. Various extracts of mullaca have demonstrated potent activity against a wide range of human and animal cancer cells, including those from breast, brain, colorectal, gastric, liver, prostate, laryngeal, and cervical cancers, as well as non–small cell lung cancer, large cell lung carcinoma, lymphoma, leukemia, osteosarcoma, melanoma, and oral squamous carcinoma.

Cancer research on mullaca began in the early 1980s with studies conducted in Thailand and the United States, which was later validated by research at the University of Taiwan in 1992. In their studies, researchers showed mullaca had significant effects against five human cancer cell lines and three animal cancer cell lines *in vitro*. In 2001, researchers at the University of Houston isolated a new compound in mullaca that exhibited remarkable toxicity against nasopharynx cancer cells, lung (adenocarcinoma) cancer cells, and leukemia in mice.

These same Taiwanese researchers had already published a separate study on mullaca's other anti-leukemic phytochemicals in 1992, reporting that two chemicals inhibited the growth of five types of acute leukemia, including lymphoid (T and B), promyelocytic, myeloid, and monocytic.

Other researchers in China and Russia independently demonstrated significant immunomodulatory effects against blastogenesis (a process triggered in leukemia) while boosting other immune functions, which might account for mullaca's anti-leukemic effects in mice seen by other researchers. Several studies in test tubes and animals and one human clinical study conducted recently in Indonesia and China report that mullaca possesses beneficial effects against fibrosis.

Fibrosis is a condition that occurs when tissues thicken, harden, or scar due to an excessive buildup of fibrous connective tissue. It can affect many different organs and tissues, including the lungs, skin, muscles, liver, and kidneys. Fibrosis can cause various diseases in those organs including scleroderma, progressive pulmonary fibrosis, and other lung diseases, as well as liver cirrhosis. Fibrosis can impact cell differentiation, proliferation, and transition, which can contribute to cancer development and are linked to skin, lung, liver, and kidney cancers.

Some of the same genes and their cascading chemical reactions operate in both fibrosis and cancer pathways; therefore, this research may suggest that it might be beneficial to prevent cancer in these higher-risk patients. See more information in this plant's "Cancer Pathways and Mechanisms of Action" section.

Mullaca grows in Indonesia and has many well-established traditional natural remedy uses; the common name for the plant there is *ciplukan*. In 2019, Indonesian researchers conducted a human clinical trial that studied 60 patients with scleroderma; 30 patients took a natural plant extract of mullaca for 12 weeks, and 30 were given a placebo. They reported there was a significant improvement of skin fibrosis in the study group taking mullaca. There was a significant reduction in skin thickness (35.9% versus 6.3%) as well as a decrease in a collagen blood test (P1NP), which is always elevated in scleroderma (17.8% versus 0.7%).

The same researchers published another study in 2024 to determine how the same mullaca extract could impact fibrosis in the lungs of mice and reported similar results. They additionally noted that "Ciplukan extract exhibited promising effects on fibrosis-related gene expressions, particularly Nox4, MMP8, and Klf4. This study suggests that the extract has the potential to intervene in fibrosis progression, offering a potential avenue for therapeutic strategies." The Chinese test-tube research is described in the next section; they studied the chemicals in mullaca recently and tested which specific chemicals had the antifibrotic action the plant extract was providing.

Chinese researchers studied a mullaca extract on oral squamous cell carcinoma and reported it highly active in very low dosages (5 parts per million). They reported in 2011: "These results strongly support an antimetastatic and anti-angiogenic activity of *P. angulata* that may contribute to the development of better chemo-preventive agents for cancer and inflammation."

ANTI-CANCEROUS PLANT CHEMICALS

Plant chemical research on mullaca reveals that it contains many types of biologically active, naturally occurring chemicals including flavonoids, alkaloids, and many different types of plant steroids, some of which have never before been seen in science. The main anti-cancer chemicals isolated in mullaca thus far include angulasteroidins A–F, choline, ixocarpanolide, physagulin A–G, physalin A–K, physalucoside A, physangulide, sitosterol, squalen-1-ol, vamonolide, withaminimin, withangulatin A, withanolide D, withanolide T, withaphysanolide, withagulides A–H, physangulide B, physaperuvin G, neophysalin A, guaiacyl-primeveroside, phyperunolide C, physalactone, physalolactone C, and perulactone.

The primary chemicals thought to be the most biologically active that relate to the traditional medicinal uses of mullaca are steroid derivatives, including physalins and withanolides. These natural plant steroids have been of great interest to researchers, and many of the documented anti-cancerous, anti-tumorous, and anti-leukemic actions of the plant are attributed to these steroids reported in many research studies. More than 40 different types of physalins and more than 40 withanolides have been isolated from mullaca so far, and they continue to discover new ones.

There are 120 species pf *Physalis* plants that are found all over the world, and all of them contain physalins and withanolides. Therefore, research has been conducted on species other than mullaca, which report the same biological activity because they share some of the same biologically active chemicals. Mullaca stands out, however, because it has more novel chemical steroids, which haven't been identified in other *Physalis* plants.

Mullaca's physalin and withanolide chemicals have also attracted the attention of cancer researchers. They have determined that withanolides can inhibit tumor cell proliferation, induce apoptosis, and suppress metastasis by targeting multiple signaling pathways involved in cancer progression. It is little wonder researchers are in the process of synthesizing these chemicals and testing analogs and derivatives in the pursuit of new cancer drugs.

A well-established research group in China seems to be the farthest along in the process and will probably be the first to create a new cancer drug (as well as a new drug for inflammatory diseases and conditions). They've produced one small-molecule drug for cancer, which they began testing in 2023 and which is still ongoing. They selected the withanolide A chemical in mullaca because it has the strongest action in very low dosages (0.08 µM). They have published several papers beginning in 2020 about how to synthesize (copy) the plant chemical and then create analogs (changing it enough to be patentable).

They report that their possible new drug will hit a newer target to treat cancer as a novel TrxR inhibitor (see chapter 5 for more information on how this enzyme affects cancer). This research group continues to study other chemicals, with an emphasis on a well-known physalin chemical, physalin F.

Withanolides: New research indicates this group of chemicals has strongly anti-cancerous, anti-tumorous, anti-inflammatory, antioxidant, antifibrotic, immunomodulatory, liver-protective, and antimicrobial actions. The *withanolides* have attracted the interest of several research groups who are studying them in China and Indonesia. Their research has continued; they discovered eight new withanolide chemicals in 2024 and named them withagulides A–H. Their study has also confirmed the antifibrotic action of these newly discovered chemicals as well as other known chemicals found in mullaca.

They reported in their test-tube study that nine withanolides showed marked antifibrotic action in liver cells (which may result in cirrhosis) by inhibiting COL1A1 expression above 50%. A physalin chemical (physalin F) was the main component in the active multiple chemical fractions. When they tested it individually, it significantly decreased (better than the other chemicals) the expression of the collagen gene and another chemical (α-SMA) in test tubes. A mechanism of action study revealed that physalin F exerted its anti–liver fibrosis effect via the PI3K/AKT/mTOR signaling pathway. More information on this pathway is shown in chapter 5.

Seven of mullaca's withanolide chemicals were studied by other university researchers in China in 2024. Most of the withanolides tested demonstrated very good GLUT1-inhibitor actions with physagulide Y showing the strongest action (more than 50% inhibition). These researchers postulated that GLUT1 inhibition could help explain and/or plays a significant role in the anti-tumorous actions seen in early animal studies. The actions of this gene for cancer can be found in the next section.

Physalins: This group of natural plant chemicals in mullaca has a good deal of research as well. Research has reported they have anti-cancerous, anti-tumorous, anti-inflammatory, immunoregulatory, antimicrobial, antimalarial, leishmanicidal, pain-relieving, and antidiabetic activities. This research has validated many of mullaca's traditional medicine uses.

Polyphenols: The main polyphenols in mullaca include caffeic acid, chlorogenic acid, and gallic acid (phenolic acids), as well as kaempferol, isoquercitrin, rutin, quercitrin, and quercetin (flavonoids). While these polyphenols are certainly contributing to mullaca's antioxidant and cellular/organ protection actions, some have cancer-preventative and anti-cancer actions; however, they haven't been used to describe mullaca's anti-cancer actions or benefits discussed herein.

CANCER PATHWAYS AND MECHANISMS OF ACTION

More complete information on these signaling pathways, cancer pathways, and new chemical targets for cancer therapy shown here can be found in chapter 5.

• Mullaca can increase reactive oxygen species (ROS) and oxidative damage in cancer cells, while acting as an antioxidant in normal cells. In addition, by inhibiting TrxR, a chemical in mullaca triggers apoptosis in cancer cells by increasing ROS as well.

• Mullaca can flip the suicide switch to restore apoptosis by restoring p53 function, as well as promote activation of pro-apoptosis proteins like Noxa, Bax, and Bak.

• Studies have shown that mullaca can trigger apoptosis in various types of cancer by activating the caspase cascade and by downregulating pro-survival proteins like c-Myc, which leads to cell death.

• Mullaca was reported to inhibit cancer cell proliferation, migration, and angiogenesis through reducing matrix metalloproteinase (MMP) activity and vascular endothelial growth factor (VEGF) expression, which results in antimetastatic properties.

- Research suggests that several of the steroidal chemicals in mullaca act on an enzyme level to selectively arrest the normal cell cycle in cancer cells, as well as cause DNA damage inside of cancer cells, which prevent them from replicating. Interestingly, it causes cell death in the G2/M cell cycle for some cancers and in the G0/G1 cell cycle in other types of cancers.
- Physalin B is a novel inhibitor of the ubiquitin-proteasome pathway, which can trigger Noxa-associated apoptosis in some types of cancer.
- Other research reports mullaca might inhibit cancer cell proliferation, migration, and angiogenesis through reducing MMP activity and VEGF expression, which results in antimetastatic properties. VEGF inhibition can also inhibit angiogenesis (the formation of new blood vessels to tumors).
- The research studying fibrosis reported that many of mullaca's steroidal chemicals inhibited COL1A1 expression by more than 50%. The COL1A1 gene is implicated in cancer, particularly in its progression, metastasis, and prognosis.
- They also reported that one physalin (physalin F) reduced collagen expression and reduced a substance named α-SMA (both are often overexpressed in ovarian cancer).
- Chemicals in mullaca have shown to inhibit IL-1β, which is necessary to promote angiogenesis (the formation of new blood vessels to tumors).
- Other chemicals in the plant are reported to inhibit AP-1, which can suppress tumor growth, induce apoptosis, inhibit metastasis, and sensitize cancer cells to chemotherapy.
- This same study also reported that this same chemical was reducing the expression of a well-known signaling pathway (PI3K/AKT/mTOR). In cancer, the signals in this pathway are often overactive, which can lead to increased proliferation and resistance to treatment. Inhibitors of this signaling pathway have been used to treat leukemia, and clinical trials are evaluating their use for other cancers. This research might help explain mullaca's previously reported benefits for leukemia.
- A 2024 study indicates that at least eight chemicals in mullaca are effective GLUT1 inhibitors. GLUT1 is a gene that regulates how much glucose is absorbed by cells. Inhibiting GLUT1 has been shown to decrease tumor cell proliferation by lowering glucose absorption needed for much higher

energy levels required by rapidly growing cancer cells. See more detailed information in the "Proliferation Pathway" section in chapter 5.

• Mullaca also inhibits ATP energy production in cancer cells, lowering their energy levels and abilities to proliferate rapidly.

• Mullaca has been reported to kill cancer cells through triggering autophagy processes.

• Mullaca has been reported to block the cyclooxygenase-2 (COX-2) enzyme. This substance is responsible for producing inflammatory chemicals that contribute to tumor growth and angiogenesis (new blood vessel formation) within the tumor microenvironment.

• Mullaca was documented with mucin-inhibitor actions. In cancer, mucins can be overexpressed and contribute to tumor growth, metastasis, and resistance to therapy.

• Mullaca was reported to modulate signaling pathways that cancer stem cells use in a manner that makes the stem cells easier to target and kill.

OTHER RESEARCHED BENEFITS THAT MAY BE HELPFUL

Many studies describe mullaca's anti-inflammatory and immune modulation actions that are also beneficial to fight cancer. Several newer studies have reported that mullaca can inhibit two crucial inflammatory signaling pathways—NF-κB and JNK/AP-1—by decreasing at least six different substances in these pathways in test tubes and animals. More information on how cancer uses the Inflammatory/Immune Pathway and these signaling pathways specifically to promote cell transformation, tumor cell survival, proliferation, invasion, angiogenesis, and metastasis is found in chapter 5. All of the anti-inflammatory and immune modulation information and research can be found in the Tropical Plant Database (see the link provided in this plant's "Online Links to More Information" section).

AVAILABILITY OF PRODUCTS

Mullaca is much better known and more widely used in Latin and South America than it is in North American herbal medicine. Mullaca is available under only a few labels, which sell liquid extracts, capsules, or powered herb.

Safety

Mullaca is a common herbal remedy in the tropics where it grows and has long been considered safe and well tolerated by the herbal healers who use it. Three small-scale human trials conducted on mullaca reported that it was well tolerated and without any toxicity. No toxicity was reported in many animal studies over the years.

Dosages

Depending on what it is employed for, generally ½ to 1 cup of a whole herb infusion one to three times daily or 1–2 mgs of a 4:1 tincture twice daily is used. If desired, 2–4 grams of powdered whole herb (depending on body weight) in tablets or capsules or stirred into water or juice twice daily can be substituted (since the active sterol chemicals are completely water soluble).

Contraindications

One animal study indicates this plant may lower blood pressure, and one test-tube study demonstrated a blood anticoagulant activity. People with blood disorders such as hemophilia, those taking heart medications or blood thinners, or those with other heart problems such as low blood pressure should not use this plant without supervision and advice of a qualified health care practitioner.

Drug Interactions

None reported; however, see aforementioned contraindications.

Summary of Benefits the Plant Has to Fight Cancer

Personally, I have used mullaca mainly in various formulas for its anti-cancerous, immune, anti-inflammatory, and/or antimicrobial actions as well as a synergist to aid absorption of other plant chemicals in a formula that might have bioavailability issues. The natural plant steroids in the aerial parts of mullaca seem to enhance digestion and uptake of many other hard-to-digest natural plant chemicals. With research reporting anti-cancer benefits on tumors, skin cancers, and blood cancers, mullaca was used as an ingredient in all three N-Tense formulas. I never used it as a stand-alone remedy, however, for anything other than parasites and microbial infections, and then only occasionally. It combines well with the other anti-cancerous plants and plays an important role in acute leukemias. In the past, I've added extra mullaca to naturopathic protocols during a blast crisis in people with leukemia and was pleased with the results.

ONLINE LINKS TO MORE INFORMATION

• Tropical Plant Database file for mullaca: https://rain-tree.com/mullaca.htm.

• Research references for this text: http://rain-tree.com/Mullaca-Cancer-Research.pdf.

PAU D'ARCO

Family: Bignoniaceae

Genus: *Tabebuia*

Species: *impetiginosa, heptaphylla*

Synonyms: *Tabebuia avellanedae, T. ipe, T. nicaraguensis, T. schunkeuigoi, T. serratifolia, T. altissima, T. palmeri, Gelseminum avellanedae, Handroanthus avellanedae, H. impetiginosus, Tecoma adenophylla, Tecoma avellanedae, Tecoma eximia, Tecoma impetiginosa, Tecoma integra, Tecoma ipe*

Common Names: Pau d'arco, ipê, ipê roxo, lapacho, tahuari, taheebo, trumpet tree, ipê-contra-sarna, tabebuia ipê, tajy

Parts Used: Bark, wood

Pau d'arco is a huge canopy tree native to the Amazon rainforest and other tropical parts of South and Latin America. It grows to 100 feet high, and the base of the tree can be 6–10 feet in diameter. The *Tabebuia* genus includes about 100 species of large, flowering trees that are common to South American cities' landscapes for their beauty. The tree also is popular with timber loggers—its high-quality wood is some of the heaviest, most durable wood in the tropics. Pau d'arco wood is widely used in the construction of everything from houses and boats to farm tools.

The common name pau d'arco (as well as its other main names of commerce, ipê roxo, taheebo, and lapacho) is used for several different species of *Tabebuia* trees that are used interchangeably in herbal medicine systems. *T. impetiginosa* is known for its attractive purple flowers and often is called "purple lapacho." It has been the preferred species employed in herbal medicine. It is often referred to by its other botanical name, *Tabebuia avellanedae*, and sometimes *Tabebuia heptaphylla*, but all three names refer to the same tree.

TRADITIONAL HERBAL MEDICINE USES

Pau d'arco also has a long history in herbal medicine around the world. In South American herbal medicine, it is considered to be astringent, anti-inflammatory, antibacterial, antifungal, and a laxative; it is used to treat ulcers, syphilis, urinary tract infections, gastrointestinal problems, candida and yeast infections, cancer, diabetes, prostatitis, constipation, and allergies. It is used in Brazilian herbal medicine for many conditions including cancer, leukemia, ulcers, diabetes, candida, rheumatism, arthritis, prostatitis, dysentery, stomatitis, and boils. In North American herbal medicine, pau d'arco is considered to have analgesic, antioxidant, antiparasitic, antimicrobial, antifungal, antiviral, antibacterial, anti-inflammatory, laxative, and anti-cancerous properties.

It is used for fevers, infections, colds, flu, syphilis, urinary tract infections, cancer, respiratory problems, skin ulcerations, boils, dysentery, gastrointestinal problems of all kinds, arthritis, prostatitis, and circulation disturbances. Pau d'arco also is employed in herbal medicine systems in the United States for lupus, diabetes, ulcers, leukemia, allergies, liver disease, Hodgkin lymphoma, osteomyelitis, Parkinson's disease, and psoriasis; it also is a popular natural remedy for candida and yeast infections.

The recorded uses in European herbal medicine systems reveal that it is used in much the same way as in the United States, and for the same conditions. Various research published over the years has validated many of these traditional remedy uses. More complete information on pau d'arco's traditional uses and this research can be found in the Tropical Plant Database (see the link provided later in this plant's "Online Links to More Information" section).

ANTI-CANCEROUS ACTIONS

The traditional medicine uses of pau d'arco were reported as early as 1873. In the United States, scientific interest in plant extracts began in the 1960s when the National Cancer Institute (NCI) systematically began researching plant extracts all over the world looking for active compounds against cancer. The NCI looked at pau d'arco in considerable detail after other researchers reported that the plant demonstrated marked anti-tumorous effects in animals.

In 1967, after reports in the Brazilian press, pau d'arco came to the attention of clinicians (and the public in general). The Brazilian news magazine *O'Cruzeiro* started reporting "miraculous" cures in cancer patients in a hospital.

Researchers decided that the most potent single chemical for this activity was a naphthoquinone chemical named lapachol, and they concentrated solely on this single chemical in their subsequent cancer research. In a 1968 study, lapachol demonstrated highly significant activity against cancerous tumors in rats. By 1970, NCI-backed research was testing lapachol in human cancer patients. The institute reported, however, that their first Phase I study failed to produce a therapeutic effect without side effects—and they discontinued further cancer research shortly thereafter. These side effects were nausea and vomiting and anti–vitamin K activity.

Interestingly, other chemicals in the whole plant extract (which showed positive antitumor effects at very low toxicity) demonstrated positive effects on vitamin K and, conceivably, compensated for lapachol's negative effect. Once again, instead of pursuing research on a complex combination of at least 100 active chemicals in a whole plant extract (several of which had antitumor effects and other positive biological activities), research focused on a single, patentable chemical—and it didn't work as well.

Over many years pau d'arco continued to demonstrate anti-tumorous and anti-cancer actions in many types of cancer at low dosages without toxicity to healthy cells. These included breast carcinoma, lung carcinoma, cervical carcinoma, and liver carcinomas with the GI50 values (corresponding to a sample concentration achieving 50% growth inhibition in human tumor cell lines) reported at 1.21, 1.03, 0.91, and 1.10 mcg/ml, respectively, using an alcohol tincture (the water infusion was not toxic to the cancer cells). This study, published in 2015, reported that there was no toxicity to healthy cells.

In other studies, it is noteworthy that pau d'arco not only displayed significant growth inhibition against various tumor cell lines *in vitro* but also prolonged the duration of survival in a number of mouse models *in vivo* including estrogen positive breast cancer, triple-negative breast cancer, cervical cancer, liver cancer, pancreatic cancer, and large cell lung cancer.

Anti-Cancerous Plant Chemicals

Despite NCI's abandonment of the early lapachol research, another group developed a lapachol analog (which was patentable) in 1975. One study reported that this lapachol analog increased the life span of mice inoculated with leukemic cells by more than 80%. In a small, uncontrolled, 1980 study of nine human patients with various cancers (liver, kidney, breast, prostate, and cervix), pure lapachol was reported to shrink tumors and reduce pain caused by them—and three of the patients realized complete remissions.

Researchers in 2013 tested lapachol, α- and β-lapachone, and 25 related synthetic 1,4-naphthoquinones derivatives and analogs against esophageal cancer cells. They reported most of the compounds exhibited enhanced cytotoxicity (IC50 1.6 to 11.7 mcg) compared to the current drug of choice, cisplatin (IC50 = 16.5 mcg). IC50 means the amount necessary to inhibit 50% of the cancer cells' growth in the test tube. Another chemical in pau d'arco, beta-lapachone, has been studied closely, and a number of patents have been filed on it. The actual natural plant chemical has been turned into a small-molecule drug (named ARQ761) and has been the subject of recent human clinical trials for cancer. It has been demonstrated in laboratory studies to have activities similar to lapachol (antimicrobial, antifungal, antiviral, anti-tumorous, anti-leukemic, and anti-inflammatory) with few side effects.

Research published from 2003 to 2005 provided important new insights into the possible molecular mechanisms of the anti-cancer activity of beta-lapachone specifically against prostate, colon, pancreatic, and lung cancers. In a 2002 U.S. patent, beta-lapachone was cited to have significant anti-cancerous activity against human cancer cell lines, including melanoma, promyelocytic leukemia, prostate, malignant glioma, colon, liver, breast, ovarian, pancreatic, multiple myeloma, and drug-resistant cell lines.

In yet another U.S. patent, beta-lapachone was cited with the *in vivo* ability to inhibit the growth of prostate tumors. Most chemotherapeutic drugs kill cancer cells by indirectly activating checkpoint-mediated apoptosis after creating nonselective damage to DNA or microtubules, which accounts for their toxicity toward normal cells. U.S. researchers showed in 2003 that β-lapachone selectively induces apoptosis in cancer cells without causing the death of nontransformed cells.

This unusual selectivity against cancer cells was preceded by activation of S-phase checkpoint and selective induction of E2F1, a regulator of checkpoint-mediated apoptosis. This study suggests direct checkpoint activation as a strategy against cancer. Checkpoint inhibitor drugs are a newer type of immunotherapy that helps the body's immune system fight cancer. They work by blocking proteins called "checkpoints" that prevent the immune system from attacking cancer cells.

β-Lapachone is also well known to inhibit an enzyme called Topo 1 (topoisomerase I) and to induce NQO1 (NAD[P]H:quinone oxidoreductase 1). Topo 1 is a newer target for new chemotherapy drugs to disrupt DNA replication and transcription, leading to cell death. NQO1 is a protein that helps protect cells (including cancer cells) from damage caused by oxidative stress. It works by turning harmful molecules called quinones into less dangerous ones, preventing cell damage.

NQO1 also helps maintain the balance of chemicals inside the cell, which affects processes like cell growth, cell death, and stabilizing important proteins like p53 and p73. NQO1 inhibitors are a new molecular target for new chemotherapy drugs. NQO1 is upregulated in many human cancers; specifically, studies have shown increased NQO1 expression in breast cancer, colorectal cancer, lung cancer, pancreatic cancer, uterine cancer, cervical cancer, and melanoma. Currently, Phase II clinical trials are being conducted for the treatment of pancreatic cancer with β-lapachone. It has also entered a human trial for the treatment of squamous cell carcinomas.

Pau d'arco has provided a handful of novel chemicals that have been turned into small-molecule drugs specifically for cancer, some of which are in human clinical trials (see chapter 3, page 29, for more information). These include (but aren't limited to) the following:

Small-Molecule Drugs
- **NSC-11905** is a direct copy of the natural lapachol plant chemical.
- **ARQ761** is a direct copy of the beta-lapachone natural molecule.
- **ARQ501** is a fully synthetic version of the natural molecule beta-lapachone, which attached a new molecule (hydroxypropyl-beta-cyclodextrin) for a new patented small-molecule drug. It successfully completed Phase I clinical trials and several Phase II human clinical trials for the treatment of pancreatic cancer, head and neck cancer, and leiomyosarcoma. It is in several Phase III trials now either as a monotherapy for advanced cancers and in combination with various frontline chemotherapy drugs.
- **BBI608** (Napabucasin) is another naphthoquinone chemical in pau d'arco (2-acetylnaphtho [2,3-b]furan-4,9-dione), which was developed into

a small-molecule drug referred to as BBI608 and then named Napabucasin. Its main mechanism of action is inhibiting STAT3, which provides cancer cell stemness inhibitor actions. Various research and trials report Napabucasin inhibits cancer cell proliferation, induces apoptosis and cell cycle arrest, and suppresses metastasis and relapse. It has completed several Phase III human clinical studies on advanced solid tumors (pancreatic, colorectal, gastric, glioblastoma, and others). Several trials added Napabucasin to other frontline chemotherapy drugs to determine if it inhibited metastasis and recurrence or prevented drug resistance.

• **NSC-95397**, also known as Cdc25 Inhibitor IV, is a potent and selective Cdc25 dual-specificity phosphatase inhibitor copied from a quinone chemical from pau d'arco. It acts by inhibiting Cdc25 phosphatases, which are crucial for regulating cell cycle progression. These types of inhibitors affect an important substance called CDK1 and are usually referred to in cancer research as checkpoint inhibitors. Cancer cells generally affect programmed checkpoints, which allow them to continue to replicate and ignore the programmed cell death. This particular new chemical inhibitor has shown to restore the apoptosis code and cause cell cycle arrest at the G2/M phase (at the intra-S checkpoint) in colon, breast, and liver cancers.

Cancer Pathways and Mechanisms of Action

More complete information on these signaling pathways, cancer pathways, and new chemical targets for cancer therapy shown here can be found in chapter 5.

• Pau d'arco flips the suicide switch to restore apoptosis by restoring p53 function.

• Pau d'arco inhibited growth of cancer cell lines and STAT3 phosphorylation activity. Furanonaphtho-quinones in pau d'arco were the key structures required to exhibit STAT3 phosphorylation inhibitory activities in the JAK-STAT pathway.

• Pau d'arco showed dose-dependent anti-proliferative effects in human estrogen-positive carcinomas by upregulating metabolism-specific and apoptosis-specific genes and by downregulating estrogen response and cell cycle regulatory actions.

- β-lapachone induces programmed necrosis through the NQO1-dependent ROS-mediated RIP1/PARP1/AIF pathway in liver cancer.
- Pau d'arco inhibited growth of non–small cell lung cancer and telomerase activity, induced apoptosis by reducing the expression of Bcl-2, increased the expression of Bax, and activated caspase-3 and caspase-9.
- Pau d' arco can make targeting and killing cancer stem cells much easier by modulating specific signaling pathways and affecting cellular metabolism.
- While beta-lapachone induces apoptosis through E2F1 checkpoint pathways, necrotic cell death can be selectively induced by beta-lapachone in a variety of cancer cells.
- Beta-lapachone exhibits DNA topoisomerase I-inhibitor actions.
- Pau d'arco has PAK1-inhibitor actions. Its involvement in growth factor signaling, metastasis, angiogenesis (blood vessel formation), and drug resistance makes PAK1 an attractive therapeutic target for cancer treatment.
- Beta-lapachone significantly inhibited the proliferation of human liver cancer by inducing apoptosis, which was associated with upregulation of pro-apoptotic Bax and downregulation of anti-apoptotic Bcl-2, Bcl-xL, and MCL-1 expression; activation of caspase-3 and caspase-9; as well as degradation of PARP protein.
- Research suggests lapachol may target pyruvate kinase M2 (PKM2), a crucial enzyme in the glycolysis pathway, which is often upregulated in cancer cells. Inhibiting PKM2 could disrupt the energy production of cancer cells and potentially slow their growth.
- Lapachol has been observed to reverse the polarization of M2-like macrophages, which are often associated with tumor growth and suppression of the immune response. By reversing this polarization, lapachol may help boost the immune system's ability to fight cancer.
- Lapachol inhibits glycolysis in melanoma cancer cells by targeting pyruvate kinase M2.
- Lapachol was reported with MMP (matrix metalloproteinases) inhibitor actions. MMPs are a group of enzymes that break down proteins and play a dual role in tumor growth and metastasis processes. MMPs are promising therapeutic targets for various diseases, and research is ongoing to develop MMP inhibitors for treating conditions like cancer and arthritis.

- Pau d'arco has NQO1-inhibitor actions. NQO1 protects cancer cells from oxidative stress that would normally instigate apoptosis and is upregulated in many human cancers.

Other Researched Benefits That May Be Helpful

Small-scale human studies showed that a pau d'arco–based preparation may help prevent oral mucositis in patients with head and neck cancer undergoing radiotherapy. Pau d'arco provides anti-inflammatory actions through various mechanisms of action. Research reports showed it to have inhibitory activity on production of the inflammatory cytokines, such as TNF-a and IL-1b. It also inhibited the production of NO and PGE2 and suppressed the mRNA levels of COX-2 and iNOS. Many types of cancer actually promote inflammation inside their cells to encourage its growth and spread. Blocking these substances may provide additional anti-cancer benefits.

Availability of Products

Pau d'arco is an important resource from the rainforest with many applications in herbal medicine. Unfortunately, its popularity and use have been controversial due to varying results obtained with its use. For the most part, these seem to have been caused by a lack of quality control—and confusion as to which part of the plant to use and how to prepare it. Many species of *Tabebuia*, as well as other completely unrelated tree species exported today from South America as "pau d'arco," have few to none of the active constituents of the true medicinal species. Pau d'arco lumber is in high demand in South America.

The inner bark shavings commonly sold in the United States are actually by-products of the timber and lumber industries. Even mahogany shavings from the same sawmill floors in Brazil are swept up and sold around the world as "pau d'arco" (due to the similarity in color and odor of the two woods). In 1987, a chemical analysis of 12 commercially available pau d'arco products revealed only one product containing lapachol—and only in trace amounts. As lapachol concentration typically is 2–7% in true pau d'arco, the study surmised that the products were not truly pau d'arco, or that processing and transportation had damaged them. Most pau d'arco research has centered on the heartwood of the tree.

Most of the commercially available products, though, contain the inner and outer bark of the tree—which is stripped off at sawmills when the heartwood is milled into lumber for construction materials. Additionally, at least 10 species of *Tabebuia* are logged commercially in South America for lumber purposes alone. When these logs arrive at lumber mills, the identifying leaves and flowers (which distinguish the tree species) are long gone—it's all just "pau d'arco." This may explain varying species of pau d'arco bark being sold as herbal products—and their resulting (diminished) quality.

Finally, many consumers and practitioners are unaware that, for the best results when extracting these particular active chemicals (even after obtaining the correct species), the bark and/or wood must be boiled at least 8–10 minutes, rather than brewed as a simple tea or infusion (lapachol and the other quinoids are not very water soluble).

It is therefore not surprising that consumers and practitioners are experiencing spotty results with commercially available pau d'arco products. With its many effective applications, however, it would behoove consumers to take the time to learn about the available products and suppliers and find a reliable source for this important medicinal plant from the rainforest.

Relatively new in the marketplace are standardized extracts of pau d'arco, which guarantee the amount of lapachol and/or naphthoquinones. In such a product, it would be unclear if other active quinones have been extracted (and to what extent) in these chemically altered products. The natural wood and bark are quite effective when the correct species is used and prepared properly. Although more expensive, the new standardized extracts may be the safer purchase for most laypersons and general consumers concerned about quality but who don't have the time to research each product.

Safety

There have been no reports of human toxicity when a whole-bark decoction or tincture of pau d'arco is used. The oral LD_{50} dosage for lapachol is reported to be 1.2–2.4 g/kg (of body weight) in rats and 487–621 mg/kg (of body weight) in mice. Good quality pau d'arco (*Tabebuia impetiginosa*) contains an average of 4% lapachol (or 40 mgs of lapachol per gram of pau d'arco bark/wood).

Dosages

The recommended dose is ½ cup to 1 cup bark and/or heartwood decoction taken orally two to four times daily. (Do not prepare an infusion/tea for this plant; it will not be as effective.) If desired, 2–3 mgs of a heartwood tincture two to four times daily can be substituted (and would be preferred).

Contraindications

There have been no reports in the literature of contraindications when a whole-bark decoction or tincture is used. At least one isolated phytochemical in pau d'arco (lapachol), however, has demonstrated abortifacient properties in animal studies. As there are no studies confirming the safety of traditional bark decoctions used by pregnant women (nor is there indication in traditional medicine systems using this plant during pregnancy), the use of pau d'arco during pregnancy is not recommended.

Large single dosages of pau d'arco decoctions (more than 1 cup) may cause gastrointestinal upset and/or nausea. Do not use in high doses unless under the advice of a qualified health practitioner; reduce dosage if nausea occurs.

Drug Interactions

None reported.

Summary of Benefits the Plant Has to Fight Cancer

Since pau d'arco's main anti-cancer chemicals are not very water soluble, I never used it as an ingredient in any of the cancer formulas I developed that were sold in capsules. I did use it for the topical product I developed for skin cancers, called N-Tense Topical. I also had a pau d'arco tincture that I would recommend for some types of cancer (small cell lung cancer and recurring/metastatic cancers) to add to other cancer formulas or protocols.

Newer research indicates pau d'arco can affect cancer stem cells, which will be beneficial in any cancer (and especially small cell lung cancer) that easily develops drug resistance and reoccurs. In fact, this action against cancer stem cells may well explain why pau d'arco has been reported with antimetastatic actions in many studies with many cancer types.

Online Links to More Information

- Tropical Plant Database file for pau d'arco: https://rain-tree.com/paudarco.htm.

- Research references for this text: https://rain-tree.com/Pau-d-Arco-Cancer-Research.pdf.

PICÃO PRETO

Family: Asteraceae

Genus: *Bidens*

Species: *pilosa*

Synonyms: *Bidens adhaerescens, B. alausensis, B. chilensis, B. hirsuta, B. leucantha, B. montaubani, B. reflexa, B. scandicina, B. sundaica, Coreopsis leucantha, Kerneria pilosa*

Common Names: Picão preto, carrapicho, amor seco, pirca, aceitilla, cadillo, chilca, pacunga, cuambu, erva-picão, alfiler, clavelito de monte, romerillo, saltillo, yema de huevo, z'aiguille, jarongan, ketul, pau-pau pasir, Spanish needles, bident herisse, herbe d'aiguille, zweizahn, bidente piloso, mozote, beggar's tick

Parts Used: Whole herb

Picão preto is a small, erect annual herb that grows to 3 feet high. It has bright green leaves with serrated, prickly edges and produces small, yellow flowers and black fruit. Its root has a distinctive aroma similar to that of a carrot. It is indigenous to the Amazon rainforest and other tropical areas of South America, Africa, the Caribbean, and the Philippines. It is often considered a weed in many places. It is a southern cousin to *Bidens tripartita*, the European bur marigold, which has an ancient history in European herbal medicine. In Brazil, the plant is most commonly known as picão preto or carrapicho; in Peru it is known as amor seco or pirca.

Traditional Herbal Medicine Uses

In Peruvian herbal medicine, picão preto is employed to reduce inflammation, increase urination, and support and protect the liver. It is commonly used there for hepatitis, conjunctivitis, abscesses, fungal infections, and urinary infections; as a weight loss aid; and to stimulate childbirth. In Brazilian herbal medicine, it is used for fevers, malaria, hepatitis, diabetes, sore throat, tonsillitis, obstructions in the liver and other liver disorders, urinary infections, and vaginal discharge and infections.

An infusion or decoction of the entire plant is often gargled for tonsillitis and pharyngitis. Externally it is used for wounds, fungal infections, ulcers, diaper rash, insect bites, and hemorrhoids. Brazilian herbalists also report using picão preto to normalize insulin and bilirubin levels in the pancreas, liver, and blood. In Mexico, the entire plant or leaf is used to treat diabetes, stomach disorders, hemorrhoids, hepatitis, nervous problems, and fever.

Many of picão preto's traditional uses have been confirmed by some kind of research. The plant has been reported with anticandidal, anti-inflammatory, anti-ulcerous, antibacterial, anticoagulant (blood thinner), antifungal, antihepatotoxic (liver detoxifier), anti-leukemic, antimalarial, antioxidant, antitumorous, antivenin, antiviral, cardiotonic (tones, balances, strengthens the heart), COX-inhibitor (typically reduces inflammation), gastroprotective (protects the gastric tract), hepatoprotective (liver protector), hepatotonic (tones, balances, strengthens the liver), hypoglycemic, hypotensive (lowers blood pressure), immunomodulator (selectively modulates overactive immune cells), and uterine stimulant properties and actions. More complete information on picão preto's traditional uses and this research can be found in the Tropical Plant Database (see the link provided later in this plant's "Online Links to More Information" section).

Anti-Cancerous Actions

The very first anti-cancer study was in 1979, and researchers reported that feeding picão preto leaves to rats reduced the size of esophageal cancerous tumors by two-thirds. More research followed in the 1980s and 1990s, which reported that various types of picão preto extracts could reduce tumor size in animals or prevent the growth of various types of cancer cells in test tubes. These included breast, cervical, colon, colorectal, esophageal, gastric, head and neck, liver, lung, nasopharyngeal, prostate, ovarian, skin, and triple-negative breast cancers, as well as glioblastoma and melanoma. Picão preto first was reported to have anti-leukemic actions in 1995.

Researchers from Taiwan reported (in 2001) that a simple hot-water extract of picão preto could inhibit the growth of five strains of human and mouse leukemia at less than 200 mcg/mg *in vitro*. They summarized their research by saying that picão preto "may prove to be a useful medicinal plant for treating leukemia." Newer research has identified the possible natural compounds in picão preto that are responsible for its anti-leukemic actions in two other studies.

Most of the research published thereafter was on chemicals in picão preto rather than the plant; however, some of this research started with verifying the anti-cancerous action of the plant, then employing varying extraction methods to extract groups of plant chemicals to test against cancer. Some of the most recently published research uses new testing methods to determine what effect the plant, various extracts, and active chemicals have on a molecular level in signaling pathways that cancer is known to affect. Researchers in Egypt reported in 2024 that picão preto reduced tumor growth of liver cancer cells in test tubes without any toxicity to healthy cells.

A Chinese research group published a study in 2018 reporting picão preta was toxic to lung, melanoma, liver, and nasopharyngeal cancer cells in test tubes as well as reduced tumor formation in mice with lung cancer effectively. They also noted no toxicity to healthy cells or toxic effects in the animals.

A glycolic extract of picão preto is produced in Brazil, which was developed as an adjuvant cancer therapy to help reduce the toxicity and inflammation to healthy cells that chemotherapy drugs cause. In one of their first studies (published in 2015) the plant extract protected healthy intestinal cells from 5-fluorouracil (5-FU)-induced intestinal damage in mice. They then combined this herbal extract with curcuminoid chemicals from another plant (turmeric) and named it FitoProt®. They published several human clinical trials in 2023 studying cancer patients taking it with chemotherapy and reported the same protective effect on healthy cells without protecting or reducing the effects the drugs had on cancer cells.

Picão preto's immune modulating actions are well known and play a significant role in the plant's benefits for cancer. IFN-γ is a protein secreted by immune cells that is crucial for activating cellular immunity, boosting antitumor responses, and modulating immune responses, including inflammation and autoimmunity. Researchers in Taiwan reported that hot-water crude extracts of picão preto increased its expression twofold in leukemia cells. Two of the chemicals in the extract (centaurein and centaureidin) increased IFN-γ activity approximately fourfold in much lower dosages. Other research reports that picão preto can increase cells in the immune system (NK cells), which are responsible to hunt down, engulf, and remove foreign cells (including cancer cells) from the body.

Anti-Cancerous Plant Chemicals

Major chemical constituents (including 301 compounds) belonging to polyacetylenes, polyacetylene glycosides, polyphenols (flavonoids, flavone glycosides, aurones, chalcones, okanin glycosides, and phenolic acids), terpenes, pheophytins, fatty acids, and phytosterols have been identified or isolated from the different parts of this plant. Many of them have been considered as the bioactive compounds that are potentially responsible for the pharmacological actions. Some of these chemicals are well known and well researched polyphenol chemicals (see chapter 2 for more information).

Acetylenes: More than 50 acetylenes have been isolated from picão preto. Some of these chemicals occur in many plants and are well documented with anti-cancer, antimalarial, and anti-diabetes activities. At least 10 polyphenols, however, are novel and only found in picão preto; some of these chemicals are now being documented with anti-cancer actions. When acetylenes are found in plants, much like protective polyphenols, they help enhance the overall resilience of plants by adapting to environmental stressors, like temperature, rainfall fluctuations/flooding, and pest attacks.

Researchers in China discovered two new natural polyacetylene isomers (7-Phenyl-2-hepten-4,6-diyn-1-ol and [Z]-7-Phenyl-2-hepten-4,6-diyn-1-ol) in picão preto in 2023. Their study first revealed the excellent antimetastatic potential of these two polyacetylenes on human gastric cancer cells and the distinctive molecular mechanisms underlying their activities. They reported the polyacetylenes inhibited the migration, invasion, and adhesion of gastric cancer cells without toxicity to healthy cells in a dose-dependent manner.

These findings suggested that they exhibited its antimetastatic activities through the reversal of the EMT process (epithelial-mesenchymal transition is a cellular process that plays a crucial role in cancer metastasis by suppressing nine chemical substances and increasing one substance in the main pathways the EMT process uses [Wnt/β-catenin and Hippo/YAP signaling pathways]).

Daucosterol: Daucosterol is an active natural sterol compound, which has anti-inflammatory, anti-cancer, and immunomodulatory activities. Daucosterol inhibits cancer cell proliferation by inducing autophagy through a reactive oxygen species (ROS)–dependent manner. It also inhibits colon cancer growth by inducing apoptosis, inhibiting cell migration and invasion, and targeting caspase signaling pathways.

Friedelan: Friedelan is a triterpenoid chemical compound documented with anti-cancer, anti-inflammatory, antioxidant, analgesic, antipyretic, and antimicrobial activities. It has shown promising anti-cancer properties, inhibiting the growth and metastasis of various cancer cell lines, including leukemia, breast, and prostate cancer cells, through mechanisms like modulating signaling pathways and inducing cell death.

Polyphenols: Like most tropical plants, picão preto is a rich source of polyphenols with a wide variety of benefits (see more information on polyphenols in chapter 2). Some researchers studying the plant reported that the high amount of one particular polyphenol (isoquercitrin) found in picão preto might relate to some of the plant's anti-tumorous actions. Isoquercitrin has been reported to inhibit tumor growth in animals and in test tubes in quite a few studies published by different researchers around the world.

A research group in China studied the anti-cancer action of many of the polyphenols in picão preto in 2024 and reported that flavonoids are one of the key active ingredients responsible for the antitumor effect of the plant. They identified 18 flavonoids and nine polyacetylenes in a methanol extract of picão preto. Their test-tube research reported that four of the chemicals exhibited potent toxicity against a panel of five human cancer cell lines.

They also revealed that 11 flavonoids and polyacetylenes exerted strong inhibitory activities on human DNA Topo I. This substance is an essential enzyme in regulating DNA during transcription and replication, as well as an important therapeutic target for new antitumor agents. In addition, three of the compounds potently arrested cell cycle at the G1/S and G2/M phases in human colon cancer cells.

p-Coumaric Acid: This polyphenol has shown to inhibit tumor cell proliferation and migration, promote apoptosis, and modulate signaling pathways involved in cancer development in lung and colon cancer in a dose-dependent manner.

Okanin: Picão preto contains a rare polyphenol (only found in the flowers of one other plant to date that shares the same plant family) called okanin. Picão preto contains 17 different metabolites of okanin. In a 2024 study, researchers in Taiwan reported okanin was toxic to four different types of oral cancer in test tubes by causing cell cycle arrest, which triggered apoptosis (programed cell death) and pyroptosis (a type of programmed cell death that's characterized by inflammation and the release of cellular contents).

When they grafted human oral cancers into mice, they reported that okanin treatment significantly delayed the growth of human squamous cell carcinoma, reducing tumor volume by approximately two-thirds in 21 days. No toxicity or weight changes were noted in the animals. Iso-okanin has also been well studied, and it is sold as a small-molecule drug used for the research of various illnesses including cancers, skin rashes, snake and insect bites, diabetes mellitus, and diarrhea.

Other well-known and studied anti-cancer polyphenols in picão preto include apigenin, chlorogenic acid, ellagic acid, kaempferol, luteolin, and rutin.

Cancer Pathways and Mechanisms of Action

More complete information on the signaling pathways, cancer pathways, and new chemical targets for cancer therapy shown here can be found in chapter 5.

- Studies in animals and humans suggest picão preto can selectively prevent oxidative damage to healthy cells, which cancer drugs cause by downregulating the expression of apoptotic markers, such as Bax and p53, without affecting damage to cancer cells.
- Other studies report that picão preto significantly downregulates the expression of apoptosis-related protein Bcl-2 and upregulates the protein expression of Bax and caspase-3.
- Picão preto was reported to reduce cancer recurrence by modulating several specific signaling pathways that cancer stem cells use to escape

detection and hide from the immune system (including the NOTCH and the Wnt/β-catenin pathways).
- Test-tube studies reported inhibitory activities against both Raf-1 and MEK-1 gene expression, as well as a significant reduction in autophagy-related genes Atg12 and LC3B, which resulted in apoptosis of liver cancer cells.
- Picão preto can increase the level of reactive oxygen species (ROS) inside of cancer cells by increasing the expression of the JNK/NF-κB pathway, which triggers cell death.
- In animals, okanin reduced tumor growth and involved pyroptosis-related markers such as CASP1, GSDMC, GSDMD, and GSDME.
- In cancer, mucins can be overexpressed and contribute to tumor growth, metastasis, and resistance to therapy. Several chemicals in picão preto inhibit mucins.
- Water extracts of picão preto arrested acute lymphocytic leukemia cells in the G1 cell cycle, and it inhibited the phosphorylation of IκB kinase β and IκBα, and NF-κB-DNA binding, in conjunction with reduction of expression of proteins involved in G1/S cell cycle transition and suppression of apoptosis.
- In liver cancer cells, picão preto and one of its natural compounds induced G2/M-phase cell arrest and apoptosis.
- Human DNA topoisomerase I (Topo-I) is an essential enzyme in regulating DNA and is an important therapeutic target for antitumor agents. Picão preto showed potent cytotoxicity and inhibitory activities on DNA Topo I. At least 12 individual plant chemicals in the plant have demonstrated Topo-1 inhibitory actions.
- Multiple chemicals in picão preto have demonstrated anti-angiogenic actions, reducing or preventing increased blood flow to tumors by modifying the expression of ERK1/2 and CREB. A novel polyacetylene significantly inhibits angiogenesis and promotes apoptosis through activation of the CDK inhibitors and caspase-7.
- Polyacetylene chemicals were reported to suppress the metastasis of gastric cancer cells by inhibiting Wnt/β-catenin and Hippo/YAP signaling

pathways. In mice with breast tumors, the polyacetylene chemicals inhibited MDSC differentiation from bone marrow to drastically impair tumor metastasis.

• Chemicals in picão preto were reported to stimulate IFN-γ. This protein is secreted by immune cells and is crucial for activating cellular immunity, boosting antitumor responses, and modulating immune responses, including inflammation and autoimmunity.

Other Researched Benefits That May Be Helpful

Many of picão preto's traditional uses have been validated in some type of scientific research that is more completely described in the Tropical Plant Database file. Cancer patients who are using conventional chemotherapy and/or radiation may notice additional benefits in reducing side effects of these traditional therapies. Picão preto has been confirmed with effective anti-ulcerous, gastric-protective, liver-protective, and heart-protective benefits and actions. As described earlier, picão preto is offered as an herbal drug in Brazil for this purpose to treat oral mucositis (mouth ulcers) and to protect the gastric system and intestines from the ulcerative effect of some chemotherapy drugs. Patients who are at risk for these side effects may want to consider preparing an herbal tea of picão preto to drink once or twice daily. See chapter 8, page 140, for more instructions.

Picão preto has also shown to have pain-relieving and anti-inflammatory actions in other research, which some may find helpful.

Availability of Products

While this rainforest plant needs much more education in the U.S. market, it is offered in a handful of products in bulk powders, capsules, and liquid extracts. Try doing an internet search using the keywords *picao preto products*, *Bidens pilosa supplements*, and *Spanish Needles products* to find all available purchasing choices.

Safety

Picão preto has long been regarded as a safe herbal remedy with little toxicity; however, it is an active remedy that deserves attention and respect to use it safely. Picão preto has long been used to treat high blood pressure and diabetes, and in therapeutic dosages in animals, it has been shown to lower blood pressure and glucose levels. One small-scale human study was conducted in Taiwan in 2015 on glucose levels in diabetics and nondiabetics. They reported better pancreatic B-cell function and insulin release in diabetic subjects but no changes in glucose levels in healthy or diabetic subjects. They reported it was safe with no obvious side effects in all subjects. In animal studies, orally administered infusions of the ground powder of picão preto aerial parts at a concentration of 100 mg/ml and at a dose limit of 2,000 mg/kg of body weight over 28 days was reported nontoxic in rats.

Dosages

In herbal medicine systems the whole plant or ariel parts are used to create natural remedies. In the tropics, generally 1 cup of a standard decoction is used one to three times daily depending on the condition that is being treated; 2–3 mgs of a 4:1 tincture twice daily or 2–3 grams of powdered herb in tablets, capsules, or stirred into water (or juice) twice daily can be substituted, if desired. See chapter 7 for dosages and recipes based on cancer types, as well as remedies for minimizing chemotherapy side effects.

Contraindications

- Picão preto has evidenced weak uterine stimulant activity in guinea pigs. As such, it should not be used during pregnancy.

- This plant contains several coumarin derivatives. Coumarins are a group of chemicals that thin the blood. This possible effect has not been confirmed in animal or human studies. Those on blood thinning medications, however, should use picão preto with caution and monitor these possible effects.

- The plant has been documented to lower blood sugar levels in several animal studies, but this has not been confirmed in humans. Those with hypoglycemia or diabetes should use picão preto under the supervision of a qualified health care professional and monitor their blood sugar levels accordingly.

- Picão preto has been documented with hypotensive activity in several animal studies, but this hasn't been confirmed in humans. People with heart conditions and those taking antihypertensive drugs should consult their doctors prior to using this plant to monitor these possible effects (as medications may need adjustment).

Drug Interactions

No clinically documented drug interactions in humans have been reported; however, based on plant chemicals and animal studies, the use of this plant may potentiate antidiabetic, anticoagulant, and antihypertensive drugs.

Summary of Benefits the Plant Has to Fight Cancer

Picão preto, one of South America's well-known medicinal plants, is widely used for numerous conditions. Many of its indigenous uses for inflammation, hypertension, ulcers, diabetes, and infections of all kinds are being validated and verified by modern research. I have long used it in various multi-herb formulas I've created over many years (for allergies, arthritis, antiaging, hypertension, infections, and supporting liver function). It was also an important ingredient in the NTense-2 formula.

In newer research, picão preto has been reported to inhibit topoisomerase type I, with more than a dozen natural compounds in the plant providing this action. In standard frontline chemotherapy drugs, the two most common topoisomerase type I inhibitors in use today are the camptothecin derivatives topotecan and irinotecan. They are used in the treatment of ovarian cancer, small cell lung cancer, and cervical and renal cell cancers, as well as leukemias and lymphomas. If picão preto can augment or enhance the Top-1-inhibitor actions of the drugs with much less toxicity to healthy cells and negative side effects, it would certainly make an attractive adjunctive natural therapy to use for a wider range of tumorous cancers that are hard to treat. Hopefully, more research will be forthcoming.

Online Links to More Information

• Tropical Plant Database file for picão preto: https://rain-tree.com/picao preto.htm.

• Research references for this text: https://rain-tree.com/Picao-Preto-Cancer-Research.pdf

SIMAROUBA

Family: Simaroubaceae

Genus: *Simarouba*

Species: *amara, glauca*

Synonyms: *Quassia simarouba, Zwingera amara, Picraena officinalis, Simarouba medicinalis*

Common Names: Simarouba, gavilan, negrito, marubá, marupá, dysentery bark, bitterwood, paradise tree, palo blanco, robleceillo, caixeta, daguilla, cedro blanco, cajú-rana, malacacheta, palo amargo, pitomba, bois amer, bois blanc, bois frene, bois negresse, simaba

Parts Used: Bark, wood, leaves

Simarouba is a medium-sized tree that normally grows 50–80 feet high (occasionally reaching 115 feet in height) with a trunk 20–30 inches in diameter. It produces bright green leaves 8–12 inches in length, small white flowers, and small red fruits. It is indigenous to the Amazon rainforest and other tropical areas in Mexico, Cuba, Haiti, Jamaica, and Central America.

TRADITIONAL HERBAL MEDICINE USES

Simarouba has a long history of use as an herbal remedy in South and Central America for diarrhea, dysentery, malaria, intestinal parasites, colitis, and other stomach and bowel disorders, and it is used externally for wounds and sores. Simarouba also grows in India, and it has long been used by natural health practitioners as a natural remedy for cancer in their Ayurveda traditional medicine system. See the Tropical Plant Database page for more information on simarouba's herbal medicine uses and other research performed on this important rainforest resource that validated its traditional uses.

Anti-Cancerous Actions

Early cancer screening performed by the National Cancer Institute (NCI) in 1976 indicated that an alcohol extract of simarouba root (and a water extract of its seeds) had toxic actions against cancer cells at very low dosages (less than 20 mcg/mg). Following up on that initial screening, scientists discovered that several of the quassinoid chemicals in simarouba (such as glaucarubinone, alianthinone, and dehydroglaucarubinone) had anti-leukemic actions against lymphocytic leukemia in test tubes and published several studies in 1977 and 1978. In 1983, researchers found that yet another simarouba quassinoid, holacanthone, also possessed anti-leukemic and anti-tumorous actions.

Researchers in the United Kingdom cited the anti-tumorous activity of two of the quassinoids, ailanthinone and glaucarubinone, against human epidermoid carcinoma of the pharynx. A later study in 1998 by U.S. researchers demonstrated the anti-tumorous activity of glaucarubinone against solid tumors (human and mouse cell lines) in test tubes, as well as multidrug-resistant mammary tumors and anti-leukemic activity in mice.

With these kinds of results, it's little wonder that research continues. More recently, scientific studies report and confirm much of the same anti-cancerous actions in test tubes and in animals. The newer research reports simarouba provides effective anti-cancerous benefits in breast, cervix, colorectal, brain (glioblastoma), ovarian, and lung cancers, as well as melanoma and several types of leukemia.

Anti-Cancerous Plant Chemicals

The main active group of chemicals in simarouba are called *quassinoids*, which belong to the triterpene chemical family. Quassinoids are found in many plants and are well known to scientists. Some of simarouba's quassinoids are unique and only found in simarouba and/or *Simarouba*'s plant family. The quassinoids found in simarouba, such as ailanthinone, canthin-6-one, glaucarubinone, glaucarubolone, and holacanthone, are considered the plant's main therapeutic constituents and are the ones documented to be toxic to cancer and leukemia cells. These natural plant chemicals have been identified in simarouba's bark, leaves, roots, and fruit seeds. Simarouba's medicinal properties and seven of its active plant chemicals appear in more than 40 patents, including its ability to treat cancer.

Glaucarubinone: One of these chemicals, glaucarubinone, has demonstrated the strongest action against cancer. Scientists have copied this chemical and have changed it enough (creating analogs and derivatives) to create a new patented anti-cancer chemical. U.S. government research has been conducted by cancer research divisions within the National Institutes of Health (NIH), including a newer department involved in the genetic research on cancer.

NIH researchers have published a handful of small studies indicating they may be working on a new cancer drug for brain cancer created from one or more of simarouba's quassinoid chemicals, including glaucarubinone. Their research published in 2011 reported that glaucarubinone was a dose-dependent AP-1 inhibitor at nontoxic concentrations to healthy cells. Oncogenic transcription factor activator protein-1 (AP-1) regulates a wide range of cellular processes in cancer cells.

AP-1: AP-1 has emerged as an actively pursued drug discovery target over the past decade by cancer researchers. Mounting data reports that it regulates the expression of downstream genes involved in various aspects of cancer biology, such as cell growth, apoptosis, angiogenesis, invasion, metastasis, and drug resistance. AP-1 has been described as being overexpressed in many tumors, including triple-negative breast cancer, colon cancer, Hodgkin lymphoma, and large cell lymphoma. AP-1 is often overexpressed in brain tumors, particularly in glioblastomas, where its increased expression is associated with tumor progression and aggressive behavior.

These researchers reported in 2009 that, when quassinoids (two found in simarouba) inhibit the activity of the transcription factor AP-1, this effect does not necessarily lead to cell death (cytotoxicity) or a reduction in protein production (protein synthesis inhibition) in healthy cells—implying that quassinoids can specifically target AP-1 function in cancer cells without causing significant overall cellular damage to normal cells.

A 2014 published study described one of the most common genetic mutations (1 in 3,000 live births), which results in cells that are deficient in a genetic substance called NF-1. This can result in NF-1 deficient cancer cells that are harder to treat. People with this genetic disorder (usually starting in childhood) develop a diverse set of tumor types, including benign neurofibromas, malignant peripheral nerve sheath tumors, brain cancer (gliomas), gastrointestinal stromal tumors, myeloid leukemia, breast cancer, and others. This study reported that in test tubes quassinoid chemicals (glaucarubinone in simarouba and ailanquassin in *Simarouba berteroana*) inhibited the growth of NF-1-deficient glioma cancer cells between 57% and 71% at 2 mcg/ml without observed toxicity.

A 2015 study by U.S. researchers reported that glaucarubinone's cancer benefits were due, in part, to affecting another important signaling pathway (PAK1) that plays a role in many of the main cancer pathways. PAK1 can promote cell survival; prevent apoptosis; enhance cell movement, proliferation, and tumor formation; and increase resistance to drug treatment. They studied the effect glaucarubinone has on PAK1 in five different types of colorectal cancers in test tubes as well as colorectal adenocarcinomas and a highly aggressive type of human colon cancer in mice. They reported that glaucarubinone significantly inhibited tumor growth without any harm to the animals. Inhibition of growth and migration was also shown against all cancer strains in test tubes as well.

In other research in the United States, scientists reported that a different quassinoid, glaucarubulone, was toxic to breast cancer cells, without any toxicity to healthy cells. In fact, they reported it worked better and at a lower dosage than two standard cancer drugs used to treat breast cancer (tamoxifen and 5-fluorouracil).

More important, research has been conducted now revealing how simarouba actually affects different cancer cells on a molecular level within the main cancer pathways. Today, we know much better how and why it is beneficial to combat cancer. This research, performed in animals and test tubes, indicates that simarouba may be working as described here.

Cancer Pathways and Mechanisms of Action

More complete information on these signaling pathways, cancer pathways, and new chemical targets for cancer therapy shown here can be found in chapter 5.

- Simarouba has been shown to inhibit angiogenesis (the formation of blood vessels to tumor cells).

- Glaucarubinone triggers apoptosis through the activation of pro-apoptosis proteins such as p53, Bax, caspase-9, and caspase-3 selectively in cancer cells without harming healthy cells. When glaucarubinone was used in combination with chemotherapy drugs, it increased the oxidative burst of the drugs, making them more effective at triggering apoptosis to kill the cancer cells.
- The plasma membrane in some cancers can promote too much of an enzyme (NADH oxidase), which contributes to uncontrolled cell proliferation. This makes its inhibition a potential therapeutic strategy for cancer that uses the enzyme to enhance proliferation. The quassinoids in simarouba inhibit NADH, which may slow down or stop the rapid growth of these types of cancers.
- Glaucarubinone was also reported to interrupt the normal cycle to create a new cancer cell (induced cell arrest in the G2/M phase), which also reduces proliferation.
- PAK1 (p-21-activated kinase 1) enhances colorectal cancer progression by stimulating Wnt/β-catenin, ERK, and AKT pathways. PAK1 also promotes cancer survival via upregulation of hypoxia-inducible factor 1α (HIF-1α), a key player in cancer survival. Research indicates that glaucarubinone inhibited colorectal cancer growth by downregulation of HIF-1α and β-catenin via a PAK1-dependent pathway.
- When combined with standard cancer drugs, glaucarubinone acted as an ABCB1 inhibitor. ABCB1 is a gene that cancer can mutate or activate to produce more protein molecules necessary to create a P-glycoprotein pump, which pumps cancer drugs out of cells. When the protein is blocked or inhibited, the cancer cell loses this defense mechanism, making the drug more effective and the cancer less likely to return as a multidrug-resistant tumor.
- In neuroblastoma, a simarouba quassinoid (NBT-272) was demonstrated to inhibit cellular proliferation and to downregulate c-MYC protein expression.
- Chemicals in simarouba have shown the ability to kill cancer stem cells by metabolic modifying actions specific to stem cells as well as to alter specific pathways that stem cells use to evade and escape detection by immune cells.

- Several chemicals in simarouba have been reported to inhibit TGF-β-associated EMT progression. Inhibiting this process has become a new target in cancer research to reduce invasiveness and metastasis of various cancers.

Other Researched Benefits That May Be Helpful

Simarouba has a long history of use, as well as preliminary research, indicating that the leaves and/or bark of the tree can help protect the gastric tract and liver from chemicals and drugs that normally harm these organs. This may provide additional benefit to cancer patients taking chemotherapy drugs that may have a toxic or harmful effect to the stomach, intestines, or liver.

Availability of Products

Simarouba bark and/or leaf products are available in bulk herb powders, capsules, and liquid extracts under several different manufacturers' labels.

Safety

Simarouba has been an effective, well-documented herbal remedy in Europe and the United States since the early 1700s. It is considered to be a safe and well-tolerated remedy without toxicity. Acute and chronic toxicity studies on simarouba were conducted in 2021 in rats where it was reported to be without toxicity even in very high dosages of 5,000 mg/kg of body weight.

Dosages

The traditional herbal remedy calls for preparing a standard decoction with the bark. A teacup full (about 6 ounces) is taken two to three times daily; 5–10 mgs of a bark or leaf tincture or 3–4 grams in capsules or tablets twice daily can be substituted if desired.

Contraindications

Avoid very high dosages. Reported side effects at high dosages (approximately three times the traditional remedy) include increased perspiration and urination, nausea, and/or vomiting.

Drug Interactions

None reported.

Summary of Benefits the Plant Has to Fight Cancer

The research on simarouba and brain tumors is compelling, especially in light of how I learned of this new research. Out of the blue, I received an email in early 2012. It was a discussion among five researchers at the National Cancer Institute (NCI), the National Institutes of Health (NIH), and a pharmaceutical company. I was carbon-copied on the email for some unknown reason. The researchers were discussing that simarouba (and several of its quassinoid chemicals) could not only treat but also cure brain tumors in children (glioblastomas and medulloblastomas).

This was stated so matter-of-factly that I was shocked. I didn't recognize any of the names in the email, but I discovered when looking them up in my company's database that the NIH researcher had ordered simarouba from my company several times. One of the researchers declared that simarouba's action against brain tumors was even greater than that of bee propolis. This was yet another known natural remedy for brain cancer, and it was another shock that no one really knew about bee propolis and brain tumors but these government researchers.

After I closed Raintree later that year, I sent a copy of this email to the Health Science Institute (HSI) so they could write an article on it (and these two natural remedies for brain tumors) in their newsletter. See the HSI article linked in this plant's "Online Links to More Information" section for more information. Simarouba has been one of the natural remedies I've long used in my naturopathic protocols for brain tumors since that time, and it has made a difference. It is also an ingredient in NTense-2 (see chapter 6, page 81).

Online Links to More Information

• Tropical Plant Database file for simarouba: https://rain-tree.com/simaruba.htm.

• Research references for this text: https://rain-tree.com/Simarouba-Cancer-Research.pdf.

• HSI article on simarouba and brain tumors: https://rain-tree.com/reports/hsi_2013_simarouba.pdf.

SUMA

Family: Amaranthaceae

Genus: *Pfaffia*

Species: *paniculata*

Synonyms: *Hebanthe paniculata, Gomphrena paniculata, G. eriantha, Iresine erianthos, I. paniculata, I. tenuis, Pfaffia eriantha, Xeraea paniculata*

Common Names: Suma, Brazilian ginseng, pfaffia, para toda, corango-acu

Parts Used: Root

Suma, also referred to as Brazilian ginseng, is a large, rambling, shrubby ground vine with an intricate, deep, and extensive root system. It is indigenous to the Amazon basin and other tropical parts of (southern) Brazil, Ecuador, Panama, Paraguay, Peru, and Venezuela. Since its first botanical recording in 1826, it has been referred to by several botanical names, including *Pfaffia paniculata, Hebanthe paniculata,* and *Gomphrena paniculata*. The genus *Pfaffia* is well known in Central and South America, with more than 50 species growing in the warmer tropical regions.

TRADITIONAL HERBAL MEDICINE USES

In North American herbal medicine, suma root is used as an adaptogenic and regenerative tonic regulating many systems of the body; as an immunostimulant; and to treat exhaustion and chronic fatigue, impotence, arthritis, anemia, diabetes, cancer, tumors, mononucleosis, high blood pressure, premenstrual syndrome, menopause, hormonal disorders, and many types of stress. In herbal medicine in Ecuador today, suma is considered a tonic and "normalizer" for the cardiovascular system, the central nervous system, the reproductive system, and the digestive system; it is used to treat hormonal disorders, sexual dysfunction and sterility, arteriosclerosis, diabetes, circulatory and digestive disorders, rheumatism, and bronchitis.

Thomas Bartram, in his book *Encyclopedia of Herbal Medicine*, reports that suma is used in Europe to restore nerve and glandular functions; to balance the endocrine system; to strengthen the immune system; for infertility, menopausal, and menstrual symptoms; to minimize the side effects of birth control medications; for high cholesterol; to neutralize toxins; and as a general restorative tonic after illness. Various research published over the years has validated some of these traditional remedy uses.

In traditional medicine systems throughout the world today, suma is considered a tonic and an adaptogen. The definition of an adaptogen is a plant that increases the body's resistance to adverse influences by a wide range of physical, chemical, and biochemical factors and has a normalizing or restorative effect on the body as a whole. In modern Brazilian natural medicine practices, suma root is employed as a cellular oxygenator and taken to stimulate appetite and circulation, increase estrogen production, balance blood sugar levels, enhance the immune system, strengthen the muscular system, and enhance memory. More complete information on suma's traditional uses and this research can be found in the Tropical Plant Database (see the link provided later in this plant's "Online Links to More Information" section).

Anti-Cancerous Actions

Research in Japan (in 2000) reported that natural suma root had anti-cancerous activity. In this *in vivo* study, an oral administration of powdered suma root (at dosages of 750 mg/kg) was reported to inhibit the proliferation of lymphoma and leukemia in mice and, otherwise, delay mortality. Notice, however, that this anti-cancerous effect slowed the growth of these cancer cells but did not eradicate them. These researchers postulated that the inhibitory effect evidenced might be due to the enhancement of the nonspecific and/or cellular immune systems.

Brazilian researchers reported in 2010 that suma root had an anti-cancer effect against liver cancer in mice, which was related to the control of cellular proliferation and apoptosis (but not to cell communication and/or connexin expression) and directly influenced by the root concentration. Other Brazilian researchers reported in 2015 that suma's anti-inflammatory actions were immune modulatory in nature and included lowering pro-inflammatory immune cells levels of IL-1β, INF-γ, TNF-α, and IL-6. Lowering these specific substances is known to have anti-cancer benefits. IL-1β can promote tumor growth and metastasis by influencing angiogenesis (formation of new blood vessels) and the tumor microenvironment.

Interferon-gamma (IFN-γ) is a key player in antitumor immunity, immune evasion, and immunotherapy response. TNF-α can encourage cancer cell growth, survival, and metastasis by promoting inflammation, which can create a favorable environment for tumor development. Interleukin-6 (IL-6), one of the major cytokines in the tumor microenvironment, is an important factor that is found at high concentrations and known to be deregulated in cancer. Its overexpression has been reported in almost all types of tumors. IL-6 is implicated in various stages of tumorigenesis, including the initiation, growth, and progression of different cancers.

Brazilian researchers reported in 2017 that suma provided significant antimutagenic (cancer-preventative) actions in animals given known drugs that create mutations, which can efficiently contribute to improvements in quality of life and recovery for people undergoing chemotherapeutic treatment. Most recently, researchers reported in 2024 that human colon cancer HCT116 and mouse breast tumor model 4T1 cells treated with methanolic extract of suma showed a significant decrease in the viability of cancer cells.

ANTI-CANCEROUS PLANT CHEMICALS

The specific saponins found in the roots of suma include a group of novel phytochemicals that scientists have named *pfaffosides*. These saponins have clinically demonstrated the ability to inhibit cultured tumor cell melanomas (*in vitro*). The pfaffosides and pfaffic acid derivatives in suma were patented as antitumor compounds in several Japanese patents in the mid-1980s. In a study described in one of the patents, researchers reported that an oral dosage of 100 mg/kg (of suma saponins) given to rats was active against abdominal cancer. The other patents and Japanese research report that the pfaffic acids found in suma root had a strong *in vitro* activity against melanoma, liver carcinoma, and lung carcinoma cells at only 4–6 micrograms of pfaffic acids.

Other anti-cancer chemicals found in suma include ecdysterone and beta-ecdysterone, calenduloside E 6'-methyl ester, daucosterol, mesembryanthemoidigenic acid, oleanolic acid 28-O-beta-D-glucopyranoside (OAG), and pfameric acid.

Oleanolic acid 28-O-beta-D-glucopyranoside (OAG): OAG has demonstrated antitumor activity and anti-cancer properties in various studies. Studies have shown that OAG can inhibit the growth of various cancer cells, including those from liver, colon, lung, ovarian, and breast cancers. It appears to exert its effects by inhibiting cancer cell proliferation, promoting apoptosis (programmed cell death), and inhibiting tumor cell invasion, migration, and angiogenesis. OAG has also shown promise as a new drug for ulcerative colitis in animal studies. As such, it may provide a protective effect against chemotherapy drugs that cause gastric ulcers and/or damage to the digestive tract.

Plant sterols: Phytosterols have been widely accepted as natural anti-cancer agents in multiple malignant tumors. Beta-ecdysone, a naturally occurring steroid hormone in suma, has shown potential as an antitumor agent, particularly in breast cancer, by inhibiting cell growth and inducing cell death. It also appears to synergize with certain chemotherapy drugs like doxorubicin, enhancing their effectiveness. Suma contains another naturally occurring steroid hormone, daucosterol, which has shown promising anti-cancer effects in various studies, primarily by inducing autophagy and apoptosis in cancer cells.

It has been investigated in relation to liver cancer, prostate cancer, lung cancer, breast cancer, and multiple myeloma. Ecdysterone, another sterol in suma, has shown potential anti-cancer effects, particularly in breast cancer and lung cancer cell lines, by inhibiting growth and inducing cell death. Studies have also revealed its ability to enhance the effectiveness of chemotherapy drugs and reduce the development of radiation-induced oral mucositis.

Polyphenols: Suma root contains some standard polyphenols found in many other plants such as protocatechuic acid, coumaryl-hexoside, caffeoylquinic acid, quercetin, rutin, and kaempferol. Some of these polyphenols have shown anti-cancerous actions in independent research.

Cancer Pathways and Mechanisms of Action

More complete information on these signaling pathways, cancer pathways, and new chemical targets for cancer therapy shown here can be found in chapter 5.

- Suma demonstrated multiple mechanisms of action against liver cancer including cycle arrest in the S phase, by CDK2 and cyclin E downregulation, p27 (KIP1) overexpression, and induction of apoptosis through caspase-3 activation.
- Suma induces cell cycle arrest and caspase-3-induced apoptosis (programmed cell death) in liver cancer cells.
- Suma has immune-modulatory actions and reduced a number of pro-inflammatory immune cells (IL-1β, INF-γ, TNF-α, and IL-6). Most types of cancerous tumors promote inflammation by increasing the production and/or expression of these same immune cells, which promote the initiation, growth, and progression of different cancers.
- Suma can inhibit IL-1β. IL-1β can promote tumor growth and metastasis by influencing angiogenesis (formation of new blood vessels) and the tumor microenvironment.
- Oleanolic acid (OA) helped stop tumor cells from growing by lowering the levels of proteins (Bcl-2, Cyclin D1, and CDK4) that support cell growth, and increasing the levels of proteins (Bax and p21) that help stop or slow down cell growth. It also activated the p53 pathway, which is known for fighting cancer.
- OA slowed the growth of human glioblastoma (brain cancer) cells by turning on the STAT3 protein in both the cancer cells and nearby immune cells (macrophages).
- Suma was shown to inhibit JAK-STAT. JAK-STAT activation can promote cancer cell growth, survival, and migration, leading to tumor progression and proliferation. The pathway can also influence immune responses, potentially suppressing antitumor immunity and allowing cancer cells to evade immune surveillance.
- OA slowed down the growth of stomach cancer cells by reducing the levels of cyclin A and CDK2, two proteins that help cells divide.

Other Researched Benefits That May Be Helpful

In other research, suma demonstrated pain-relieving and anti-inflammatory activities in various *in vivo* rat and mouse studies. The anti-inflammatory actions also provide an anti-cancer benefit. Animal studies indicate that suma has gastroprotective and anti-ulcer effects, which may be helpful for those taking chemotherapy drugs that cause mucositis and gastric problems. In fact, researchers in Brazil conducted a study with mice in 2017 that suggested suma "can efficiently contribute to improvements in quality of life and recovery for people undergoing chemotherapeutic treatment, or those looking for health and preventive habits." They also reported that suma evidenced antimutagenic (cancer-preventative) actions.

Availability of Products

Suma is now widely available in the United States. It is available under various labels in bulk powders, capsules and tablets, teabags, and various liquid extracts. Simply do an internet search using the keywords *suma root products*.

Safety

Toxicity studies with humans indicated no toxicity at an oral dosage of 1.5 grams of the root. Another orally administered toxicity study with rats also reported no toxicity—even when suma root represented 50% of the rats' food supply for 30 days. Mice injected subcutaneously with the equivalent of 5 g/kg (in an ethanol extract), however, evidenced sedation, drop in body temperature, and loss of motor coordination; mortality was observed at 10 g/kg (again, in an ethanolic extract) when injected in mice.

One animal study reported that levels of the sex hormones estradiol-17beta, progesterone, and testosterone were clearly higher for mice that drank *P. paniculata* root-enriched water than for mice that drank plain water. They also reported that no adverse reactions were seen in mice within 30 days of oral intake, so consumption of suma for long periods of time appears safe.

Dosages

The Brazilian traditional remedy calls for preparing a standard decoction with 10 grams of suma root boiled in a liter of water; 2 cups of the decoction are generally taken daily. Herbalists and health practitioners also employ suma root powder in capsules (the decoction tastes quite bitter) with the reported dosage being 2–4 grams daily depending on body weight and health condition; this daily dosage is usually taken in two or three divided dosages throughout the day. For standardized or liquid extract products, follow the labeled dosage instructions.

Contraindications

• Suma has been documented to contain a significant amount of plant sterols including a significant amount of beta-ecdysterone and small amounts of stigmasterol and beta-sitosterol. These sterols might have estrogenic properties or activities and/or cause an increase in estrogen and/or testosterone production (not clinically proven in humans). As such, it is advisable for those with hormone-positive cancers (breast and prostate) to check with their doctors before using suma.

• One animal study (mice) reports suma may reduce male fertility. While this has not been confirmed in humans, those seeking pregnancy should probably avoid taking suma.

• The root powder has been reported to cause asthmatic allergic reactions if inhaled. When handling raw suma root powder or preparing decoctions with root powder, avoid inhalation of the root powder/dust.

• Ingestion of large amounts of plant saponins in general (naturally occurring chemicals in suma) has shown to sometimes cause mild gastric disturbances including nausea and stomach cramping. Reduce dosages if these side effects are noted.

Drug Interactions

None reported.

SUMMARY OF BENEFITS THE PLANT HAS TO FIGHT CANCER

Suma is one of the ingredients in the NTense-2 formula and N-Tense Topical. It has long been considered a very safe natural remedy, even when consumed in large dosages, which have been confirmed in animal toxicity studies.

ONLINE LINKS TO MORE INFORMATION

• Tropical Plant Database file for suma: https://rain-tree.com/suma.htm.

• Research references for this text: https://rain-tree.com/Suma-Cancer-Research.pdf.

VASSOURINHA

Family: Scrophulariaceae

Genus: *Scoparia*

Species: *dulcis*

Synonyms: *Scoparia grandiflora, Scoparia ternata, Capraria dulcis, Gratiola micrantha*

Common Names: Vassourinha, ñuñco pichana, anisillo, bitterbroom, boroemia, broomweed, brum sirpi, escobilla, mastuerzo, piqui pichana, pottipooli, sweet broom, tapixava, tupixaba, licorice weed

Parts Used: Leaves, aerial parts, roots

Vassourinha is an erect annual herb in the foxglove family that grows about 18 inches high. It produces serrated leaves and many small, white flowers. It is widely distributed in many tropical countries in the world and is found in abundance in South America and the Amazon rainforest. It can be found as far north as the southern United States, including Texas, Florida, and Louisiana. The plant is called escobilla in Peru and vassourinha in Brazil, and here in the United States, the plant is known as sweet broomweed or licorice weed. In many areas, the plant is considered an invasive weed.

TRADITIONAL HERBAL MEDICINE USES

Vassourinha is employed in herbal medicine throughout the tropics. In Peru, a decoction of the entire plant is recommended for upper respiratory problems, biliary colic or congestion, menstrual disorders, and fever; the leaf juice is still employed externally for wounds and hemorrhoids. In

Brazilian herbal medicine, the plant is used to reduce fever, lower blood sugar and blood pressure, and relieve coughs and lung congestion. A tea is prepared from the leaves or aerial parts of the plant for fevers and urinary tract diseases, upper respiratory disorders, bronchitis, coughs, menstrual disorders, and hypertension.

The leaf juice or a decoction of the leaves is also employed topically for skin ulcers and erysipelas. In Ayurvedic herbal medicine systems in India, a leaf tea is widely used for diabetes. Various research published over the years has validated some of these traditional remedy uses. More complete information on vassourinha's traditional uses and this research can be found in the Tropical Plant Database (see the link provided later in this plant's "Online Links to More Information" section).

Anti-Cancerous Actions

In addition to its tested anti-cancerous chemicals, a methanol extract of vassourinha leaves also showed toxic actions against cancer cells (with a 66% inhibition rate) by Japanese researchers. These findings fueled more research on the chemicals in this plant and their activities that is still ongoing today. In fact, the majority of research published in the last 10 years has studied the known anti-cancer chemicals found in vassourinha rather than a whole plant extract.

One exception is research published in Thailand in 2019, which studied a whole plant extract of vassourinha against a rare cancer called cholangiocarcinoma (CCA). While the disease is rare in most countries, Thailand has the highest incidence rate of all countries for this hard-to-treat lethal cancer. They tested two different strains of CCA cancers in test tubes and reported the vassourinha plant extract significantly inhibited the growth of the strains by percentages of 56.06 and 74.76. They additionally reported that the ability to inhibit CCA cell growth was through the induction of apoptosis.

Anti-Cancerous Plant Chemicals

Chemical screening of vassourinha has shown that it is a source of novel phytochemicals in the flavone and terpene classification, some of which have not been seen in science before. Many of vassourinha's active biological properties, including its anti-cancerous properties, are attributed to these phytochemicals. The main chemicals being studied are scopadulcic acids A and B; scopadiol; scopadulciol; scopadulin; scopanolal; scoparic acids A, B, C, D, and E; neo-dulcinol; dulcinodiol; dulcinodal; dulcidiol; betulinic acid; friedelin; and acteoside/verbascoside.

Scopadulcic acid B and betulinic acid: Scientists began trying in the mid-1990s to synthesize several plant chemicals found in vassourinha, including scopadulcic acid B and betulinic acid, for their use in the pharmaceutical industry. The anti-tumorous activity of scopadulcic acid B was demonstrated in a 1993 study, and antitumor activity against various human cancer cell lines was reported again in 2001. Betulinic acid is another phytochemical that has been the subject of much independent cancer research (beginning in the late 1990s).

Many studies report that betulinic acid has powerful anti-cancerous, anti-tumorous, and anti-leukemic properties. This potent phytochemical has displayed selective cytotoxic activity against malignant brain tumors, bone cancer, and melanomas (without harming healthy cells). Today, 62 betulinic acid derivatives have been created and tested against just human ovarian cancer alone.

Acteoside: Acteoside (also called verbascoside) has wide-spectrum, therapeutic anti-cancer actions and has been the subject of a large amount of research. Iso-dulcinol, 4-epi-scopadulcic acid B, dulcidiol, scopadulciol, scopanolal and scopadiol have been reported with toxic actions against various types of cancers without harming healthy cells.

Polyphenols: Japanese researchers isolated a polyphenol in vassourinha (7-dihydroxy-3040,6,8-tetramethoxyfavone) and tested it against two types of cervical cancer in test tubes. They reported in 1988 that it inhibited the growth of cervical cancer at very low dosages (ID50 values of 0.097 and 0.14). Other polyphenols in vassourinha that have shown anti-cancer actions in various research over the years include apigenin, chlorogenic acid, caffeic acid, catechin, ferulic acid, p-coumaric acid, hispidulin, gentisic acid, kaempferol, luteolin, mannitol, naringin, quercetin, rutin, and scutellarein.

CANCER PATHWAYS AND MECHANISMS OF ACTION

More complete information on these signaling pathways, cancer pathways, and new chemical targets for cancer therapy shown here can be found in chapter 5.

- Scoparic acid A is reported to be a β-glucuronidase inhibitor that may increase the safety and tolerability of anti-cancer agents and chemotherapy drugs. For example, research suggests that inhibiting gut bacterial β-glucuronidase enzymes can reduce the gastrointestinal toxicity caused by irinotecan, a cancer drug that treats colorectal and pancreatic cancers.
- Acteoside mitigates cell proliferation and aggressiveness of prostate cancer by the downregulation of TGF-β-associated EMT progression through HMGB1/RAGE suppression.
- Acteoside exerts an antitumor effect through its upregulation of p53 levels as well as inhibition of KLK expression and angiogenesis.
- Acteoside attenuates tyrosinase activity and inhibits melanin biosynthesis by activating ERK signaling and downregulating the expression of MITF, tyrosinase, and TRP-1 in melanoma.
- In colorectal cancers, acteoside inhibits the proliferative activity of colorectal cancer (IC50 = 117 mcg), induces G1 cell cycle arrest, and increases cell apoptosis by modifying PI3K/AKT signaling.
- Acteoside inhibits metastasis and promotes cell apoptosis and autophagy by let-7g-5p/HMGA2/Wnt/β-catenin signaling.
- In prostate cancer, acteoside decreases HMGB1/RAGE/TGFβI/II/Smad2/3 and inhibits EMT.
- In oral squamous cell carcinoma, acteoside inhibits metastasis by decreasing NF-κB/MMP-2 signaling and promotes cell apoptosis by affecting Bcl-2/Bcl-XL.
- Acteoside increases p53 expression and decreases KLK-1, -2, -4, -9, and -10 expression in liver cancer. Acteoside also inhibits expression of AXL, FGFR, BRAF, TIE2, and RAF1.
- Acteoside inhibits CDC42 via the HMGB1/RAGE axis in esophageal cancer.

Other Researched Benefits That May Be Helpful

Vassourinha is considered an effective pain reliever, which may be helpful for some types of cancer.

Availability of Products

Vassourinha is available in bulk powder, capsules, and tinctures from various companies. Just do an internet search using the keywords *vassourinha products* to find them.

Safety

Vassourinha has a long history of use in traditional medicine systems in the tropics. It is considered a safe remedy with no toxicity that is well tolerated. In toxicity studies, water and ethanol extracts given to mice at up to 2 g/kg of body weight showed no toxicity, and none of the animal studies published on vassourinha reported any animal deaths or signs of toxicity at any dosages given. Even when vassourinha (up to 2 g) was injected into mice, there was no toxicity noted.

Dosages

The reported therapeutic dosage generally used in South America is 2–3 grams twice daily or 1 cup of a standard infusion twice daily.

Contraindications

• The traditional use as an abortive and/or childbirth aid warrants that vassourinha should not be taken during pregnancy.

• Avoid combining with antidepressants or barbiturates unless under the supervision of a qualified health care practitioner (see drug interactions later in this section).

• A vassourinha extract recently demonstrated hypoglycemic activity, significantly lowering blood sugar levels in rats. While this has not been confirmed in humans, this plant is probably contraindicated in people with hypoglycemia. Diabetics should monitor their blood glucose levels closely if they use vassourinha to monitor these possible effects.

Drug Interactions

One human study documented that an ethanol extract of vassourinha inhibited radioligand binding to dopamine and serotonin. Another study reported that a water extract given intragastrically to rats potentiated the effects of barbiturates. As such, it is possible that vassourinha may enhance the effect of barbiturates and selective serotonin reuptake inhibitor antidepressants.

Summary of Benefits the Plant Has to Fight Cancer

Vassourinha and its active plant chemicals have a broad-spectrum action against a wide variety of cancer cells including brain, breast, cervical, colorectal, esophageal, gastric, liver, lung, oral, ovarian, prostate, renal, and skin cancers, as well as leukemia and melanoma. Unbelievably, all of the published research reports that it is selectively toxic to just cancer cells and nontoxic to healthy cells. It employs different ways to affect different types of cancers, but the end result is generally that it turns back on or restores the apoptosis (cell death) code through various communication/signaling pathways. This stops the cancer from replicating uncontrollably and triggers cell death by apoptosis.

Vassourinha is an ingredient in all three N-Tense formulas I developed for cancer.

Online Links to More Information

• Tropical Plant Database file for vassourinha: https://rain-tree.com/vassourinha.htm.

• Research references for this text: https://rain-tree.com/Vassourinha-Cancer-Research.pdf.

CONCLUSION

Our knowledge about cancer has grown exponentially over the last decade or so. Thankfully, new research on the important medicinal plants of the Amazon rainforest and how they interact with cancer has kept pace. This book's goal is to put these two areas of important research together in a fashion that will arm cancer patients, faced with life and death decisions, with new knowledge and tools in their fight to survive. For many, it is so frustrating waiting for discoveries to result in new drugs. From the time an effective anti-cancer chemical is isolated from a natural plant and eventually turned into a new chemotherapy drug, it can take anywhere from 30 to 50 years to get it approved for use. And all too often, that new single-chemical drug has toxicity and side effects.

When you really look at the process, you come to realize that the whole 30-to-50-year process is all about how to establish a patentable drug, so that a pharmaceutical company can profit from its "discovery." Of course, the original discovery typically came from the traditional medicine derived from the plant and the results it achieved from its uses. The preliminary research on such plants identifies which natural chemicals in the plant were achieving those results. In a more perfect world, the actual natural remedy could then be validated with research and promoted for those uses. Think how much time and money would be saved! Better yet, think of how many lives could have been saved. As I see it, Big Pharma considers these natural remedies as competition with the potential of reducing their profits. The real problem is that there is no one crazy enough to fund the expensive research to validate a natural remedy if it could never be patented and promoted to fight cancer under our current rules and regulations governing drugs and dietary/herbal supplements.

Years ago, when I was still in Austin, Texas, a large, well-respected cancer research hospital in Houston, Texas, offered to do a clinical trial on N-Tense

CONCLUSION

and to publish the results of their testing it in cancer patients. All I had to do was provide them with the product, and they would pay for everything else. After careful consideration, I respectfully declined. The two oncologists making the offer were well intentioned and saw many of their patients coming into their office with bottles of N-Tense. They had already seen some of the remarkable results in their patients. I explained that the herbal supplements I sold were, by law, prohibited "to treat, cure, diagnose, mitigate or prevent any disease." As soon as such a trial would begin using my formula, the Food and Drug Administration (FDA) could remove the product from the market by declaring it an unapproved drug. (They could also shut down my company, confiscate all my products, and fine me hundreds of thousands of dollars—all for selling an "unlicensed drug.") By my giving this formula to the doctors to test on their patients, it would prove that I knew it was being used to treat a disease like cancer.

Those rules and regulations are still in place today. That's why it is important that I share the knowledge I have of these natural remedies and plants in this book. None of the companies that sell herbal supplements using these plants and formulas can share this information with their customers, share the research, or provide guidance on their intended uses. It is up to independent authors, like myself, to get the factual knowledge out there, so it can be used to positively affect people's health.

There are already about a dozen experimental cancer drugs created from the chemicals found in the plants featured in this book, with another 10 or so drugs in the pipeline under development. Unfortunately, I'll probably not live long enough to see any of them approved as new chemotherapy drugs by the time they become available. The good news is that these plants are here today, and they can be used now as natural remedies.

The researchers at Big Pharma have known for years that some substances in these plants work against cancer. So why shouldn't we use them to help us fight cancer today? All of these plants have a very long history of safe use in traditional medicine systems throughout the world. Unlike single-chemical prescription drugs, chemically rich plants have the ability to specifically target and eliminate cancer cells in multiple ways without harming healthy cells or creating the same side effects and toxicity as drugs do.

As I said from the very start of this book, everybody is different. What works for one person may not work the same way in another. Each cancer is different, and how each of us responds to that cancer—and how we choose to treat it—may be different. Our genetics, lifestyles, risk factors, diets, and much more determine how drugs and natural remedies might work on an individualized basis. My sincere hope is that you have found the information in this book compelling enough to consider using rainforest plants in your fight against cancer—and that they work for you, as they have for so many others. If you would like, you are welcome to share your results using these plant remedies at my blog at https://leslie-taylor-raintree.blogspot.com.

RESOURCES

Rainforest Herbal Supplements

Health Food Stores

Many larger health food stores that carry herbal supplements will have several rainforest plants that are featured in this book. Some of the major rainforest plants of commerce that are found in health food stores (online and walk-in retail stores) include anamu, bitter melon, cat's claw, chanca piedra, graviola, and pau d'arco.

Herbs America Company

PO Box 446
Murphy, OR 97533
(541) 846-6222 | https://herbs-america.com

This company offers a small line of rainforest herbal extracts and bulk herbs under the name brand Amazon Therapeutics.

Rainforest Pharmacy

16300 SW 137th Avenue, Unit 115
Miami, FL 33177
(305) 235-9880 | https://rainpharm.com

This company manufactures and sells many of the manufactured products and formulas that Raintree Nutrition once sold (as well as others) under the Rainforest Pharmacy name brand. These include the three N-Tense products mentioned in this book. They also sell bulk plant powders by the kilogram (2.2 pounds) and some of the Amazon Support Formulas referred to in this book. I now get my personal rainforest supplements from them.

Raintree Products
1344 Disc Drive, Suite 5023
Sparks, NV 89436
(800) 553-4657 | https://raintree.com
In London, England: https://raintree.com/uk

    This company opened shortly after Raintree Nutrition closed, specifically to capitalize on selling the Raintree products. They originally named their company Raintree Formulas. Leslie Taylor, Raintree Nutrition, and Leslie's Raintree website have no affiliation whatsoever with Raintree Formulas.

    If you choose to order any of their products, especially the N-Tense formulas and Amazon Support Formulas, check the ingredients, both online and on their product labels. Make sure they are still using the same formulas. At one point, they had reformulated these products and added other ingredients or deleted some ingredients. The people who own the company are located in London, England, and they set up contract manufacturing and order fulfillment services for distribution in the United States. They have a separate UK website for products distributed in the United Kingdom and other European countries.

Whole World Botanicals
PO Box 322074
Ft. Wash. Station
New York, NY 10032
(877) 885-5517 | https://wholeworldbotanicals.com

    This company sells a small line of rainforest herbal supplements in capsules and extracts.

BULK HERB SUPPLIERS

Tropilab Inc.
PO Box 48164
St. Petersburg, FL 33743
(727) 344-7608 | https://tropilab.com/plantlist.html

    This company sells cut/sifted rainforest plants by the pound for teas and decoctions. They also sell some tinctures for some plants. If you live in a tropical to semitropical area and want to grow any of these rainforest plants, they also sell seeds to plant. Some small plants (like chanca piedra, mullaca, picão preto, and bitter melon) can be grown and harvested as annuals in nontropical areas easily.

Monterey Bay Herb Company
241 Walker Street
Watsonville, CA 95076
(800) 500-6148 | https://www.herbco.com

This company sells bulk plants in powders and cut/sifted forms by the quarter pound and pound. They also sell empty capsules and manual capsule machines.

Mountain Rose Herbs
PO Box 50220
Eugene, OR 97405
(800) 879-3337 | https://mountainroseherbs.com

This company sells bulk plants in powders and tea-cut forms, some prepared liquid extracts, and vegetable glycerin.

Supplies for Filling Capsules

Herb Affair
700 N Sacramento Boulevard, Suite 210
Chicago, IL 60612
(866) 445-9040 | https://www.herbaffair.com/products/capsule-it-capsule-filler

This company sells a wide variety of capsule-filling machines.

Monterey Bay Herb Company
241 Walker Street
Watsonville, CA 95076
(831) 722-3400 | http://www.herbco.com

In addition to selling herbs in bulk, this company sells empty capsules and smaller manual capsule fillers.

Swanson
4075 40th Avenue S
Fargo, ND 58104
(800) 824-4491 | https://www.swansonvitamins.com/capsule-connection

In addition to nutritional supplements, Swanson sells capsule machines and empty capsules.

OTHER RECIPES/PRODUCTS

The following links will take you to my website, which will provide you with the recipes for four products mentioned in this book. These formulas may be available to purchase from the companies that sell the N-Tense formulas.

Amazon Bowel Support: https://rain-tree.com/amazon-bowel-support.htm.

Amazon Immune Support: https://rain-tree.com/amazon-immune-support.htm.

Amazon Liver Support: https://rain-tree.com/amazon-liver-support.htm.

Amazon Prostate Support: https://rain-tree.com/amazon-prostate-support.htm.

In chapter 6, we discussed a drink to help stimulate your lymphatic flow in order to clean out your lymphatic system. Here is a drink you will find both helpful and refreshing.

Lymphatic Flush Natural Remedy
Ingredients

- 1 whole unpeeled organic lemon, quartered
- 3 cups filtered water
- 2 tablespoons organic olive oil
- 2 tablespoons raw honey
- 1 inch knob of fresh peeled ginger or 1 teaspoon dried powdered ginger
- Dash of cinnamon

Instructions

Add all ingredients, besides cinnamon, to a blender or food processor. Blend on high until everything has broken down, about 1 minute. Pour through a strainer. Enjoy in ½-cup dosages with a dash of cinnamon on top once daily. Refrigerate any remainder.

Other Books

Information and purchasing links for the author's other books on rainforest medicinal plants can be found on the Rain-Tree website at https://rain-tree.com/books.htm.

Here is the full list:

Acerola: Nature's Secret to Fight Free Radicals

Avenca: Nature's Secret for Weight Loss

Camu Camu: Nature's Secret for Disease Prevention

Chanca Piedra: Nature's Secret for Kidney Stones

The Healing Power of Rainforest Herbs

Hibiscus Flower: Nature's Secret for a Healthy Heart

REFERENCES

The information and recommendations presented in this book are based on more than 1,000 scientific studies, academic papers, and books. If the references for all these sources were printed here, they would add considerable bulk to the book and make it more expensive as well. For this reason, the publisher and author have decided to present a complete list of references, categorized by chapter and topic, on the author's website. This format has the added advantage of enabling us to make you aware of further important studies and papers as they become available. You can find the references under the listing of my book at https://rain-tree.com/fighting-cancer-references.pdf.

INDEX

ABCB1. *See* P-glycoprotein inhibitors
acetogenins, 53, 54, 256–59, 261, 262, 263
acetylenes, 297–98
acteoside, 320, 321
activator protein-1 (AP-1) inhibitors, 212, 234, 271, 280, 281; about, 59, 306; simarouba as, 306
adenosine triphosphate (ATP) inhibitors, 53, 253
Amazon Bowel Support, 102–3
Amazon Immune Support formula, 86, 206
Amazon Liver Support, 112–13, 237
Amazon Prostate Support, 128
Amazon rainforest plants. *See* plants; *specific plants*
anamu, 192; anti-cancerous actions of, 199–201; botanical overview, 198; brain cancer and, 199–200; breast cancer and, 75, 98, 99, 199, 200; cancer pathways and mechanisms of action for, 203–4; cell cycle arrest and, 62; endometrial cancer and, 104; gastric cancer and, 108; leukemia and, 199–201; lung cancer and, 115–16; lymphoma and, 199–200; N-Tense homemade recipes with, 138; ovarian cancer and, 124; for pain-relief, 204; pancreatic cancer and, 126; plant chemicals in, 75, 201–2; polyphenols in, 202; safety and dosages, 205–6; signaling pathways impacted by, 75, 203–4; sourcing, 204–5; summary of use, 206; traditional medicine uses, 198–99

angiogenesis: cancer use of, 30, 60, 76–77; inhibitor drugs, 60, 76–77; picão preto and, 300; pristimerin impact on, 247; simarouba and, 307; suma and, 313; vassourinha and, 321
antibacterials, 9, 10, 11; bitter melon, 215–16; graviola, 265; pau d'arco, 285; picão preto, 295; pristimerin, 242
antibiotics, 11
antidepressants: graviola and, 265; vassourinha and, 323
antifungals, 9, 10, 285, 295
anti-inflammatories, 10, 12; cat's claw, 220–21; diets high in, 21; espinheira santa, 248; graviola, 257–58; mullaca, 281, 282; picão preto, 301; polyphenols as, 15, 20
antioxidants: body natural production of, 17–18, 19, 20; cat's claw, 222; chanca piedra, 228–29; defined, 17; plant polyphenols with, 18–19; ROS impacted by, 17; in vitamins and minerals, 28
antiparasitics, 9, 10, 11, 282, 285
antivirals, 9, 10; bitter melon, 211, 212
AP-1 inhibitors. *See* activator protein-1 inhibitors
apoptosis (programmed cell death): cancer cells avoiding, 36, 46–47; checkpoint inhibitors and, 287–88; drugs inducing, 37; extrinsic pathway, 45, 50–52; function of, 44–45; genes and chemicals involved in, 47–52; intrinsic pathway, 45, 46–50; lymphatic system

333

role in, 45–46; mullaca impact on, 279; oxidative stress cell death and, 45–46; pristimerin impact on, 246; simarouba and, 308; vassourinha and, 319, 321, 323
artichoke extract, 26–27
astilbin, 202
ATP inhibitors. *See* adenosine triphosphate inhibitors
autophagy, 314, 321; about, 74–75; anamu and, 203; bitter melon and, 209, 213; cancer pathways and, 74–75; chanca piedra and, 233, 234; picão preto and, 298, 300; pristimerin impact on, 247
Ayurveda, 304, 319

bacteria: as carcinogens, 32; "shotgun" approach with, 11. *See also* antibacterials
Bak activation, 49–50, 261
Bartram, Thomas, 312
Bax activation, 49, 261
Bcl-2 inhibitors, 315; about, 48, 49; anamu as, 204; espinheira santa as, 239–40, 245; graviola as, 73, 256, 261; pau d'arco, 290; picão preto as, 299; vassourinha as, 321
BCL-xL inhibitors, 48, 290, 321
bee propolis, 310
beta-lapachone, 287–88
β-glucuronidase inhibitors, 68, 321
betulinic acid, 320
Biobank, 39
biological carcinogens, 32–33
bitter melon, 192; anti-cancerous actions, 208–10; as antiviral, 211, 212; botanical overview, 207; breast cancer and, 62, 98, 208, 209, 212, 213; cancer pathways and mechanisms of action for, 212–13; cell cycle arrest and, 62; diabetes and, 208, 215, 216; leukemia and, 208–9, 211; liver cancer and, 62, 212; lung cancer and, 213; mechanisms of action, 126, 183, 208–10; melanoma and, 208; as MMP-inhibitor, 72, 209; N-Tense homemade recipes with, 137; pancreatic cancer and, 126, 209–10, 213, 216; plant chemicals in, 210–12; polyphenols in, 211–12; prostate cancer and, 62, 208, 209, 212; safety and dosages, 214–16; sourcing, 214; summary of use, 216; testicular cancer and, 131; traditional medicine uses, 207–8
bladder and kidney cancer: about, 90; chanca piedra and, 91, 237; homemade recipe for, 143–45; picão preto and, 91, 303; plans and remedies, 90–91, 143–45
blood cancers. *See* leukemia; lymphoma; multiple myeloma
blood pressure: chanca piedra and, 235, 236; graviola and, 265; picão preto for, 301–2
blood-thinning drugs, 224
blood vessel formation. *See* angiogenesis
body weight, 56
bone cancer and sarcomas: about, 92; chanca piedra and, 93, 234; homemade recipe for, 145–47; plans and remedies, 92–93, 145–47; vassourinha and, 320
bowel cancer. *See* colorectal cancer
brain cancer: about, 93–94; anamu and, 199–200; bee propolis and, 310; espinheira santa, 244; guacatonga and, 268; homemade recipe for, 147–49; plans and herbal remedies, 93–95, 147–49; simarouba and, 95, 306–7, 310; vassourinha and, 320
breast cancer: about, 96, 97, 99; anamu and, 75, 98, 99, 199, 200; bitter melon and, 62, 98, 208, 209, 212, 213; cat's claw and, 97, 219–20, 221, 225; chanca piedra and, 98, 233; EDCs and, 34; espinheira santa and, 242, 244; graviola and, 254, 256, 262; guacatonga and, 268; HER2-positive, 99–100; homemade recipes for, 150–54; hormone-negative, 97–98; hormone-positive, 96–97; pau d'arco

INDEX

and, 97, 98, 99, 286; picão preto and, 99, 301; plans and remedies for, 96–100, 150–54; simarouba and, 307
brominated vegetable oil (BVO), 34

cancer: cell traits distinct from normal cells, 42–43; common types of, 1; deaths globally from, 1; defensive and recurrence mechanisms of, 76–77, 87–88; differences and similarities between types of, 30–31; genetic changes with, 28, 35–36, 39; man-made carcinogens relation to, 34–35; plant chemicals methods of impacting, 2–3; stages of development, 21; synergistic actions of plant-based medicines for, 29; understanding, 32–41, 76–77. *See also specific cancers and topics*
The Cancer Genome Atlas (TCGA), 39
cancer industry, xv–xvi
cancer mortality: diet relation to, 4; from drug side effects, 36–37; global statistics of, 1
cancer pathways, 5; angiogenesis pathway and, 30, 60, 76–77; autophagy and, 74–75; energy inhibitors and, 53–55; extrinsic apoptosis and, 45, 50–52; inflammation/immune, 55–59; intrinsic apoptosis and, 45, 46–50; multiple-plant formulas impact on, 30, 133–34; overview of, 42–43; plant medicines impacting, 30; plant research on rainforest plants relation to, 195–96; proliferation pathway and, 60–74. *See also specific plants*
cancer plans and remedies: bladder and kidney, 90–91, 143–45; bone and sarcoma, 92–93, 145–47; brain, 93–95, 147–49; breast, HER2-positive, 99–100, 153–54; breast, hormone-negative, 97–98, 151–53; breast, hormone-positive, 96–97, 150–51; cervical, 100–101, 155–56; colorectal, 101–3, 156–58; endometrial, 103–4, 158–59; esophageal, 104–7, 160–62; gastric (stomach), 107–8, 162–64; laryngeal and nasopharyngeal, 108–10, 164–66; leukemia, 110–12, 138, 166–68; liver, 112–13, 168–69; lung, non-small cell, 115–16, 169–71; lung, small cell, 113–15, 171–73; lymphoma, 116–18, 138, 173–74; melanoma, 118–19, 175–76; multiple myeloma, 119–20, 138, 176–78; oral, 121–22, 178–79; ovarian, 122–24, 179–81; pancreatic, 124–26, 182–84; prostate, 127–28, 184–86; skin, 128–30, 138, 186–87; testicular, 130–31, 188–89; thyroid, 132–33, 189–91

cancer prevention and risk: bitter melon and, 209; chanca piedra and, 228–29; diabetes type 2 and, 124, 182; diet relation to, 4, 21, 33–35; inflammation relation to, 4; polyphenols impact on, 15, 20–21

cancer stem cells, 132; autophagy impact on, 74; chemotherapy failures with, 87–88; defense mechanisms of, 82, 106; drugs for, 63; N-Tense formulas impact on, 88, 98, 114, 131, 170, 183, 188, 190; pancreatic, 210; pau d'arco and, 293; plants targeting, 64, 106, 109, 120, 152, 161, 165, 177, 203, 213, 221, 234, 271, 281, 293, 299, 308; pristimerin impact on, 246; proliferation pathway and, 63–64; simarouba and, 308; Wnt/β-catenin pathway and, 70, 221

cancer survivor, author as, v, ix
cancer treatment: cancer stem cells and, 63–64, 87–88; diet change as part of, 21, 35; evolution of, 36–38; gene research informing, 4, 38–41; hybrid approach to, x, xiv; individualized approach to, x, 325–26; new chemical targets for, 5; N-Tense formulas with conventional, 85; "one cure for all" paradigm, x, xiv, 76, 78; polyphenols in, 20–22, 87; single-chemical

335

approach in, 1, 24–25, 27, 75, 76, 78; targeted therapy approach to, 29–30, 31. *See also* cancer plans and remedies; chemotherapy; natural remedies; pharmaceutical drugs; *specific cancers and plants*

capsules: preparation of, 140; pros and cons, 139

carcinogens: man-made chemical, 33–35; types of, 32–33

caspase-3 activation, 256, 299, 308; about, 51; anamu, 203–4; cat's claw, 222; espinheira santa, 245; graviola, 261; pau d'arco, 290; suma, 315

caspase-8 activation, 51–52, 222, 261

catechins, 211–12, 244

cat's claw, 192; anti-cancerous actions, 218–20; botanical overview, 217; breast cancer and, 97, 219–20, 221, 225; cancer pathways and mechanisms of action for, 221–22; cell cycle arrest and, 62; with chemotherapy, 218–19, 222, 225; colorectal cancer and, 221; EU botanical drug with, v; for immune support, 86, 218–19, 224; leukemia and, 220, 222, 225; liver cancer and, 221; lymphomas and, 220; for multiple health conditions, 25; N-Tense homemade recipes with, 137–38; plant chemicals in, 24, 220–21; polyphenols in, 220–21; safety and dosages, 223–24; for side effects, 218–19; sourcing, 222–23; summary of use, 224–25; synergy of chemicals in, 24; traditional medicine uses, 217–18

celastrol, 244

cell cycle: arrest, 62–63; checkpoints, 61–62, 287–88; phases of, 62

cell death. *See* apoptosis

cellular signaling. *See* signaling pathways

cervical cancer, 286, 303; about, 100; carcinogens in, 32; homemade recipe for, 155–56; plans and remedies, 100–101, 155–56

chanca piedra, 192; anti-cancerous actions, 227–29; bladder and kidney cancer and, 91, 237; bone cancer and, 93, 234; botanical overview, 226–27; breast cancer and, 98, 233; cancer pathways and mechanisms of action for, 232–34; cancer prevention and, 228–29; cell cycle arrest and, 63; with chemotherapy, 229, 237; diabetes and, 236; leukemia and, 63, 111–12, 233; liver cancer and, 63, 228, 233, 237; lung cancer and, 115–16; melanoma and, 119, 234; as MMP-inhibitor, 72; oral cancer and, 122; ovarian cancer and, 63, 124, 233; plant chemicals in, 229–32, *231*; polyphenols in, 230; prostate cancer and, 234; safety and dosages, 235–36; for side effects, 237; skin cancer and, 228; sourcing, 234–35; summary of use, 236–37; thyroid cancer and, 132–33; traditional medicine uses, 227

chemical carcinogens, 32–35

chemical synthesis, of plants, xvi–xvii

chemotherapy: benefits of plants with, xiv, 3; cancer stem cells and, 87–88; cat's claw with, 218–19, 222, 225; chanca piedra with, 229, 237; drug resistance issues with, 2, 37; espinheira santa with, 251; failures of, 1–2, 87–88; gene research informing, 40; graviola with, 259, 262; intrinsic apoptosis pathway and, 45; N-Tense formulas used with, 85; picão preto with, 296, 301; polyphenols reducing impact of, 22; pristimerin with, 243; pump therapy method, 37–38; simarouba with, 309; suma with, 315–16; targeted therapies compared with, 29, 30

Chinese Traditional Medicine, 242, 244

cholangiocarcinoma, 319

chondrosarcoma. *See* bone cancer and sarcomas

chronic inflammation. *See* inflammation

c-Met inhibitors, 67, 213

INDEX

c-Myc inhibitors, 271, 279, 308; about, 65
coffee, 14
COL1A1 inhibitors, 69, 278, 280
colorectal cancer: about, 101–2; carcinogens in, 32; espinheira santa and, 239–40, 245; graviola and, 254–55, 256, 262; guacatonga and, 268, 273; homemade recipe for, 156–58; picão preto and, 298; plans and remedies, 101–3, 156–58; simarouba and, 307; vassourinha and, 63, 321
computer models, xviii, 40
contraindications, 196–97. *See also specific plant or remedy*
copaiba, 81, 138–39
coumarins, 299, 302
Curzerenone (SF-1603), 260
cynarin, 26
cytokines, 56, 57, 244, 291, 313

database, of plants. *See* Tropical Plant Database
daucosterol, 298
diabetes: bitter melon and, 208, 215, 216; cancer risk and type 2, 124, 182; chanca piedra and, 236; picão preto for, 301–2; vassourinha and, 323
dibenzyl trisulfide, 200, 201–2, 203, 204
diet, 56; cancer prevention and risk relation, 4, 21, 33–35; cancer treatment and changes in, 21, 35, 86–87; cleaning up, 35; free radicals in highly processed, 16–17; Mediterranean, 21; plant chemicals in, 4, 10; polyphenols inclusion in, 15
Dietary Supplement Health and Education Act of 1994 (DSHEA), vi–xiii
DNA, 35; cancer changes to, 42, 61; free radicals impact on, 20, 21, 55; PARP inhibitors and, 52; picão preto action on, 298; proliferation pathway and, 60–61; small-molecule drugs and, 29; testing method advances, 39
drug manufacturing: process of plant-based, 4, 25; same plant with different methods of, 27–28. *See also* pharmaceutical industry
drug resistance: bitter melon aiding, 209–10, 212; with chemotherapy, 2, 37; pancreatic cancer and, 209–10; pau d'arco and, 293. *See also* multidrug resistance
drugs, pharmaceutical. *See* multidrug resistance; pharmaceutical drugs; small-molecule drugs
DSHEA. *See* Dietary Supplement Health and Education Act of 1994
dysentery, 10–11

EDCs. *See* endocrine disruptor chemicals
EGCG, 106, 161
EGFR inhibitors, 204, 213, 262; about, 65–66
electrons: in cellular signaling, 16; free radicals and, 15–16, 17; inhibitors and, 54, 258
endocrine disruptor chemicals (EDCs), 34, 35
endometrial cancer: about, 103; homemade recipe for, 158–59; plans and remedies, 103–4, 158–59
energy inhibitors: cancer pathways relation to, 53–55; function of, 53
Epstein-Barr virus, 32, 109, 164
esophageal cancer: about, 104–5; green tea and, 106, 161; homemade recipe for, 160–62; plans and remedies, 104–7, 160–62; pristimerin impact for, 247; vassourinha and, 321
espinheira santa, 192; anti-cancerous actions, 239–40; botanical overview, 238; brain cancer, 244; breast cancer and, 242, 244; cancer pathways and mechanisms of action for, 245–47; cell cycle arrest and, 63; with chemotherapy, 251; colorectal cancer and, 239–40, 245; leukemia and, 242, 250; liver cancer and, 239–40, 245; lung cancer and, 114–15; lymphomas and, 250; melanomas and, 242;

337

as MMP-inhibitor, 73; N-Tense homemade recipes with, 137–39; plant chemicals, 240–45; polyphenols in, 244–45; pristimerin benefits found in, 242–44, 245–47; safety and dosages, 249–50; for side effects, 242, 248; skin cancer and, 239; sourcing, 248–49; stomach ulcers and, 247–48; summary of use, 250–51; traditional medicine uses, 238–39
European Union (EU), v, 34, 39
Ewing sarcoma. *See* bone cancer and sarcomas
ex vivo studies, 201, 254

fast food, 16
FDA. *See* Food and Drug Administration
fibrosis, 276, 278, 280
Food and Drug Administration (FDA): enforcement procedures, xi–xii; gene therapy approved by, 40; herbal supplements regulations under, vi–xiii, xi–xii, 28, 325; small-molecule drugs approved by, 29; standard cancer treatment protocols under, xv; targeted therapies approved by, 30; third-party documentation and, vii, xi–xii
free radicals: creation and impact of, 15–17; DNA damage from, 20, 21, 55; inflammation and, 55; types of, 15. *See also* reactive oxygen species
friedelan, 298
friedelin, 243–44

gastric (stomach) cancer: about, 107; carcinogens in, 32; homemade recipe for, 162–64; picão preto and, 108, 300–301; plans and remedies, 107–8, 162–64
gemcitabine, 209–10
genes: angiogenesis pathways, 77; cancer-driver, 39; cancer impact on, 28, 35–36, 37, 46–47, 61; cancer treatment advancements with research of, 4, 38–41; chemotherapy and research of, 40; extrinsic apoptosis, 50–52; GLUT1 inhibitors and, 55; HGP collaboration and road map of, 38; immunotherapy drugs and, 40, 43; inflammation/immune pathway, 55–56, 58; intrinsic apoptosis, 47–50; NIH research on cancer and, 306; proteogenomics research and, 41; simarouba and cancer, 306–7; testing for specific cancers, 40; testing methods, 38. *See also* DNA
gene therapy, 40
gene transfer, 40
Germany, 25–26
glaucarubinone, 305, 306, 307–8
glioblastomas. *See* brain cancer
Global Traditional Medicine Centre (GTMC), 12
GLUT1-inhibitor, 55, 278–79, 280–81
glycerin extracts: homemade, 142–43; pros and cons, 139
glycolysis inhibitors, 53–54
graviola, xiv, 192; acetogenins in, 53, 54, 256–59, 261, 262, 263; anti-cancerous actions, 253–56; Bak activation and, 50; as Bcl-2 inhibitor, 73, 256, 261; botanical overview, 252; breast cancer and, 254, 256, 262; cancer pathways and mechanisms of action for, 260–62; cell cycle arrest and, 63; with chemotherapy, 259, 262; colorectal cancer and, 254–55, 256, 262; leukemia and, 111–12; liver cancer and, 253, 256, 259, 261; lung cancer and, 114–15, 259; lymphoma and, 117–18; as MMP-inhibitor, 73; N-Tense homemade recipes with, 137; ovarian cancer and, 253–54; pancreatic cancer and, 255–56; plant chemicals, 256–60; polyphenols in, 259–60; products and distribution of, x–xi; regulatory hurdles with, xi–xii; research obstacles, viii–ix; safety and dosages, 263–65; for side effects, 262; sourcing, 262–63; summary of use,

INDEX

265–66; traditional medicine uses, 252–53. *See also* N-Tense formula
green tea: esophageal cancer and, 106, 161; polyphenols in, 14–15
GTMC. *See* Global Traditional Medicine Centre
guacatonga, 192; anti-cancerous actions, 268–69; botanical overview, 267; brain cancer and, 268; breast cancer and, 268; cancer pathways and mechanisms of action for, 270–71; cell cycle arrest and, 63; colorectal cancer and, 268, 273; leukemia and, 268, 270; liver cancer and, 268; melanoma, 268; N-Tense homemade recipes with, 137; for pain-relief, 268–69; plant chemicals, 269–70; polyphenols in, 270; safety and dosages, 271; for side effects, 271–72; sourcing, 272; summary of use, 272–73; traditional medicine uses, 267–68
gut microbiome: plant chemical bioavailability and, xvii; research on, 39

head lice, xi
Health Science Institute (HSI), 310
heat shock proteins (Hsp) inhibitors, 68, 204
Helicobacter pylori infections, 32, 107, 163
hepatitis, 32, 112, 113, 168, 169
herbal remedies. *See* cancer plans and remedies; homemade recipes; natural remedies
HGP. *See* Human Genome Project
Homeland Security Act (2002), xii
homemade recipes: for bladder/kidney cancer, 143–45; for bone cancer and sarcomas, 145–47; for brain cancer, 147–49; for breast cancer, 150–54; for cervical cancer, 155–56; for colorectal cancer, 156–58; for endometrial cancer, 158–59; for esophageal cancer, 160–62; for gastric cancer, 162–64; for laryngeal and nasopharyngeal cancer, 164–66; for leukemia, 138, 166–68; for liver cancer, 168–69; for lung cancer, 169–73; lymphatic flush, 330–31; for lymphoma, 138, 173–74; for melanoma, 175–76; for multiple myeloma, 138, 176–78; for N-Tense formulas, 137–39; for oral cancer, 178–79; for ovarian cancer, 179–81; for pancreatic cancer, 182–84; preparation types, 139–42; pros and cons, 135, 191; for prostate cancer, 184–86; for skin cancer, 138, 186–87; for solid tumors, 137; sourcing plants and products for, 135–36; storage of plant materials for, 136–37; for testicular cancer, 188–89; for thyroid cancer, 189–91
HPV. *See* human papillomavirus
HSI. *See* Health Science Institute
Hsp inhibitors. *See* heat shock proteins inhibitors
Human Genome Project (HGP), 38–41, 43, 75
human papillomavirus (HPV), 32, 100, 105, 155, 160
human studies, xviii
hypertension/hypotension. *See* blood pressure
hypoglycemia/hyperglycemia. *See* diabetes

ICGC. *See* International Cancer Genome Consortium
IFN-γ stimulant, 255, 296–97, 301, 313; about, 74
IL-1β inhibitors, 57, 280, 313, 315
IL-6: inhibitors, 57, 256, 313, 315; signaling pathways and, 43–44
imatinib, 30
immune pathway and support: anamu impact on, 204; cat's claw impact on, 86, 218–19, 224; chanca piedra impact on, 230, 232; espinheira santa impact on, 248; formulas and protocols for, 85–86, 206; about inflammation and, 55–59; picão preto and, 296–97, 301

immunotherapy, 270; genes and, 40, 43
infections, causing cancer, 32–33
inflammation and inflammation pathway: about, 43, 55–59, 204; anamu impact on, 204; cancers relation to, 4, 21, 55–56; chanca piedra impact on, 231–32, 233; cytokines and, 56, 57, 244, 291, 313; diseases linked to, 19–20; genes and, 35–36; mullaca impact on, 281; from oxidative stress, 19–20, 56; pristimerin impact on, 246–47
infusions/teas: preparation of, 140–41; pros and cons, 139. *See also* green tea
in silico (*INS*) research, xviii, 40, 255
interleukins, 57–58, 212, 313. *See also* IL-1β inhibitors; IL-6
International Cancer Genome Consortium (ICGC), 39, 40
in vitro (*IVT*) research, xviii, 23
in vivo (*IVA*) research, xviii, 23
IVT. See in vitro research

JAK/STAT3 inhibitors, 58, 289
JNK signaling pathway, 56, 233, 247, 281, 300

Keplinger, Klaus, 218–19
kidney cancer. *See* bladder and kidney cancer

lactate dehydrogenase-A (LDH-A) inhibitors, 54–55, 221, 261
lapachol, 286–87, 288, 290
laryngeal cancer: about, 108–9; homemade recipe for, 164–66; plans and remedies, 108–10, 164–66
LDH-A inhibitors. *See* lactate dehydrogenase-A inhibitors
leukemia: about, 110–11; anamu and, 199–201; bitter melon and, 208–9, 211; cat's claw and, 220, 222, 225; chanca piedra and, 63, 111–12, 233; espinheira santa and, 242, 250; guacatonga and, 268, 270; homemade N-Tense remedy for, 138; homemade recipes for, 138, 166–68; mullaca and, 275–76, 280, 283; picão preto and, 63, 296, 297, 300; plans and remedies, 110–12, 138, 166–68; simarouba and, 305; suma and, 312; vassourinha and, 320
lifestyle: cancer relation to, 33; cancer treatment and changes in, 86–87; free radicals created by, 17; weight loss and, 56. *See also* diet
liver cancer: about, 112; Amazon Liver Support for, 112–13, 237; bitter melon and, 62, 212; carcinogens in, 32; cat's claw and, 221; chanca piedra and, 63, 228, 233, 237; espinheira santa and, 239–40, 245; graviola and, 253, 256, 259, 261; guacatonga and, 268; homemade recipe for, 168–69; pau d'arco and, 286; picão preto and, 63, 296; plans and remedies, 112–13, 168–69; remission, 237; suma and, 63, 312–13
lung cancer: about, 113–14, 115; bitter melon and, 213; graviola and, 114–15, 259; homemade recipes for, 169–73; mullaca and, 275; pau d'arco and, 114–15, 286; picão preto and, 114–15, 296; plans and remedies for non-small cell, 115–16, 171–73; plans and remedies for small cell, 113–15, 169–71; vassourinha and, 63
lymphatic flow, 43, 45–46
lymphatic system: apoptosis pathway and, 45–46; drink for cleansing, 330–31
lymphoma, 32; about, 116–17; anamu and, 199–200; cat's claw and, 220; espinheira santa and, 250; homemade N-Tense remedy for, 138; homemade recipes for, 138, 173–74; plans and remedies, 116–18, 138, 173–74; suma and, 312

MAP-30, 211
MAPK pathway. *See* mitogen-activated protein kinase pathway
matrix metalloproteinases (MMPs) inhibitors: bitter melon as, 72, 209,

INDEX

212; chanca piedra as, 72, 234; defined, 72, 207; espinheira santa and, 73, 247; graviola as, 73, 261; lapachol as, 72; mullaca as, 73, 279–80; pau d'arco (lapachol) as, 73, 290; pristimerin impact on, 247; vassourinha as, 73, 321

maytansine/maytansinoids, 239, 241–42, 244

maytenin/maitenin, 242

MCL-1 inhibitors. *See* myeloid cell leukemia-1 inhibitors

MDR. *See* multidrug resistance

mechanisms of action: N-Tense remedies and, 93, 126, 146; rainforest plants multiple, 87, 195–96; of small-molecule drugs, 29. *See also specific plants*

medicinal plants. *See* natural remedies; plant chemicals; *specific plants*

Mediterranean diet, 21

melanoma: about, 118; bitter melon and, 208; chanca piedra and, 119, 234; espinheira santa and, 242; guacatonga, 268; homemade recipe for, 175–76; plans and remedies, 118–19, 175–76; vassourinha and, 320, 321

metabolism: free radicals and, 16; polyphenols and, 18

metformin, 54

microtubule inhibitors (MTIs), 64, 203

milk, EDCs in, 34

minerals, 28

mitocans, 200–201

mitochondrial complex I inhibitors, 53–54, 258

mitogen-activated protein kinase (MAPK) pathway, 58; bitter melon impact on, 212; pristimerin affecting, 246

MMPs. *See* matrix metalloproteinases inhibitors

mouth ulcers, 301

MTIs. *See* microtubule inhibitors

mTOR inhibitors, 69–70, 261

mucin inhibitors, 73–74, 281

mullaca, 50, 193; anti-cancerous actions, 275–77; botanical overview, 274; cancer pathways and mechanisms of action for, 279–81; cell cycle arrest and, 63; fibrosis and, 276, 278, 280; leukemia and, 275–76, 280, 283; lung cancer and, 275; as MMP-inhibitor, 73, 280; nasopharynx cancer and, 275; N-Tense homemade recipes with, 137–39; oral cancer and, 277; plant chemicals, 277–79; polyphenols in, 279; safety and dosages, 282; sourcing, 281–82; summary of use, 282–83; traditional medicine uses, 275

multidrug resistance (MDR): ABCB1 inhibitors and, 308; graviola and, 258–59, 260–61; P-glycoprotein and, 73, 212, 233, 259; pristimerin help for, 243; simarouba and tumors with, 305

multiple myeloma: about, 119–20; homemade N-Tense remedy for, 138; homemade recipes for, 138, 176–78; plans and remedies, 119–20, 138, 176–78

mutamba, 81, 138–39, 157, 169, 185, 189, 190

myeloid cell leukemia-1 (MCL-1) inhibitors, 48–49

myeloma. *See* multiple myeloma

NADH oxidase inhibitors, 69, 257, 308

NAD(P)H:quinone oxidoreductase 1 (NQO1) inhibitors, 288, 291; about, 68–69

nasopharyngeal cancer: about, 109; carcinogens in, 32; homemade recipe for, 164–66; mullaca and, 275; plan and remedies, 108–10, 164–66

National Cancer Institute (NCI): pau d'arco research by, 285, 286; plants for cancer screening by, xvii, 3, 10, 239, 253, 305; proteogenomics research under, 41

National Cancer Society (NCS), 33

National Institutes of Health (NIH), 306, 310

341

National Library of Medicine, PubMed Database of, 194
natural remedies: ability and underlying mechanisms of, 2–3; angiogenesis pathway, 60; for cancer cell cycle arrest, 62–63; cancer drugs compared with, 23–31; cancer drugs to market timeline compared with, xiv; cancer pathways impacted by, 30; chemically synthesizing, history of, xvi; chemotherapy drugs use with, xiv; energy inhibitors, 53–55; format for listing of, 6; global prevalence of, 25–26; Homeland Security Act stopping shipments of, xii; for immune support, 85–86; inflammation/immune pathway, 57–59; intrinsic apoptosis pathway, 47–50; layout for use of, 78–79; multiple plant chemical benefits in, 23, 75, 76, 87–88, 133–34; NCI findings on anti-cancerous, 3, 10; "no medical claims" stipulation in U.S., xvi, 4, 26–27, 28; for oxidative burst, 46; plant chemicals number in, xvii; prescription drugs based on, 26; proliferation pathway, 62–74; regulations in U.S. on, vi–xiii, xvi, 26–27, 28, 325; scope of use in U.S. and globally, 12; "shotgun" approach with, 11; signaling pathways and, 47, 72, 75; sourcing products for making, 135–36; synergistic actions of multi-plant, 29, 78; synergy with, 28–29; unique characteristics of rainforest, 8–13. *See also* cancer plans and remedies; homemade recipes; plant chemicals; *specific plants*
naturopathic protocols: development of, 5; how to use, 5–6; layout for, 78–79; for N-Tense formulas, 80–85. *See also* cancer plans and remedies
NCI. *See* National Cancer Institute
NCS. *See* National Cancer Society
neuroblastoma, 65, 308

new biological testing methods, xviii, 245
NF-1 genetic mutation, 306–7
NF-κB. *See* nuclear factor-kappaB
NIH. *See* National Institutes of Health
Notch signaling pathway, 234; inhibitors, 67–68
Noxa protein, 50, 279, 280
NQO1 inhibitors. *See* NAD(P)H:quinone oxidoreductase 1 inhibitors
N-Tense formulas: for bladder and kidney cancer, 91; for brain cancer, 95; for breast cancer, 96–100; cancer pathways impacted by, 30, 133–34; for cervical cancer, 100–101; for colorectal cancer, 102–3; contraindications with, 84–85; with conventional treatments, 85; for endometrial cancer, 103–4; for esophageal cancer, 105–7; for gastric cancer, 107–8; homemade recipes using, 137–39; for laryngeal and nasopharyngeal cancer, 109–10; for leukemias, 111–12, 138; for liver cancer, 112–13, 237; for lung cancer, 114–16; for lymphomas, 117–18; for melanomas, 119; for multiple myeloma, 120; for oral cancer, 121–22; origins, ix, 80; for ovarian cancer, 123–24; overview of, 81; for pancreatic cancer, 125–26; preparation types and, 139–43; for prostate cancer, 128; protocols for using, 80–85; regulatory hurdles with, xi–xii, 324–25; for skin cancer, ix, 129–30, 138; sourcing of, 81; for testicular cancer, 131; for thyroid cancer, 132–33
nuclear factor-kappaB (NF-κB): about, 56, 58; espinheira santa and, 244–46; graviola and, 255, 260, 262; inhibitors, 58, 73, 221, 233, 244–46, 255, 260, 262, 281, 300, 321; ROS impacting, 46

obesity, 56
okanin, 299, 300
oncologist: cancer-free diagnosis from, 39; protocols followed by, xv–xvi

INDEX

online resources, overview, 192–93, 197
oral cancer: about, 121; homemade recipe for, 178–79; mullaca and, 277; plans and remedies, 121–22, 178–79
osteosarcoma. *See* bone cancer and sarcomas
ovarian cancer: about, 122–23; chanca piedra and, 63, 124, 233; graviola and, 253–54; homemade recipe for, 179–81; plans and remedies, 122–24, 179–81; vassourinha and, 320
oxidative stress: cell death/oxidative burst through, 45–46, 308; chronic inflammation from, 19–20, 56; defined, 19, 45; polyphenols impact on, 22
oxygen, free radicals and, 16

P2X7 inhibitors, 204, 220, 221; about, 64–65
p21-activated kinase 1 (PAK1) inhibitors, 64, 213, 290, 307, 308
P53 (tumor suppressor protein), 47, 289, 321
pain-relief, xvi, 12; anamu for, 204; guacatonga for, 268–69; picão preto for, 301; suma for, 315; vassourinha for, 321
PAK1. *See* p21-activated kinase 1 inhibitors
pancreatic cancer: about, 124–25; bitter melon and, 126, 209–10, 213, 216; drug resistance and, 209–10; graviola and, 255–56; homemade recipe for, 182–84; plans and remedies, 124–26, 182–84; vassourinha and, 321
Parkinson's disease, 263, 264
PARP inhibitors. *See* Poly(ADP-ribose) polymerase cleavage
pau d'arco, 193; anti-cancerous actions, 285–86; botanical overview, 284–85; breast cancer and, 97, 98, 99, 286; cancer pathways and mechanisms of action for, 289–91; cervical cancer and, 100–101, 286; esophageal cancer and, 106–7; laryngeal and nasopharyngeal cancers and, 109–10; liver cancer and, 286; lung cancer and, 114–15, 286; as MMP-inhibitor, 73; multiple myeloma and, 120; N-Tense homemade recipe with, 138–39; ovarian cancer and, 124; pancreatic cancer and, 125–26; plant chemicals, 286–89; prostate cancer and, 287; safety and dosages, 292–93; for side effects, 291; small-molecule drugs, 288–89; sourcing, 291–92; summary or use, 293; traditional medicine uses, 285
p-coumaric acid, 299, 302
P-glycoprotein (ABCB1) inhibitors, 73, 208, 212, 233, 259
pharmaceutical drugs: angiogenesis pathway, 60, 76–77; apoptosis inducing, 37; blood-thinning, 224; for cancer stem cells, 63; in cancer treatment evolution, 36–38; energy inhibitors, 53–55; gene research and new, 40, 41; healthy cells impacted by, 36–37; immunotherapy, 40, 43; inflammation/immune pathway, 57–59; intrinsic apoptosis pathway, 47–50; N-Tense formulas used with, 85; oxidative burst, 46, 308; plant chemicals aiding effectiveness of, 12–13; plant chemical synthesis relation to, xvi–xvii; plant medicines compared with, 23–31; proliferation pathway, 62–74; protocols, 1–2; research for plant drugs compared with, 27–28; single-chemical, realities, 1, 23, 24–25, 27, 75, 76, 78; small-molecule, 29, 31, 77–78; time to market, xiv, 75, 324; U.S. approach to, 26–27. *See also* chemotherapy; multidrug resistance; small-molecule drugs
pharmaceutical industry: agenda in, 27, 324, 325; in China, 202, 242; drugs time to market in, xiv, 75, 324; patents in, 24, 26; profits driving, ix, 26, 27–28, 324; single-chemical approach of, 24–25, 27, 78; traditional medicine knowledge use by, 12

physalins, 279
physical carcinogens, 32
PI3K/AKT signaling pathway, 46, 74, 278, 321; espinheira santa and, 246, 247; inhibitors, 69–70, 72, 204, 232, 233, 234, 246, 280
picão preto, 193; anti-cancerous actions, 295–97; bladder and kidney cancer and, 91, 303; for blood pressure, 301–2; botanical overview, 294; breast cancer and, 99, 301; cancer pathways and mechanisms of action for, 299–301; cell cycle arrest and, 63; cervical cancer and, 100–101, 303; with chemotherapy, 296, 301; colorectal cancer and, 298; for diabetes, 301–2; esophageal cancer and, 106–7; gastric cancer and, 108, 300–301; laryngeal and nasopharyngeal cancers and, 109–10; leukemia and, 63, 296, 297, 300; liver cancer and, 63, 296; lung cancer and, 114–15, 296; N-Tense homemade recipes with, 138; ovarian cancer and, 124; for pain-relief, 301; plant chemicals, 297–99; polyphenols in, 298; safety and dosages, 301–3; sourcing, 301; summary of use, 303; traditional medicine uses, 295
plant-based remedies. *See* natural remedies
plant chemicals: anti-cancerous, identification of, 3, 10, 195; bioavailability importance, xvii; cancer drugs effectiveness aided by, 12–13; creation and role of, 3–4, 8–10; cynarin, 26; defensive, 9–10, 18; list and documented impacts, *231*; mechanisms of action complexity relation to, 195–96; multiple, benefits of, 23, 75, 76, 87–88, 133–34; number in rainforest plants, 8, 195; number of, xvii, 2; into small-molecule drugs, 29; specific cancers relation to, 2; synergy of, xvii, 24, 25, 78. *See also* polyphenols; *specific plants and chemicals*

plants: adaptations in rainforest conditions, 9–10; diversity of rainforest, 8; format and sections for, 193–97; list of anti-cancer, 192–93; multiple mechanisms of action for, 87, 195–96; NCI screening for anti-cancerous, xvii, 3, 10, 239, 253; new research on rainforest, 12–13; plant chemicals scope in rainforest, 8, 195; polyphenol-rich, 14–15; polyphenols in cultivated compared with rainforest, 10, 22; research and books on, v–vi; research on synergistic nature of, 28–29; research on synergy of, 28–29; sourcing, for homemade remedies, 135–36; storage of bulk, 136–37; survival adaptations, 8–10; tea-cut compared with powders of, 136; traditional medicine systems using, 10–12; unique characteristics of rainforest, 8–13. *See also* natural remedies; *specific plants*
plastics, 34, 35
Poly(ADP-ribose) polymerase (PARP) cleavage, 52, 212, 213, 245, 290
polyphenols: in anamu, 202; as anti-inflammatories, 15, 20; antioxidants in plant, 18–19; in bitter melon, 211–12; cancer risk lowering action of, 15, 20–21; in cancer treatment, 20–22, 87; in cat's claw, 220–21; in chanca piedra, 230; in espinheira santa, 244–45; in graviola, 259–60; in guacatonga, 270; high heat impact on, 15; lack in diet, 4; in mullaca, 279; number of unique, 19; oxidative stress reduction with, 20; in picão preto, 298; plants rich in, 14–15; power of, 4, 13, 14–22; in rainforest compared to cultivated plants, 10, 22; ROS suppression by, 19; in vassourinha, 320
pregnancy: anamu and, 205; bitter melon and, 215; cat's claw and, 224; chanca piedra and, 235–36; graviola and, 265; guacatonga and, 272; N-Tense

INDEX

contraindications with, 84; pau d'arco and, 293; picão preto for, 302; suma and, 317; vassourinha and, 323
preparation types: capsules, 140; considerations, 139; glycerin extracts, 142–43; infusions/teas, 140–41; tinctures, 141–42
prevention. *See* cancer prevention and risk
pristimerin, 242–44, 245–47
profits: cancer industry focus on, xv; pharmaceutical industry, ix, 26, 27–28, 324; research driven by, xvi, 27–28, 245
programmed cell death. *See* apoptosis
proliferation pathway: cancer stem cells and, 63–64; cell cycle arrest and, 62–63; cell cycle checkpoints and, 61–62, 287–88; function of, 60–61; inhibitors, 64–74
prostate cancer: about, 127; bitter melon and, 62, 208, 209, 212; chanca piedra and, 234; homemade recipe for, 184–86; pau d'arco and, 287; plans and remedies, 127–28, 184–86; pristimerin impact for, 247; vassourinha and, 321
proteins (in cells): ABCB1 inhibitors and, 73, 208, 212, 233, 259; activation of, 51–52; anti- and pro-apoptotic, 46–47; Bcl-2, 48; BCL-xL, 48; MAPK pathway and, 59; Noxa, 50, 279, 280; P53 tumor suppressor, 47; proliferation pathway and, 60–61; TGF-β inhibition and, 213, 233, 309, 321. *See also* activator protein-1 inhibitors; caspase-3 activation; caspase-8 activation; matrix metalloproteinases inhibitors
proteogenomics, 41
proto-oncogenes, 36
published studies, xvii–xviii
PubMed Database, of National Library of Medicine, 194

quassinoids, 305–8

radiation: cat's claw for side effects of, 219; pau d'arco for side effects of, 291

Rainforest Medicinal Plant Database. *See* Tropical Plant Database
rainforest plants. *See* plants; *specific topics*
Raintree Nutrition Inc.: evolution into Rain-Tree Publishers, xiii; founding of, v, vi, 224–25; regulations journey, vi–xiii
Rain-Tree Publishers, origins, xiii
Raintree website resources, xvii
reactive oxygen species (ROS): antioxidants impact on, 17; defined, 15–16; diet and lifestyle factors in, 16–17; mullaca impact on, 279; of plants, 18; polyphenols impact on, 19; pristimerin affecting, 246; signaling pathways affected by, 46
recipes. *See* homemade recipes
recurrence: cancer defense mechanisms and, 76–77, 87–88; after remission, 82–83
regulations, on herbal supplements: caution around research and, 324–25; FDA and DSHEA, vi–xiii; "right to try" law on, xiv; in U.S., vi–vii, 26–27
remission: cancer plan after, 83; "cured" compared with, 38; leukemia relapses in, 166; liver cancer, 237; multiple myeloma cycles of, 119–20; recurrence after, 82–83
renal failure, 242
research: animal studies and confirmation of, xviii; on anti-cancerous actions of rainforest plants, 194–95; on anti-cancerous plant chemicals, 3, 10, 195; background of, v–vi; chemically synthesizing plants and, xvi–xvii; computer models used in, xviii, 40; of genes informing cancer treatment, 4, 38–41; on gut microbiome, 39; NCI, 3, 285, 286; new rainforest plant, 12–13; new testing methods for, xiii–xiv; overview of plant listings relation to, 194–97; for pharmaceutical compared with plant-based drugs, 27–28; on polyphenols, 13, 14; profits driving, xvi, 27–28, 324–25;

345

proteogenomics, 41; published studies, xvii–xviii; on rainforest plants relation to cancer pathways, 195–96; Raintree website inclusion of, xvii; regulations on providing consumer with, vi–vii; safety, 196–97; study types, xviii; on synergistic nature of plants, 28–29; on synergy of medicinal plants, 28–29; Tropical Plant Database aiding, xii–xiii; in U.S. compared globally, 4, 28; WHO funded, 12. *See also specific plants*

review articles, xviii, 260

risk. *See* cancer prevention and risk

ROS. *See* reactive oxygen species

RSK1 inhibitors, 71–72

safety, 196–97. *See also specific plant or remedy*

sangre de grado, 81, 138–39

sarcoma. *See* bone cancer and sarcomas

scopadulcic acid B, 320

SF-1603 (Curzerenone), 260

"shotgun" approach, 11

side effects, xiv; cat's claw for, 218–19; chanca piedra for, 237; chemotherapy pump therapy and, 37–38; death from cancer drug, 36–37; espinheira santa for, 242, 248; graviola for, 262; guacatonga for, 271–72; lapachol, 286; pau d'arco for, 291; plant medicine aiding cancer drug, xiv, 13, 29; simarouba for, 309; suma for, 315–16

signaling pathways: aberrant, 61; anamu impacting multiple, 75, 203–4; cancer action on, 30, 44, 61; cancer drugs targeting, 29, 43–44, 47; cancer stem cells, 63; defined, 1, 16, 43; JAK/STAT3, 58, 289; JNK, 56, 233, 247, 281, 300; MAPK, 59, 212, 246; mTOR, 69–70, 261; mucin inhibitors and, 74; natural remedies targeting, 47, 72, 75; Notch, 67–68, 234; picão preto impact on, 299–300; pristimerin impact on, 246–47; ROS impacting, 46; Wnt/β-catenin, 70–71, 221. *See also* angiogenesis; apoptosis; autophagy; cancer pathways; immune pathway and support; inflammation and inflammation pathway; PI3K/AKT signaling pathway

simarouba, 193; anti-cancerous actions, 305; botanical overview, 304; brain cancer and, 95, 306–7, 310; breast cancer and, 307; cancer pathways and mechanisms of action for, 307–9; cell cycle arrest and, 63; with chemotherapy, 309; colorectal cancer and, 307; leukemia and, 305; plant chemicals, 305–7; safety and dosages, 309; for side effects, 309; sourcing, 309; summary of use, 310; traditional medicine uses, 304–5

skin cancer: about, 128–29; carcinogens, 32; chanca piedra and, 228; espinheira santa and, 239; homemade N-Tense remedy for, 138; homemade recipes for, 138, 186–87; N-Tense topical for, ix, 128–29, 138; plan and remedies, 128–30, 138, 186–87. *See also* melanoma

small-molecule drugs, 29, 31, 49–50; mainstream use of plant-based, 77–78; mullaca, 278; okanin, 299; pau d'arco, 288–89

snakebites, 271

sourcing products, 327–30; for capsule making, 140; for glycerin extracts, 143; for infusion/tea making, 141; N-Tense formulas and, 81; raw plant materials and, 135–36. *See also specific plants*

spices, with polyphenols, 15

stem cells. *See* cancer stem cells

steroidal chemicals, 277, 280, 282, 314

stomach cancer. *See* gastric cancer

stomach ulcers, 247–48, 271–72

storage, of plant materials, 136–37

suma, 193; anti-cancerous actions, 312–13; botanical overview, 311; cancer

INDEX

pathways and mechanisms of action for, 314–15; cell cycle arrest and, 63; with chemotherapy, 315–16; hormone-positive cancers and, 317; leukemia and, 312; liver cancer and, 63, 312–13; lymphoma and, 312; N-Tense homemade recipes with, 138–39; for pain-relief, 315; plant chemicals, 313–14; safety and dosages, 316–17; for side effects, 315–16; sourcing, 316; summary of use, 316–17; traditional medicine uses, 311–12

survival instincts, 8–9

synergy: cat's claw example of whole plant, 24; defined, 24; pharmaceutical drugs failures around, 25; of plant chemicals, xvii, 24, 25, 78; research on medicinal plant, 28–29

targeted therapies, 29–30, 31

TCGA. *See* Cancer Genome Atlas

teas. *See* green tea; infusions/teas

telomerase inhibitors, 234, 246, 290; about, 66–67

testicular caner: about, 130–31; homemade recipe for, 188–89; plans and remedies, 130–31, 188–89

Texas Department of Health, x, xi, xii

TGF-β inhibition, 213, 233, 309, 321; about, 71

Thioredoxin NADPH Reductase (TrxR) inhibitors, 52, 278, 279

third-party documentation, vii, xi–xii

thyroid cancer: about, 132; homemade recipe for, 189–91; plans and remedies, 132–33, 189–91

tinctures: homemade, 141–42; pros and cons, 139

tingenone, 242

TNF inhibitors. *See* tumor necrosis factor inhibitors

TOP2A inhibitors. *See* topoisomerase II alpha inhibitors

topoisomerase 1 (TOPO I), 66, 288, 298, 300, 303

topoisomerase II alpha (TOP2A) inhibitors, 66, 262

traditional herbal medicine systems: Ayurvedic, 304, 319; Chinese, 242, 244; evidence of ancient, 11–12; rainforest plants in, 10–12, 194; WHO support of, 12. *See also specific plants*

treatment. *See* cancer plans and remedies; cancer treatment

triterpenoids and triterpenes, 210, 232, 270, 298; espinheira santa, 240, 242, 243–44; simarouba and, 305–6

Tropical Plant Database, 197; FDA regulatory obstacles for, xi–xiii; origins, v, x; plant list and links for, 192–93; research aided by, xii–xiii; on traditional medicine systems, 11, 194

TRxR inhibitors. *See* Thioredoxin NADPH Reductase inhibitors

tumor growth: angiogenesis relation to, 30; apoptosis pathway and new, 46; espinheira santa and, 242–43, 246; graviola and, 253, 255–56, 258; guacatonga and, 269–70; homemade recipe for, 137; inflammation and, 56; lapachol on, 287; MMPs and, 209; mullaca and, 280–81; normal cells in, 42–43; P53 and, 47, 289, 321; picão preto and, 295–96; plants for arresting, 62–63; process of, 36; simarouba and, 305, 307; treatment for, 36–38; vassourinha and, 320

tumor necrosis factor (TNF) inhibitors, 57, 244, 256, 291, 313, 315; about, 50–51

United States (U.S.): cancer cases and deaths in, 1; herbal supplement use in, 12; man-made chemical carcinogens used in, 33–35; plant-based drug manufacturing in, 4; regulations on herbal supplements in, vi–xiii, 26–27; "right to try" law for herbal remedies in, xiv. *See also* Food and Drug Administration

uterine cancer. *See* endometrial cancer

347

vassourinha, 193; anti-cancerous actions, 319; bone cancer and, 320; botanical overview, 318; brain cancer and, 320; cancer pathways and mechanisms of action for, 320–21; cell cycle arrest and, 63; cholangiocarcinoma and, 319; colorectal cancer and, 63, 321; diabetes and, 323; esophageal cancer and, 321; leukemia and, 320; lung cancer and, 63; melanomas and, 320, 321; as MMP-inhibitor, 73; N-Tense homemade recipes with, 137–39; ovarian cancer and, 320; for pain-relief, 321; pancreatic cancer and, 321; plant chemicals, 319–20; polyphenols in, 320; prostate cancer and, 321; safety and dosages, 322; sourcing, 322; summary of use, 323; traditional medicine uses, 318–19

viruses: as carcinogens, 32; Epstein-Barr, 32, 109, 164; HPV, 32, 100, 105, 155, 160; survival instinct of, 8

vitamins, 28

weight loss, 56
WHO. *See* World Health Organization
withanolides, 277, 278–79
Wnt/β-catenin signaling pathway, 70–71, 221
World Health Organization (WHO), 12

ABOUT THE AUTHOR

Leslie Taylor, ND, is considered one of the world's leading experts on rainforest medicinal plants. Dr. Taylor founded, managed, and directed the Raintree group of companies from 1995 to 2012, and was a leader in creating a worldwide market for the important medicinal plants of the Amazon rainforest.

Having survived a rare form of leukemia only because of alternative health and herbal medicine, Dr. Taylor has been researching, studying, and documenting alternative healing modalities—including herbal medicine—for more than 30 years. A dedicated herbalist and naturopath, she developed many herbal formulas and remedies for her companies, for practitioners, and for individuals needing help. In 1995, while researching alternative AIDS and cancer therapies in Europe, she became aware of a medicinal plant from the Peruvian rainforest called cat's claw. This research took her to Peru to gain firsthand knowledge of this new medicinal plant. Upon her return, she founded Raintree Nutrition Inc. to make this rainforest plant and others available in the United States.

After that first trip, Dr. Taylor returned to the Amazon numerous times, continuing to research and document more medicinal rainforest plants. In these endeavors, she worked directly with indigenous Indian shamans and healers, learning about their use of healing plants, as well as with indigenous tribal communities and other rainforest communities. She also worked with phytochemists, botanists, ethnobotanists, researchers, and alternative and integrative health practitioners to document, research, test, and validate rainforest medicinal plants.

In 2012, with many other companies selling the rainforest plants that she had introduced to the United States, Dr. Taylor decided to close her business and devote herself to educating people about the benefits of medicinal plants.

She freely shared all of her proprietary formulas by posting them on her Raintree website so that anyone could make and use them.

Dr. Taylor remains a trusted source of information about rainforest medicinal plants and continues to update her Tropical Plant Database for these purposes. A practicing board-certified naturopath for many years (now retired), she has lectured and taught classes in naturopathic medicine, herbal medicine, and ethnobotany, as well as environmental and sustainability issues in the Amazon. She is the author of *Herbal Secrets of the Rainforest* and the best-selling *The Healing Power of Rainforest Herbs*, as well as the highly popular and extensively referenced Raintree Tropical Plant Database (http://www.rain-tree.com/plants.htm), which has been online since 1996.

More information about Leslie Taylor and her other books can be found online at http://rain-tree.com. She also has a personal blog where you can ask questions and share cancer stories and strategies with others at http://leslie-taylor-raintree.blogspot.com.

The Healing Power of Rainforest Herbs: A Guide to Understanding and Using Herbal Medicinals

Leslie Taylor, ND

"Extraordinarily well researched, superbly written, and absolutely the best reference work on rainforest herbs." —Review, *Making Scents Magazine*

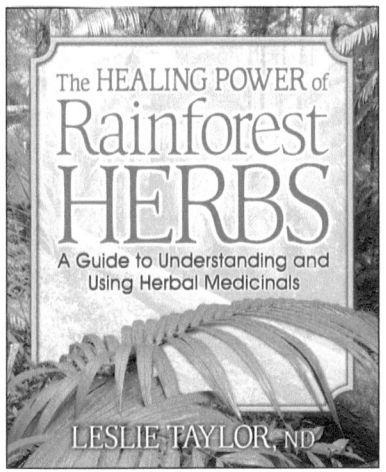

Rainforests contain an amazing abundance of plant life—over half of the planet's vegetation. For centuries, tribal shamans have successfully used these botanicals as remedies for various health disorders. Scientists have begun to uncover the medicinal qualities of these plants, which offer new approaches to health and healing. *The Healing Power of Rainforest Herbs* is a unique guide to these herbs and their uses.

Detailing more than seventy rainforest botanicals, this book presents the history of the herbs' uses by indigenous peoples and describes current use by natural health practitioners throughout the world. Discover Amazon healers' traditional knowledge as well as the clinical studies that support what shamans have known for ages. Essential dosage and preparation methods are provided, while at-a-glance tables help you locate the best botanicals for each disorder. *The Healing Power of Rainforest Herbs* is a unique book that offers a blend of ancient and modern knowledge in an accessible reference format.

---

528 pages • 7.5 x 9.13 quality paperback • ISBN 978-0-7570-0144-4

Avenca: Nature's Secret for Weight Loss

Leslie Taylor, ND

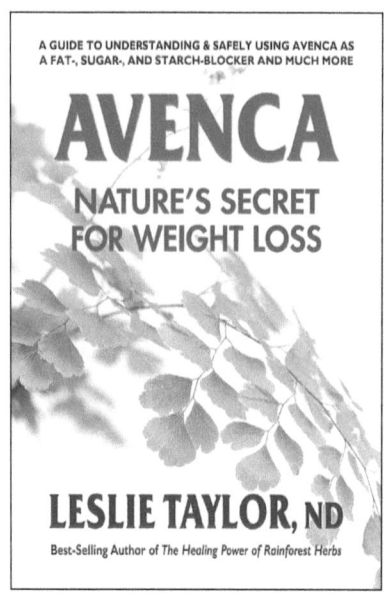

While there may not be any perfect formula for people to lose weight, nature may have created one that comes very close to being perfect. Avenca is a plant that grows in forests throughout the world, and for centuries it has been safely used as an herbal remedy for numerous aliments. Recently, however, new research has shown that along with its healing benefits, avenca can also prevent fats, sugars, and starches—the very elements responsible for weight gain—from being absorbed during digestion. Based on Dr. Taylor's research and testing, her book provides a complete guide to understanding how avenca works and how it can be used to lose those unwanted pounds. And considering that over seventy million Americans are classified as obese, the timing could not have been better.

With avenca, it's no longer about counting calories, since you can eat what you normally eat. It's about your body no longer absorbing fats, sugars, and starches. And interestingly enough, you are likely to feel fuller quicker. Yes, avenca will be a game changer, but as a consumer you will find that the information in this book will help you ask the right questions, become a savvy shopper, and, most important, allow you to reach your ideal weight.

---

192 pages • 6 x 9 quality paperback • ISBN 978-0-7570-0191-9

www.ingramcontent.com/pod-product-compliance
Ingram Content Group UK Ltd.
Pitfield, Milton Keynes, MK11 3LW, UK
UKHW041844240426
5401IPUK00002B/20